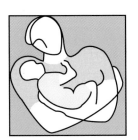

Complementary Therapies for Pregnancy and Childbirth

Edited by

Denise Tiran RGN RM ADM MTD PGCEA
Principal Lecturer – Complementary Therapies/Midwifery,
School of Health, University of Greenwich, London, UK

and

Sue Mack MSc CQSW Ad Dip Counselling
Therapist, Charter Nightingale Hospital, London, UK

SECOND EDITION

Baillière Tindall

EDINBURGH LONDON NEW YORK PHILADELPHIA ST LOUIS SYDNEY TORONTO 2000

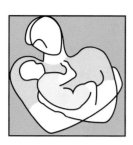

BAILLIÈRE TINDALL
An imprint of Harcourt Publishers Limited

© Baillière Tindall 1995
© Harcourt Publishers Limited 2000

✤ is a registered trademark of Harcourt Publishers Limited

First edition 1995
Second edition 2000

ISBN 0 7020 2328 0

British Library Cataloguing in Publication Data
A catalogue record for this book is available from the British Library

Library of Congress Cataloging in Publication Data
A catalog record for this book is available from the Library of Congress

Note
Medical knowledge is constantly changing. As new information becomes available, changes in treatment, procedures, equipment and the use of drugs become necessary. The editors, contributors and the publishers have, as far as it is possible, taken care to ensure that the information given in this text is accurate and up to date. However, readers are strongly advised to confirm that the information, especially with regard to drug usage, complies with the latest legislation and standards of practice.

Printed in China

Contents

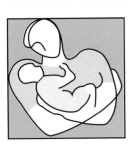

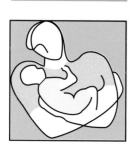

Contributors

Sarah Budd Dip AC BPhil MBAcC RGN RM
Midwifery Sister and Acupuncturist, Maternity Unit, Derriford Hospital, Plymouth, UK

Penelope L. Conway DO PGDip
Registered Osteopath, London, UK

Bridget Cummings RGN RM LCH MCH RSHOM
Independent Midwife/Homeopath, Enniskerry, Republic of Ireland

Dianne Garland SRN RM ADM PGCEA
Senior Midwife – Practice and Research, Maidstone Hospital, Maidstone, UK

Elise M. Johnson BSc mBAc mRSS
Shiatsu Therapist and Acupuncturist, Fryerning, UK

Sue Mack MSc AdDipCoun
Therapist, Charter Nightingale Hospital, London, UK

Fiona Mantle BSc(Hons) RN RHV CertEd RNT
Independent Clinical Nurse Specialist and Lecturer in Complementary Therapies, New Malden, UK

Helen Stapleton MSc RGN SCM MNIMH
Research Midwife, Women's Informed Childbearing and Health Research Group, School of Nursing and Midwifery, University of Sheffield, Sheffield, UK

Dianne Steele BSc(Hons) RGN RM ADM PGCEA Aquanatal ENB Level I & II
Senior Lecturer, School of Health, University of Greenwich, London, UK

Tone Tellefsen BSc DC
Chiropractor, Godalming Chiropractic Clinic, Godalming, UK

Denise Tiran RGN RM ADM PGCEA
Principal Lecturer – Complementary Therapies/Midwifery, School of Health, University of Greenwich, London, UK

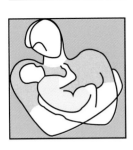

Acknowledgements

Chris Mack of Starlight Productions for the photographs of osteopathy and shiatsu.

Nursing Times for the use of photographs of Denise Tiran.

Carola Beresford-Cooke for the boxed quotation at the foot of p. 194.

All the midwives, mothers and doctors who gave their help and especially those who agreed to be photographed.

Denise Tiran

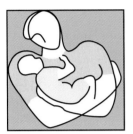

Chapter 1 **Incorporation of Complementary Therapies into Maternity Care**

Complementary and alternative medicine is one of the fastest growing areas of healthcare for both consumers and professionals. Over one in three people in the United Kingdom has sought help or advice from a complementary therapist (Consumers' Association, 1995) and certain areas of alternative medicine have become highly successful commercial enterprises, notably the aromatherapy and herbal medicine fields. Medical practitioners are increasingly acknowledging the benefits of many areas of complementary medicine. Since the publication of the British Medical Association's report (1993) *Complementary Medicine: New Approaches to Good Practice* in which there was a tacit acceptance of some of the more widely used therapies, there has been improved communication leading to greater understanding and collaboration between conventional and complementary practitioners. General practitioners are more willing to refer patients for treatment from therapists such as osteopaths and chiropractors, particularly since their national regulation under the Osteopaths Act of 1993 and the Chiropractors Act of 1994. Increasing numbers of GPs are adding to their skills by learning acupuncture or homeopathy and then selecting whichever is the most appropriate system of care for an individual. Midwives, nurses and health visitors in particular are incorporating various therapies into their existing practice or are interested in extending their role and learning more about the alternatives. Indeed, a recent report

(NHS Confederation, 1997) identified midwives as the professional group most likely to use complementary therapies, with 34% of midwives from a survey in Leicestershire having utilised one or more therapies in their work. Complementary practitioners too are evolving improved education at undergraduate and postgraduate levels for both initial registration and ongoing practice and recognising the need for research and evidence-based practice.

Whilst preparing the Report (1993) the British Medical Association's working party set out to identify exactly how many complementary and alternative therapies exist, and emerged with a list of over 140 different therapies! Today this number is probably nearer 180 and growing constantly, although many are so newly developed or so obscure that they have no real academic, research-based background and are generally disregarded by orthodox practitioners, while others are considered to be aspects of conventional care such as counselling and relaxation techniques or, in specialities such as mental health, art, music or drama therapy. The BMA listed what they considered to be the 'top ten' therapies, with the 'big five' (homeopathy, osteopathy, chiropractic, acupuncture and medical herbalism) being those discrete systems of medicine which are nationally regulated, or in the process of becoming so, having defined criteria for education and training, codes of conduct and a sound body of evidence to support them. The other five therapies are thought of as 'supportive' and include those which may be used alongside either conventional treatments or other complementary practices: massage, aromatherapy, reflexology, shiatsu/acupressure and hypnotherapy.

The move towards integrated care It is interesting to note the changes in terminology which have occurred in previous years, from 'witchcraft' or 'fringe medicine', with the underlying implication of something un-acceptable, to 'alternative' and 'complementary'. Therapies may still of course be considered as alternatives to current surgery, medicine or other orthodox treatment regimes, or they may be used as an adjunct to other forms of care. The British Medical Association report (1993) referred to 'non-conventional' therapies, although what is conventional within con-temporary healthcare may not be so in the future, nor was it necessarily so in the past.

Many people refer to 'natural' remedies, although this can lead to the mistaken belief that 'natural' means 'safe'. Indeed there have been reports of deaths and severe complications from the inappropriate use of natural substances (Beccara, 1995; Hartnoll et al., 1993). Neither is the term 'non-pharmaceutical' strictly accurate, for although some herbal and aromatherapy remedies may be absorbed into the body, metabolised and excreted in ways similar to synthetic pharmaceutical preparations, this is not true of all therapies.

The accelerating pace of change in the acceptance of complementary and alternative therapies has hitherto resulted in the evolution of a new phrase—integrated medicine—implying a 'coming together' of the two systems of healthcare, which are, after all, merely two ends of the same spectrum.

In 1997 the Foundation for Integrated Medicine was launched to promote the further integration of complementary medicine into conventional healthcare, and its report (FIM, 1997) focused specifically on the areas of education and training, research, regulation and delivery of services. A conference in London in 1997, hosted by the Foundation and attended by its Patron, HRH the Prince of Wales and the Secretary of State for Health, brought together a vast range of expertise from the conventional and complementary fields to discuss the way forward for integrated healthcare.

Why then has there been such an explosion of interest in complementary medicine in recent years? The boom may be due in part to increasing demands from consumers to be more actively involved in their care, to act in partnership with professionals and no longer merely to accept the belief that 'doctor knows best'. Within maternity care this fact was highlighted in the Department of Health *Changing Childbirth* report of 1993 in which it was recommended that women should have 'choice, control and continuity', and much work has been done to develop innovative initiatives for pregnant and childbearing women around the country. The incorporation of complementary therapies into conventional maternity care expands choices for women and helps them to feel in control of their own wellbeing. There is also a growing acknowledgement that conventional or allopathic medicine does not have all the answers and is not appropriate for all illnesses—take for example the difficulties of treating HIV infection or myalgic encephalitis (ME). For pregnant women there have always been physiological symptoms which have not been treatable with drugs, either because the drugs are potentially teratogenic or because resistant symptoms simply fail to respond to the medicines which can be used.

One of the advantages of complementary medicine is that therapists possibly have more time to talk to their clients than many of their colleagues in the National Health Service, mainly due to workload differences, although as complementary practices become more widespread the time allocation per client may be forced to be reduced. Patients and clients dislike the 'conveyor belt' system which operates in the National Health Service, and want to be treated as individuals working in partnership with their care givers.

However, the fundamental difference between conventional and complementary medicine is the philosophy underpinning each system. Orthodox medicine views the body in a reductionist manner, as an engine which can be dismantled, mended and reassembled, irrespective of temperament, personality, emotions or external influences. Complementary medicine is based on an understanding of the interaction between body, mind and spirit, and a recognition of each person as an individual in the wider context of the environment. Advice and counselling is central to the philosophy of complementary therapy, an integral part of a partnership between therapist and client, in which the latter has as much responsibility for involvement in their treatment as the former. Midwives pride themselves on practising a profession which incorporates an holistic approach to care of pregnant and newly delivered women and their families, yet they are constrained by time, money and politics, which often prevents them from providing truly integrated care of body, mind and spirit.

There can be said to be an over-reliance, in some areas of orthodox healthcare, on technology, although the outstanding advances which have been made must also be applauded. Conversely, complementary medicine frequently receives negative reports in the media, for example the cancer patient who rejects conventional treatment known to work and who subsequently dies. Perhaps the pertinent point is that any element of treatment must be used appropriately, whether it be high technology or natural remedies. It will also, of course, depend on whether therapies are used as an alternative, i.e. instead of, or as a complement, i.e. an adjunct to, conventional practices. The World Health Organization (1993) recommended that in the Western world there should be a return to more natural methods of pain relief in labour and less dependence on high technology. Certainly within obstetrics, and to a lesser extent within midwifery, there is an element of defensive practice, the 'just in case' syndrome, on which some professionals base a more technology-dependent style of care, one which restricts flexibility, and consequently maternal choice.

Fortunately the meteoric rise of popularity of complementary therapies appears to have 'given permission' to consumers to broach the subject with their GPs, midwives or other care givers. However, this does remain sporadic and is affected by opinions, experiences and knowledge of individuals in local maternity units. The very fact that women may have previously used remedies or consulted complementary therapists, or may wish to self-administer herbal, homeopathic or aromatherapy treatments during pregnancy and labour, means that conventional healthcare professionals cannot be complacent or dismissive about their use. It is far better that women are given correct advice and feel that they can discuss uses of complementary therapies openly than that they should continue to administer them covertly, with the possible risks of problems such as drug interactions or exacerbation of pathological conditions. Ideally the subject should be broached at the very first meeting between the mother-to-be and the midwife and recorded as part of the booking history.

Research The focus of maternity care on the normal physiological process of pregnancy, parturition and the puerperium and the consequent reluctance to submit women to pharmacological preparations to relieve symptoms facilitates the use of more natural remedies in the sometimes mistaken belief that they can do no harm. However it is important to remember that where a remedy has the power to do good it also has the potential to do harm if used inappropriately or inaccurately. It is therefore incumbent on all health professionals to ensure that the advice or treatment they offer to women, be it conventional or complementary, is 'based on sound principles and all available contemporary knowledge' (UKCC, 1994), which, where possible, should be evidence-based.

It remains one of the problems of the relationship between conventional and complementary medicine that until recently there appears to have been little research to demonstrate either the effectiveness or the safety of alternative therapies, and sceptical medical staff use this as an argument not to become involved. However, it makes no sense on the one hand to dismiss complementary therapies as being of no use and on the other to reject them because of the perceived harm they may do to patients. It should also be pointed out that some medical practices have been introduced and continue to be used without adequate preparatory investigation into their safety and true worth. Furthermore the current lack of scientific data does not automatically mean that complementary therapies are of no value. Hitherto research into alternative therapies was either not published or was improperly written up in non-peer reviewed journals or was published only in non-English language journals which were often inaccessible. This situation is slowly changing and a much improved dialogue of discussion is taking place in mainstream respected journals such as the *British Medical Journal*, *The Lancet* and the American medical journals. There has also been a disregard by the medical establishment for anything other than randomised, double-blind controlled clinical trials, but this is not always an appropriate methodology for complementary medical research. Whilst this issue has not yet been resolved it has initiated collaborative discussion about methodologies which can bring only positive outcomes for the future.

Research findings on complementary therapies can be accessed via the Internet from a variety of database sources including Cinahl, Medline, Extract (the Exeter Traditional Medicine, Pharmacology and Chemistry Project initiated at Exeter University) and various worldwide complementary medicine databases. The Research Council for Complementary Medicine, set up in 1983, offers a telephone service for enquirers to request literature searches on any aspect of complementary medicine.

Education and training In England and Wales, under English Common Law, it is perfectly acceptable for anyone to set themselves up in private practice as a complementary therapist without a recognised qualification, so long as they do not do anything which is against the law, for example guarantee to cure cancer, treat tuberculosis or pose as a professional whose role is defined by law such as a doctor or midwife. However, training and education for the 'top ten' therapies has become far more formalised and academic with minimum criteria laid down, and many courses are university based, offering a firm grounding in biological sciences as well as the philosophy and practice of the individual therapy. Similarly preparatory and post-basic courses for practitioners of conventional healthcare now include at least an introduction to complementary medicine, in line with the proposals of the report of the Foundation for Integrated Medicine (1997).

It is vital that all practitioners are adequately and appropriately educated. It is not acceptable, for example, for a doctor to assume that because he or she has completed six or more years' training in *conventional* medicine, they can add a complementary therapy such as acupuncture to their skills by undertaking a short six week course. Neither should a complementary therapist presume that a generic qualification in a specific therapy entitles them to specialise in treating pregnant and labouring women without further in-depth training in the relevant physiology and a knowledge and understanding of conventional maternity care.

Some of the supportive therapies such as aromatherapy and reflexology have pursued the idea of key competencies and National Occupational Standards. Others, for example herbal medicine, acupuncture and hypnotherapy, require initial qualifications at undergraduate and postgraduate level. There is also an increasing number of complementary medical studies being undertaken as part of Masters or PhD level courses.

Regulation of complementary therapies Although some of the more obscure therapies remain largely unregulated, the 'top ten' have moved increasingly towards national regulation. The osteopaths and chiropractors chose to go down the statutory regulation pathway and the process of standardising requirements and updating long-experienced practitioners is under way to ensure protection of the public from inadequately trained therapists. Other therapies have selected a system of voluntary self-regulation, such as the acupuncturists and herbalists, and while homeopaths currently retain two 'camps' they do at least identify those who are medically qualified and those who are lay homeopaths.

Other therapies continue to have several regulating bodies, although most aromatherapy organisations belong to the Aromatherapy Organisations Council and reflexologists are in the process of developing a similar system.

A number of over-arching regulatory bodies for complementary medicine exist, such as the British Complementary Medicine Association, the Institute for Complementary Medicine and the Council for Complementary and Alternative Medicine, all of which constitute the expert group accepted by the government to debate complementary medicine. Other organisations, such as the Guild of Complementary Practitioners, provide regulation in the form of registration, subject to defined minimum criteria, disciplinary codes of conduct and requirements for regular updating, thus enabling practitioners to obtain personal professional indemnity insurance.

Issues for healthcare professionals incorporating complementary therapies into their practice There are several issues which midwives and other practitioners of conventional maternity care need to consider when utilising complementary therapies, whether they use the therapies within their own practice, offer advice to women wishing to self-administer remedies such as Bach Flower or homeopathic remedies, aromatherapy or herbal substances, or recommend women to therapists outside mainstream services.

Education and training As mentioned previously, the therapist must be adequately and appropriately educated. For midwives and others registered with the United Kingdom Central Council this does not necessarily mean that they must be fully qualified therapists, but that they must be able to justify their actions. It is therefore acceptable for a midwife to use, for example, one aromatherapy essential oil if they are fully familiar with it, even if they are not qualified aromatherapists, or to apply acupressure wristbands to the P6 wrist points to relieve nausea, so long as they have the relevant underpinning knowledge and understanding.

For midwives wishing to train in a particular therapy it is important to select a course which will fulfil their long-term aims in relation to integrating that therapy into midwifery practice. For example the choice of therapy may depend on personal interest but will also need to be considered in the context of the individual's place of work. Aromatherapy and reflexology are perhaps more easily incorporated into everyday midwifery practice than acupuncture or homeopathy, which may be viewed by medical staff with scepticism, derision or fear (although these reactions are usually based on lack of knowledge). Demand from local women will also play a part, for instance a demand for information on herbal remedies or homeopathy may prompt the funding to train a midwife in the relevant therapy.

Issues to consider when choosing a course include the entry criteria, length, cost and intended qualification from the course, knowledge, skills and experience of the lecturers, relevance to the client group, assessment strategies, supervision and ongoing education policies of the institution. Individual midwives may additionally need to consider whether or not they can obtain funding from their employers, scholarships or a grant and the extent of support from their managers in terms of both time off and moral support.

There are several sources of funding available to midwives wishing to undertake complementary therapy courses, including most of the scholarship schemes supported by the Royal College of Midwives; one in particular, The Pregnancy Shop, specifically directs a proportion of its profits towards complementary therapy education for midwives.

Where women wish to access complementary therapy services not provided by the NHS, midwives should advise them to ensure that any independent practitioner is adequately and appropriately trained and experienced, preferably specialising in treating pregnant and childbearing women, that they are registered with one of the principal regulatory organisations and that they possess personal professional indemnity insurance.

Accountability and obligations Any practitioner must abide by the parameters laid down by their own regulating body. Midwives are accountable for their practice and should be guided by the UKCC documents on issues related to good practice.

Rule 40 of the *Midwives' Rules and Code of Practice* (UKCC, 1998) states that a midwife should not undertake any practice for which she has not been adequately and appropriately trained, although *The Scope of Professional Practice* (UKCC, 1992) states that the emphasis is not on collecting certificates but rather places responsibility for professional accountability firmly with the individual midwife. The midwife must therefore be able to justify her/his actions and recognise personal parameters of practice.

The Midwives' Rules and Code of Practice (UKCC, 1998) acknowledges that certain new skills may become integral to the role of some, but not all, midwives and specifically identifies complementary therapies as an area for consideration. The Code emphasises the need for sound contemporary knowledge, client consent and their right to self-administer substances such as herbal and homeopathic preparations.

The *Guidelines for Professional Practice* (UKCC, 1996) document examines the issue of accountability in relation to advertising of complementary therapy services by nurses, midwives and health visitors and the use of their UKCC registration to enhance the perception of acceptability of a therapy. It also reflects on the boundaries of practice for each profession: in the case of a midwife who practises a complementary therapy independently she must acknowledge when she is working as a midwife and when she is working as a therapist. It would not be acceptable, for example, to be working as a therapist but to provide care to a pregnant client if that care would normally be within the remit of midwifery practice, unless the therapist had notified her intention to practise as a midwife in a private capacity.

Advocacy and rights Women have the right to administer to themselves or to refuse when complementary remedies are offered, although if the midwife believes that the mother's choice of remedy may be detrimental to her care she should discuss the matter with a 'relevant expert practitioner' (UKCC, 1998). On the other hand midwives should act as the mothers' advocate in cases of conflict between clients and other professionals in order to facilitate choices.

Communication and collaboration It is vital to liaise with colleagues when midwives are caring for women who wish to self-administer natural remedies, or when the midwife is utilising aspects of complementary therapy in her work. This includes written and verbal communication as appropriate with other midwives, obstetricians, paediatricians, physiotherapists, general practitioners, independent complementary therapists and, of course, with the women and their families. A facilitative attitude based on sound knowledge, research-based practice and mutual respect must lead to enhanced care for the women.

Consent/record keeping Mothers offered complementary therapies by midwives or doctors must give their consent, having been offered all available information on which to base their decision. This does not necessarily need to be in writing, although comprehensive records must be kept. The mother has the right to refuse complementary treatments in the same way as any others but health professionals must take care not to prejudice her decision because of their own beliefs or biases. As with all care, detailed records must be kept and it may be appropriate to devise a form specifically for complementary therapy treatments.

Policies and protocols It is not acceptable for midwives who are qualified in complementary therapies simply to incorporate them into their practice without the knowledge of their supervisor of midwives. Within the NHS this will mean also obtaining permission to utilise the therapy; failure to work within trust policies may invalidate personal professional indemnity insurance and will certainly mean that the individual is not covered by the vicarious liability of the health authority.

Policies and protocols protect both the clients and the professionals and can be used very constructively to expand practice. Policies may be developed in relation to individual therapies, individual practitioners or aspects of therapies, such as in the form of a 'standing order' for a specific aromatherapy essential oil. However, it should be remembered that it is not appropriate to request an approval signature for the 'standing order' from someone such as the senior obstetrician unless he or she is qualified to sanction the use of the therapy.

Ideally policies should be devised in conjunction with midwife clinicians, managers, educators and supervisors, medical and other staff and possibly representative consumers. Individual policies may identify acceptable complementary therapy qualifications or training of midwives wishing to use them, named members of staff on a 'live' register, which therapies can be used for which conditions, contraindications, precautions and any other restrictions.

Evaluation and audit Monitoring of statistical data, efficacy and other relevant information can be a useful means of developing further the complementary therapy service offered within a maternity unit. Midwives initially struggling to establish a therapy could devise a proposal to carry out a short-term trial on identified areas of the therapy in order to demonstrate its efficacy, safety and cost-effectiveness. This may be, for example, the use of lavender oil to ease perineal discomfort, acupressure wrist bands for nausea and vomiting, Rescue remedy to reduce phlebotomy phobia, reflex zone therapy to treat postnatal retention of urine or homeopathic arnica for bruising. Audit may also take the form of assessing the satisfaction of the women who have used complementary therapies during their pregnancies.

In summary, the following issues are relevant to the use of complementary therapies by midwives:

- Midwives should have received some form of training in the therapy they wish to practise and recognise the limitations of that practice.
- The practice of complementary therapies should be based on sound knowledge and available research findings.
- Written and verbal communications with colleagues and parents must be maintained in order to achieve optimum care for the client.
- The use of complementary therapies must not be at the expense of normal midwifery responsibilities, nor should it conflict with conventional medical care.
- Midwives must seek informed consent from the client and respect the rights of individuals to decline treatment on moral or religious grounds.
- Employed midwives should gain approval from their managers before embarking on incorporating complementary therapies into their practice.
- All midwives are subject to the normal parameters of control by supervisors of midwives.

Pregnancy and childbirth are normal physiological, psychological, sociological life events for generally fit and healthy women and their families, and complementary therapies can usefully be used as an adjunct to conventional maternity care. They offer increased choice and control to women and fewer side-effects than many of the pharmaceutical options, and enable the mother to achieve not only a safe delivery of a healthy child but also to experience a satisfying, significant episode in her life.

Mothers and midwives are looking to complementary therapies to avoid the risks of drugs to the unborn baby, to provide more natural advice for the relief of common discomforts of pregnancy and the postnatal period and to seek alternative forms of pain relief in labour. Midwives are qualifying as acupuncturists and reflex zone therapists and utilising massage, aromatherapy and herbal remedies in their work. Women are seeking advice on homeopathy, learning hypnotherapy or being attended in labour by an osteopath or shiatsu practitioner. The demand from women has resulted in a massive rise in interest from healthcare professionals and the establishment of the Complementary Therapies in Maternity Care National Forum which brings together all professionals involved in using or investigating these therapies for pregnancy and childbirth in an attempt to improve the integration of the two systems of care.

This book is not intended as a 'how to' guide, although many simple remedies such as dietary measures can be safely suggested to mothers. There are many excellent texts on each of the therapies discussed, some of which are recommended for further reading at the end of each chapter. In addition, useful addresses are included to enable midwives wishing to pursue training in one of the therapies to find out more. The identification of priorities for midwives involved in using complementary therapies, either directly or indirectly, is essential. The issue of professional accountability is considered to be paramount and is addressed throughout.

It is not the purpose of the book to denigrate the medical or pharmaceutical professions, both of which have vital but different roles to play in the care of childbearing women and their families. Any perceived disparagement is merely a factor in discussions regarding the current nature and status of complementary therapies in relation to conventional care. Indeed it is hoped the text may go some way towards improving the relationship between midwives, doctors and complementary therapists in order to extend the range of treatments available to our clients.

It is the intention to offer an introduction for midwives into the potential uses, and abuses, of complementary therapies for childbearing women. An exploration of some of the commoner therapies with which midwives might come into contact is provided. Mothers may request advice about specific therapies or aspects of complementary medicine, and midwives should be equipped to furnish them with adequate information to make a decision about their uses. Interested midwives may wish to undertake training in a certain therapy to enhance their care of women throughout pregnancy, labour and thepuerperium. Clients may be receiving treatment from therapists outside the conventional system and maternity staff should have an understanding of the interrelationship between all carers.

All professionals need to work in harmony in order to provide the best quality and the most appropriate care for expectant and newly delivered mothers and their families. Mothers have a right to choose whatever they perceive as best for their individual situation and should be assisted in so doing by knowledgeable, expert, experienced practitioners who work in collaboration with each other and with women.

References

Beccara M D 1995 Melaleuca oil poisoning in a 17-month old. *Veterinary and Human Toxicology* 37(6): 557–8

British Medical Association 1993 *Complementary medicine: new approaches to good practice*. Oxford University Press, Oxford

Consumers' Association 1995 Healthy choice. *Which?* November 8–13

Department of Health 1993 *Changing Childbirth: report of the Expert Maternity Group*. HMSO, London

Foundation for Integrated Medicine 1997 *Integrated Healthcare: a way forward for the next five years?* FIML, London

Hartnoll G, Moore D and Douek D 1995 Near fatal ingestion of oil of cloves. *Archives of Diseases in Childhood* 69: 392–393

NHS Confederation 1997 *Complementary medicine in the NHS: managing the issues*. NHS Confederation, Birmingham

United Kingdom Central Council 1992 *The Scope of Professional Practice*. UKCC, London

United Kingdom Central Council 1996 *Guidelines for Professional Practice*. UKCC, London

United Kingdom Central Council 1998 *Midwives' Rules and Code of Practice*. UKCC, London

Wagner M 1993 *The Birth Machine*. Temple University Press, Philadelphia

Further reading

Journals
Complementary therapies in nursing and midwifery. Churchill Livingstone, Edinburgh

Complementary therapies in medicine. Churchill Livingstone, Edinburgh

Books
Mitchell A, Cormack M 1998 *The therapeutic relationship in complementary health care*. Churchill Livingstone, Edinburgh

University of Exeter 1997 *Professional organisation of complementary and alternative medicine in the UK*. Centre for Complementary Health Studies, Exeter

Bridget Cummings, Denise Tiran

Chapter 2

Homeopathy for Pregnancy and Childbirth

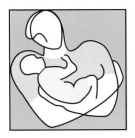

Introduction

Homeopathy is a pharmacological system of medicine using set principles and laws for administering specially prepared medicinal substances to correct individuals' disease. Homeopathy offers a safe, gentle and effective method of preventative, as well as curative, medicine. It promotes normal physiological processes and can stimulate the body's defences, in order for it to heal or correct itself. Health is seen as the well-being of mind, body and spirit. Ill-health is seen as disharmony within the whole person shown by the symptoms expressed. Its holistic and individualised approach can obviate weak areas of health and help remove these tendencies, optimising the health potential of the unborn baby whilst treating the mother.

Choudhury (1988) considered susceptibility to be the primary cause of disease and certainly the state of the mother and baby plays an enormous part in the progress of the pregnancy, birth and puerperium. Mental and emotional health as well as the mother's approach to birth is also included in her 'susceptibility'. To treat susceptibility ideally both parents would benefit from homeopathic consultation preconceptionally.

During pregnancy, labour and the postpartum period homeopathy can be used safely and effectively to treat common ailments. Provided there are no irreversible mechanical problems, homeopathy can promote a normal labour with minimal pain and discomfort. The specially prepared minute dose of the remedy ensures elimination of its toxicity whilst enhancing its curative effects. It is so dilute that no molecules of the original substance remain. Women are most commonly attracted to homeopathy during childbearing for this aspect alone.

Homeopaths do not prescribe when the progress of the pregnancy and birth is normal and healthy. Like midwives, homeopaths believe in nature and letting it work when things are going well. It is only when nature shows itself to be in need of assistance, in the form of symptoms expressed in the mother and observed by the carers, that a remedy is prescribed.

This shows the importance of knowing what 'normal' is. Birth is a normal physiological process and midwives view birth as normal until proven otherwise.

The midwife is the expert in normal birth and has an important role to play in the enhancement of primal health. When a carefully selected remedy is prescribed, homeopathy can help avoid obstetric intervention or drugs, and hence 'side-effects'; iatrogenic disease or adverse reactions from orthodox medicine are prevented. The remedy addresses an imbalance, whether emotional or physical. It works on an energy level and can stimulate vitality and the ability of the mother to cope. A knowledge and understanding of the principles and laws of homeopathy increases the sensitivity and perception of the midwife to the needs of the mother choosing this model of health and disease.

Midwives are trained under traditional 'medicine' and may find it difficult to accept homeopathy. Dr Donald Foubister (1989) found the ignorance about homeopathy in the medical profession hard to believe. This was especially noticeable in the education of medical students, where direct chemical or physical effects of drugs alone are taught.

Treating birth as a physical science, examining the biochemistry and biophysics, ignores the fact that birth is inseparable from its mental, emotional and social aspects. Obstetrics can intervene on a physical level, using fluids, drugs and instruments, but if the root cause is mental or emotional then this approach can be very traumatic (Tew, 1990).

The midwife is in a position to allow free expression of anxieties and other emotions and to allay fears. If her skills, support and nurturing are not enough to change the situation then homeopathy is an ideal, non-interventionist therapeutic tool. Rather than ignoring the mental and emotional symptoms, homeopathy uses them as the most important indicators as to the selection of a necessary remedy. Homeopathy can be incorporated successfully alongside sensitive midwifery care, by appropriately trained carers.

Peter, a first baby, was born naturally at home. He screamed and fretted at the breast and did not latch on. All 'calming' and encouraging methods were used to little or no effect.

This continued for a week, at which point expertise from

La Leche League was also sought. The mother was expressing her milk and feeding Peter using a spoon. Sometimes Peter would 'drip feed' at the breast. After discussion Anne, the mother, realised that the initial breastfeed after the birth had been extremely tense, so much so that Anne had screamed 'in pain'. This had happened at the next attempt also. It was concluded that Peter was frightened at the breast and it was this emotion which needed to be cured. Anne agreed to try Aconite 30 c. One tablet was crushed and given to the baby and the mother also had a dose. The result was immediate in that Peter calmed down, slept for a long stretch and awoke to latch on perfectly. The baby breastfed beautifully from then on.

The foundations of homeopathy

Dr Samuel Hahnemann (1755–1845) of Germany was the founder of homeopathy. He chose the name from the Greek words *homois*- 'similar' and *pathos*- 'suffering'. Whilst translating a medical text (Cullen, 1789) he was sceptical about the given reason why the Peruvian Bark (from which quinine is made) brought on the symptoms of malaria. These symptoms disappeared as soon as he stopped taking the Peruvian Bark. He realised that the drug that was known to cure malaria also produced symptoms like malaria! He gathered together many other examples of cures and in each case found that the drug used could also produce symptoms similar to those that it had cured (Handley, 1990). Hahnemann had discovered the principle that 'like cures like' or the 'Law of Similars'. In the fifth century BC Hippocrates had found that there were two ways of healing—by 'opposites' and by 'similars'. Hahnemann made the law of similars practical.

Orthodox medicine uses 'opposites'. For example, in constipation a medicine will be given which produces diarrhoea. Homeopathy uses 'similars'. For example, a remedy known to produce constipation in its crude form would cure the constipation if given in a small dose.

The symptoms caused by too much of a substance are the symptoms that can also be cured with a small dose of that substance, for example too much radium causes cancer whilst a small dose cures cancer.

Another instance from everyday life is seen when cutting a strong onion. An acrid runny nose, a particular soreness in the throat and stinging, running eyes may be experienced. A homeopath will prescribe *allium cepa* (the remedy made from onion) for the person who has a cold and bad throat with those particular symptoms. Similarly, strong coffee can give headaches and unusual activity of the mind and body. It is often drunk to 'keep us going!' A homeopath may prescribe *coffea* where there is insomnia of that nature. In relation to childbirth, a crude dose of *Ipecacuanha* (Ipecac root) will produce constant nausea and vomiting, with much saliva but a clean tongue. A minute dose of *Ipecacuanha* will relieve vomiting during pregnancy if the symptoms match.

Hahnemann went on to discover that minute doses of homeopathic remedies were safer and in fact more effective. Many years were spent experimenting and verifying the Law of Similars. In order to discover the curative potential of medicines, Hahnemann concluded that they should be tested on healthy people; these 'provings' (see Glossary) or drugs tests are still being done today amongst homeopathic students and practitioners but to a far lesser degree, as the information recorded by the early homeopaths is still applicable today. Homeopathy stands strong on its original foundations. Women continue to look for a more natural method of healing. The interest shown during pregnancy and birth suggests a reflection of the desire to keep in control and be active in the childbearing process.

Homeopathy has been, since 1948, the only complementary therapy to be part of Britain's National Health Service, although this situation is now changing. In 1952, the Faculty of Homeopathy in London was established by an Act of Parliament and recognised homeopathy as a safe alternative form of medical treatment.

The Medicines Control Agency licenses the manufacturers of homeopathic medicines. Following the Thalidomide disaster, the Medicines Act 1968 was brought in to legislate for the safety, control and regulation of medicines. Homeopathic remedies are included under this Act.

The general public can of course buy homeopathic medicines over the counter at pharmacies, health food shops and natural medicine centres. These can be useful in acute situations. However, it must be noted that although these are termed 'homeopathic' they cannot be so called until the remedies have been prescribed according to the law of similars. Then and only then is the medicine truly 'homeopathic'. Hence, although safe for women, if the remedy is inappropriately prescribed results will be non-existent. Here, it is the prescriber who is at fault, not homeopathy. This shows the importance of accuracy of prescription and appropriate advice for women. How much easier it would be for women to consult their midwife for an accurate and precise prescription, or at least a referral to a centre for homeopathic advice or consultation. The fear of the homeopath failing to recognise abnormal states in parturient women can be allayed by the fact that women normally attend routine antenatal care (Dhunny, 1993). For chronic prescribing, an in-depth study of homeopathy and its applications is necessary; therefore this is the area where an experienced homeopath should be consulted for the best treatment.

Joanne, a 32-year-old gravida 4, suffered from haemorrhoids from 30 weeks' gestation. She was emotionally very sensitive and often irritable. The 'piles' were very painful and she was also constipated. The urge to open her bowels was ineffectual and the 'piles' were large and protruding. She enjoyed coffee to drink mostly, and spicy foods. In all of her pregnancies she had haemorrhoids and described the pain with them postnatally as 'the worst part'.

The midwife gave an acute prescription of nux vomica 30 c (poison nut) to be taken in the morning and evening for a few days. She was advised to stop taking the nux vom. when there was an improvement. Both the midwife and the mother were expecting temporary relief, recognising that treatment would have been useful before this pregnancy. The report from the mother was that the piles reduced and 'went'. They were expected to return after birth but this did not happen! Constipation was also relieved.

Remedy sources

Sources of homeopathic remedies, and a few examples, are listed in Table 2.1.

There are also metals, such as gold (aurum, *aur.*) and imponderables, such as X-rays and magnetism.

Homeopathy is wide ranging and continues to develop. Like Hahnemann who continued his research and improvements on his work until his dying day, his successors continue to make valuable discoveries, so diversifying the *Materia Medica*, whilst its laws and principles remain the same. This makes medicinal help more likely for most people. More than two thousand

Table 2.1. Sources of homeopathic remedies

Type of source	Example	Remedy abbreviated
Animal kingdom	*Apis* (bee)	
	Cantharis (Spanish fly)	*Canth.*
	Sepia (cuttle fish)	
	Lachesis (snake)	*Lach.*
Plant kingdom	*Arnica montana*	*Arn.*
	Belladonna	*Bell.*
	Chamomilla	*Cham.*
	Pulsatilla nigrens	*Puls.*
Mineral kingdom	Calcarea carbonate	*Calc. carb.*
	Silica	*Sil.*
	Natrum muriaticum (salt)	*Nat. mur.*
	Phosphorus	*Phos.*
Disease products (nosodes)	Tuberculinum koch exotoxin	*Tub.*
	Diphtherium	*Diphth.*
	Pyrogen (pus)	*Pyog.*
Healthy tissues and secretions (sarcodes)	Thyroid	
	Pituitrin	
	Ooverinum	

remedies are now recognised by the homeopathic pharmacopoeia; recent provings include chocolate, granite, hydrogen and scorpion.

Releasing the medicinal properties from the inert substance

Hahnemann originally gave measured doses of the drugs without further processing but he found the reaction either too marked or excessive, or inadequate due to poor preparation. He aimed to process drugs to give better results by reducing toxicity whilst enhancing their curative ability. He also considered the individual and varied sensitivity and reaction to drugs.

He developed a step-by-step dilution and succussion (vigorous shaking) processing method which he called potentisation or dynamisation. Hahnemann wrote that homeopathic dynamisations genuinely bring to life the medicinal properties which lie hidden in natural solids when these are in a crude state (Hahnemann [1821], 1987).

Potentisation

After initial preparation of the raw material, the remedies are made by serial dilution and succussion in a solution of alcohol and water. This is done a few (three to four) times or up to many thousand times. The liquid dilution is then used itself as a remedy or soaked into tablets or granules for convenience. The diluted remedies are described as being 'potentised', in recognition of the dynamic healing power they can stimulate. Hahnemann described the self-healing energy of the person and that which his dynamic remedies stimulate as the vital force (see Glossary). Frequently, the remedy dilution is so great that no chemical trace of the original substance remains.

The process of dilution and succussion apparently imprints the characteristic energy pattern, or blueprint, of the original substance onto the water in which it is diluted. This may be likened to the transmission of television signals, where the original scene is converted into an electromagnetic energy pattern (a signal) which can then be broadcast to your receiver (Society of Homeopaths, undated).

Evidence in support of microdoses One of the more controversial aspects of homeopathy is the fact that infinitesimal doses (microdoses) of a substance – so diluted that no molecules of the original substance remain – can have any impact on a person receiving such a homeopathic dose.

Sceptical people will always point to the placebo effect as an explanation for the homeopathic success stories they have encountered. Whilst homeopaths and their clients know that this medical science is certainly no placebo, it is well worth recording scientific evidence of microdoses working on biochemicals, plants, bacteria, animals and minerals, none of which are known for falling prey to the placebo.

The use of minute quantities is recognised outside of homeopathy in the field of hormonal treatments; for example, the concentration of free thyroid hormone in the blood is one part per 10 000 million parts of blood plasma. Coulter (1981) cited evidence for the infinitesimal dose as below.

Biochemical investigations William Boyd's experiments, published in 1954, were intended to show if a microdilution of mercury chloride added to flasks containing starch, distilled water and diastase would affect the rate of hydrolysis of the starch. The amount of mercury chloride was 61x or 10^{-61} (see 'Potency scales', p. 20). In theory, this should appear to be just distilled water. The outcome, after several rigorous repetitions and attention to detail to avoid error and bias, was that the mercury chloride 61x accelerated the rate of hydrolysis.

The *Pharmaceutical Journal* (September 1954) quoted the President of the London Faculty of Homeopathy that this 'would prove to be one of the greatest medical advances recorded'. Reports also appeared in the British newspapers.

Botanical investigations In 1968 Wannamaker conducted experiments to test the effect of sulphur microdilutions on the growth of onion plants. The microdilutions were found to have a significant effect on the weight and dimensions of the onion bulbs and seedlings and also their calcium, magnesium, potassium and sodium content.

Bacteriological investigations Junker investigated the effect of microdilutions of various substances (including caffeine, lemon juice, hydrochloric acid, and copper sulphate) on paramecia cultures and found they affected the degree of daily growth of the cultures.

Zoological investigations J. and M. Tetau experimented with thuja intoxication of rats. The rats were first taught a conditioned reflex and then injected with thuja until so intoxicated that there was a loss of reflex. A test group of these rats was then injected with thuja in microdilution (9 c) and returned to their normal state more rapidly than the remaining control group.

Investigations using physics Gay and Boiron found that the dielectric index of distilled water (a measurement of electrical charge of the water) was altered by adding to it a small amount of sodium chloride 27 c. By dielectric testing they were able to select the bottle with the microdilution of sodium chloride out of 99 other bottles containing only distilled water.

Drug quality is determined by quantity Maupertuis, an eighteenth-century French mathematician, discovered the 'Law of Least Quantity' which has been accepted in science as a fundamental principle of the universe. He describes it thus: 'The quantity of action necessary to effect change in nature is the least possible.' The prescriber in homeopathy applying the Law of Similars must use the 'minimum dose' to achieve good results without aggravating the patient's symptoms and so avoid unwanted effects (Close, 1981).

Homeopathic remedies cannot cause side-effects or addiction. This area of the infinitesimal dose is the most controversial aspect of homeopathy, along with the principle that the medicinal power of a substance increases with the dilution and succussion.

Fincke (1821–1906), a homeopath, said:

> The quality of action of a homeopathic remedy (i.e. one which has been selected according to the rules of homeopathic prescribing) is determined by its quantity'. 'Thus the Law of Least Action must be acknowledged as the posological principle of homeopathy.' (Close, reprinted 1981.)

With reference to birth, in particular during labour where erratic contractions lead to obstetric augmentation using oxytocic drugs, the minimum dose of such drugs seems appropriate. Available data so far do not show that augmentation using oxytocics is beneficial to mother and baby but that simple measures such as mobility, eating and drinking are just as effective (Enkin et al., 1990). Where this does not work, researchers of effective care in pregnancy and childbirth have recommended a mode of care not dissimilar to homeopathy. 'Logic would dictate that, in such circumstances, the smallest effective drug dose should be given, in the most effective manner' (Enkin et al., 1990).

Individual sensitivity to oxytocin varies from woman to woman and it is unclear how large the initial dose or the increments should be and at what interval they should be implemented. Solid research evidence is lacking. Homeopathy avoids these risks by using the minimum dose of an individualised prescription based on the law of similars and the fixed principles of homeopathic medicine. The specially prepared potency and number of doses is determined by the physician according to the needs of the individual.

Potency scales

Remedies may be prescribed in a number of different strengths, or potencies. The lower potencies have been subjected to less dilution and succussion than the higher ones and are not, broadly speaking, as powerful and long lasting in their effects. It is the lower potencies, such as the sixth (e.g. arnica 6), which are found and bought over the counter. These lower potencies are most useful for self-care situations. They can be repeated as often as necessary in an acute situation. High potency remedies are usually prescribed by experienced, qualified homeopaths. The higher potencies are used more in chronic cases and are not suitable for self-prescribing.

The two most commonly used scales likely to be met by the midwife are as follows.

The decimal scale is shown by the letter 'x' after the amount of dilutant, for example 6x. This scale 'x' means that the first dilution is of one part of the original substance with nine parts of alcohol and water to make ten parts, i.e. $1 \pm 9 = 10$ dilution. So 6x (scale 'x') means that the medicine was diluted one part to nine parts (:9), then shaken (succussed), diluted again 1:9 and shaken and this procedure was repeated six times.

The centesimal scale is shown by the letter 'c' after the number of dilutions, e.g. 30 c. This means that the medicine was diluted one part to 99 parts to make 100 parts, i.e. $1 + 99 = 100$, then shaken; then diluted again 1 : 99 and shaken; and this was repeated 30 times.

Experienced homeopaths may use further scales. The M scale refers to a dilution of 1 : 1000 and when a medicine is labelled LM, it was diluted / 1 : 50 000.

The midwife will most commonly come across the 6x, 12x, 6 c, 30 c and 200 c potencies.

Principles of prescribing

Successful prescribing is achieved through following the principles of homeopathy laid down by Hahnemann in the sixth edition of *The Organon of Medicine* published in 1842 (Dudgeon, 1921). These principles require in–depth study.

Homeopathy treats the person as a whole and as an individual. The practice of homeopathy convinces the prescriber to view the body as more than the sum of its parts. All symptoms of the expressed complaint or condition, mental, emotional and physical, are regarded as evidence of a natural effort to resolve an inner disturbance and regain the balanced state of health. The aim of homeopathic medicine is to stimulate autoregulation and is chosen in relation to the way the individual reacts.

In acute situations the symptoms are easy to prescribe on because they are clearly defined, such as in earache or measles. Chronic disease is more complicated and so professional homeopathy is advised, whereby the root cause of the problem is treated and not just the 'named' disease.

Labour and the birth process is considered to be an 'acute' situation. The similar remedy given will stimulate the concerted effort of the body to promote a physiological and emotional process as best it can. Midwives supporting women through natural childbirth may view homeopathy as yet another intervention. This would be a misconception of a fundamental principle of homeopathy. A remedy is a stimulus only and gives nothing material to the mother nor detracts from her achievement. Midwives and homeopaths aim for a healthy baby to be born to an alert, nurturing and healthy mother whose recovery is speedy. Supporting women to achieve their own physiological potential is part of this. Homeopathy can only work with what is already there, in the person. It adds nothing and can be a great stimulus.

In order to aid communication between families, their midwife and their homeopath, the principles of homeopathy are outlined below.

Principles of homeopathy

The law of similars There are natural examples of the law of similars, such as frostbite treated with snow, sadness relieved by hearing of a worse case, phobias treated with facing the object, a cup of tea on a hot day. There are small areas where orthodoxy uses the principle of 'like cures like' without acknowledging it.

Examples include:

- the use of pollen extracts, housedust, etc. to reduce and eliminate sensitivity
- nitroglycerine (*Glonoine*), first introduced by a homeopath for cardiac symptoms and to treat angina. A century later, doctors and homeopaths use it in the management of angina pectoris
- metallic gold (*aurum*), used by homeopaths for rheumatic complaints and introduced in 1935 to orthodox medicine to treat rheumatoid arthritis
- ergot—homeopathic provings revealed circulatory difficulties, and so homeopaths used it to treat gangrene and Raynaud's disease: in 1933 doctors successfully used it to treat Raynaud's disease and later inter-mittent claudication and peripheral vascular disease. The provings revealed headaches, and in the nineteenth century homeopaths pioneered its use. Now doctors use it in migraine preparations.

To apply the law of similars, the individual symptoms of the person must be obtained and not a named collective disease concept. The individual clinical picture is matched with the symptoms obtained in drugs tests that are most similar. So 'painful contractions', 'hypertension' and 'failure to progress in labour' are the diagnosis or result of disease and as such are a name for but not the details of the external expression of the internal disease. The 'totality of symptoms' is the sole guide to the selection of a remedy and includes the physical, mental and emotional responses. It need not include every symptom but the principal signs and symptoms, usually mixed together to reveal an essence or style of what is truly going on. It does not ignore useful information obtained from the carers either, including pathology, or the use of conventional drugs or surgery as needed. In fact, the skills of the midwife with her observations and assessment can be crucial in the selection of the most similar and therefore most accurate remedy. The participation of the mother is obviously encouraged, although distur-bance is avoided, as much information is obtained without asking her a single question, particularly in labour.

The single remedy Only one remedy should be given at a time. This single remedy is the most similar remedy at any one time.

Prescribing the single remedy on the totality of symptoms generates experience of the remedy action and is of further learning value. Giving different remedies for different areas of the mother will confuse this issue and the practitioner will have difficulty evaluating the case. Hahnemann wrote, 'It is wrong to employ complex means when simple will suffice' (Dudgeon, 1921). A single remedy is enough to stimulate correction of the whole person.

The minimum dose The smallest dose possible is all that is needed to stimulate a reaction in the self-corrective power of the person. Safety encourages this principle.

Provings (drug tests) The law of similars is a method whereby the medicinal action of the remedy can be verified. So, each time this principle is applied and the remedy works, it is further evidence of the capabilities of medicines and verification of the law of similars. Also, it is not enough to look at 'poisonings' from substances to gain knowledge of the potential remedy's capabilities. 'Provings' need to be carefully done. These are the homeopathic 'drug tests'.

A minute dose of the substance is given to a group of healthy people in repeated doses sufficient to elicit symptoms but not damage. In this way, the symptoms can be noted down and a 'symptom picture' of the remedy will appear. No detail is spared but these tests are obviously limited to the subtoxic range. Symptoms noted are largely subjective and show the changes experienced by each 'prover'. Data are also obtained from toxicology and pharmacology. Organic lesions and profound functional disorders are noted from deliberate and accidental poisoning.

'Provers' today will display exactly the same symptoms as those of the nineteenth century when given the same remedy. So symptoms in people are unchanging, whilst the modern orthodox medical model of health and disease produces new theories of the causes of disease from year to year and is continually researching ever more complicated pathological and/or biochemical processes. Alongside this continual movement of medical thought and discoveries, modern industries are always researching new drugs or medicines to assist in healing the sick.

Homeopathic drug tests, principles and laws are unchanging. Homeopathy applies the law of similars scientifically and systematically, using carefully tested medicines.

The results of provings are published and form the *Materia Medica*. Each remedy's 'symptom picture' is listed. In order to match the symptoms of the patient with a symptom picture of a remedy, often a repertory is used. The *Repertory* alphabetically lists symptoms of disease, with the remedy names applying to each symptom. It is thus a cross-reference for the *Materia Medica*. Vast volumes of *Materia Medica* and repertory works are now available on computer.

The law of cure   Homeopaths are able to evaluate their work, especially in chronic cases, through time and observation of the totality of symptoms. This is done anatomically as well as historically. By using the law of cure formulated by Konstantin Hering (1800–80) it is possible to assess that healing took place in response to the remedy and not in spite of it.

Natural healing begins by removing the 'disease' away from the vital centres and towards the less vital areas until it is removed. Experience has shown that cure takes place:

- in reverse order of the appearance of symptoms;
- from above to below;
- from within to without;
- from more vital to less vital organs.

The most important of these is the reverse order of appearance.

It can be deduced that onset or exacerbation of an illness will appear as the opposite of the above, with completely new symptoms or more complicated chronic suffering.

The midwife needs to understand this aspect of homeopathy because she may be with a mother who is having professional homeopathic treatment. In this respect, a skin eruption in pregnancy, for example, could be a positive sign of healing from within to without and thus must not be tampered with. It may be an example of how the mother is eliminating, via the skin, a disturbance originally on a deeper level, such as 'wheeziness' of the chest. This eruption will be a passing phase of a curative stimulus. It may also be noted that the skin eruption disappears from above downwards. This is commonly seen in evidence in a measles case, where the spots disappear from the upper body first and then downwards to the extremities.

Homeopathy—
the more
'scientific'
medicine

The criticism of homeopathy is theoretical. In order to judge whether it works or not, the homeopathic method needs to be applied to see if sick or 'diseased' persons get well.

Homeopaths do not follow the orthodox method of defining a disorder and then prescribing a remedy to counteract the process. Nor do they justify their method in terms of cause and effect, or 'explain' in physiological terms, as does orthodox medicine. Practice is justified by practice and the drug tests are pure experiments. The selection of a homeopathic remedy is based on the symptoms in the provings. Homeopathic practice has not changed for nearly 200 years and is based on fixed principles and laws. The orthodox 'reductionist' view of explaining disease and drug actions at the cellular, microbiological or biochemical level will always be beyond the grasp of the researcher. This is because the living human being is more than the sum of its parts or just a collection of specialised cells.

Coulter (1981) writes how the reductionist view was accepted in all sciences in the early nineteenth century and has now been discarded by everyone except 'orthodox' physicians. 'Orthodox' medicine lacks a precisely structured doctrine. Coulter suggests that homeopathy is the more 'scientific' method of medicine due to its rigour and the precision of its principles. The laws of application and the principles can be seen as a unified hypothesis. Homeopathic treatment tests this hypothesis and the noted successes give the hypothesis validity. The outdated cause and effect relations of orthodox medicine have not been formulated into an operational theory governed by principles.

This is where the difficulty lies, in that orthodox medicine condemns homeopathy because it does not conform to their views of what is 'scientific'. The main requirement for a clinical trial from an orthodox point of view is to assemble homogeneous groups of people with the same 'named disease'. The treated and untreated cases are then matched.

Homeopathy has always maintained that there are no diseases but diseased individuals, and that each person is different so group homogeneity is almost impossible. Despite having to observe inappropriate 'orthodox' protocols for clinical trials, homeopathic remedies have been shown to be effective in such trials. In 1980 a group of doctors and homeopathic physicians in Glasgow treated 46 patients with rheumatoid arthritis. Half were treated with conventional anti-inflammatory medications, together with placebo. The other half were treated with the same anti-inflammatory medications together with the indicated homeopathic remedies. The patients on homeopathic remedies showed significant improvement over those on placebo.

The research evidence supporting homeopathy seldom elicits a response from orthodox medicine, despite its publication. Foubister (1989) quotes Dr Charles Wheeler in an address to the British Medical Association:

> To say that the vast body of medical opinion for a hundred years has rejected homeopathy is true, but to imply that it has rejected it after trial and investigation is a gross fallacy. Each successive decade has handed its prejudice and ignorance onto the next and the simple tests which would have settled the matter once and for all have never been made, save by the few, who, in consequence, have maintained the heresy.

The midwife can make herself familiar with the published research and consider conducting a trial within the maternity unit. In recent years there have been positive research findings published but not as yet, relating to homeopathy within midwifery practice (Kleijnan et al., 1991). This author knows of one trial being conducted by midwives with regard to the use of arnica for perineal trauma.

The public are well informed and are disappointed with what 'science' has to offer. The holistic perspective of homeopathy is attractive as it has a more comprehensive approach to promote and improve health rather than eradicate disease or ailment (Patel, 1987a). Patel also suggests that there is a need for other ways of evaluating homeopathy. He recommends that emphasis be placed on value for money, that is the improvement of health in an effective and low cost manner (Patel, 1987b).

The homeopath's approach towards disease

The homeopath's approach towards disease is very different from that of the orthodox doctor. For example, doctors view cancer as the disease which needs to be fought. Homeopaths view cancer as the product or result of disease and that it is the underlying disease cause that needs to be cured.

Some obstetricians view birth as normal only in retrospect. Homeopaths, like midwives, view birth as normal until shown not to be.

Aetiology There is a general view of aetiology in orthodox medicine but homeopaths consider every fact, incident or accident, connected with the onset or origin of the presenting ailment. If it is realised that the trouble started after a disappointment, grief, sunstroke, getting wet, over-exertion, loss of sleep, etc., then each factor will give clues to the practitioner as regards the person's susceptibility. This helps in the selection of the remedy because it shows how that person has reacted and may give an accurate description of a remedy. So the first question asked is: 'How did it start?'

In labour, a well-taken case history antenatally would be invaluable but largely the mother's mental and emotional state will show a remedy picture if there is a reason to prescribe. For example, 'since disappointment with her partner or relative she has wanted to be alone and not touched'. In labour, the contractions are erratic, very painful and stop when people or relatives enter the room. The aetiology of disappointment is to be cured—remedy such as *ignatia* may be prescribed to improve the birth process. The emotions may surface during the birth and be productive.

The concept of aetiology in homeopathy is thus not confined to age, sex, race, diet or smoking, for example, nor is the offending microbe searched for and given priority.

How homeopaths prescribe The homeopath is guided by the fixed principles of homeopathy as well as noting the individual susceptibility and energy level. Any symptoms of disease or pain reflect how that person is coping with stress on all levels of the physical, mental and emotional body, as well as the spiritual and sociological.

The 'totality of symptoms', not a disease label, is looked for via observation and questioning at interview. The homeopath will sort through the symptoms to get a picture of the 'whole' individual with the disease. Then, after grading and finding the symptoms in the *Repertory*, an elimination process is begun. This is to use the cross-referencing of symptoms to eliminate certain remedies that do not apply to all symptoms. The remedies left are looked up in the *Materia Medica* to find the one that is most similar. In order to individualise not only the remedy for the person but also its dose and potency, the energy or vitality is assessed to match the energy stimulus of the remedy.

This may at first appear a lengthy process but it is worthwhile when a carefully selected remedy proves later to be the most similar one and thus gives speedy relief. This is especially noticeable in an acute situation.

Case taking Time spent at the initial consultation is not just writing notes or selecting remedies. It can be a powerful healing experience on its own. The mother will be encouraged to tell her story in its entirety without interruption. In order to remind her that the totality of symptoms is being sought the question 'anything else?' can be repeated (Moskowitz, 1992).

The mother's own words, where significant, are noted and objective observations also. The consultation will follow the lines of a medical history, family history and past history. The art of interpersonal skills is essential in the formation of a relationship between midwife and mother. The midwife also needs to be aware of questioning techniques to influence greatly the information obtained in response.

In acute or first aid prescribing, such as during a birth, 'case-taking' is simplified as the mother will be able to describe clearly how she feels and show obvious signs of discomfort in her body language. Her behaviour will show if she is hot or cold, comfortable, coping, tiring rapidly, approaching second stage or becoming distracted too much to be able to surrender to the birth process. The observations of a midwife can be almost intuitive and, through experience, the midwife is an expert at assessing the state of the mother. This is very helpful to a homeopath.

The information needed includes: signs and symptoms; locality; sensations; aetiology; what makes it better or worse, whether there are any symptoms that accompany it; is she crying, shouting, restless, motionless, thirsty or thirstless; nauseous but not relieved by vomiting; is the os uteri rigid; are the contractions too close, too far apart, too strong or too weak?

The midwife could note exactly what the mother says, listening and watching carefully. She should use all her senses to observe and to describe the mother. For example, the midwife's sense of touch is an immensely useful diagnostic tool—used to assess contractions, temperature, sweat and consistency of the cervix—all without asking a question.

It needs to be remembered that at a birth, for example, symptoms must appear exaggerated, unusual or that which is *individual* to the mother in order to prescribe. Pain is normal in birth, therefore there is no remedy for pain, but remedies for exaggerated, individualised expression of that pain. Ineffectual contractions are abnormal and need treatment.

The symptoms point the way to the remedy needed. The aim is not to remove symptoms or 'cover them up'. Symptoms providing the information such as aetiology, location, sensation, concomitants and modalities (see Glossary) are used to find the most similar remedy. This in turn is aimed at the root cause (most commonly on the mental and emotional level) to stimulate self-regulation. Thus, as the *Organon* stated, the aim is 'the rapid, gentle and lasting restoration of health' (Dudgeon, 1921).

The three-legged stool A complete symptom picture is necessary for accurate prescriptions and this involves four areas of enquiry:

- the nature of the sensation;
- the special conditions or modalities of time, temperature, etc. that make it better or worse;
- the aetiology;
- the location.

If the prescriber has at least three of the above and can match the symptoms with those proved in drug testing to be of the nature of a remedy, then a safe prescription can be made. The stool with three legs can stand securely. With four legs, it can stand even more firmly (Koehler, 1986).

Louise suffered with mastitis 7 days postnatally.
Breastfeeding advice was expertly given, but the pain and discomfort remained. It started suddenly about 3 p.m.; the right breast was hot, red and throbbing. The skin of the affected area was shiny and taut and the heat was felt even before touching the breast. Louise started to feel feverish. The midwife was aware that not all 'mastitis' cases are infective and whilst the conventional treatment would be in the form of antibiotics or anti-inflammatory drugs, the mother chose homeopathy first. So the complete symptom picture was looked for:

- *the aetiology was unknown;*
- *the location was the right breast;*
- *the sensation was hot and throbbing;*
- *the modalities were that it suddenly started at 3 p.m.*

A dose of belladonna *30 c gave relief whilst addressing the imbalance, to cure and prevent recurrence. The provings of* belladonna *show the sudden onset of symptoms, that the affected parts are burning hot, the pain is throbbing and the right side is often affected.* Belladonna *has been proven to have the time modality of 3 p.m. This observation is relevant because it can be used as a measure for the peaks and troughs of body rhythm that are individually presented and helps differentiate the remedies (see Glossary).*

Practicalities of prescribing

'Dosage' in homeopathy refers to the number of repetitions. This is because it is a stimulus and not a chemical measure. So, if by accident a whole bottle of tablets was ingested, this would still only be one 'dose' or stimulus.

Remedies can be prescribed in different ways. Sometimes they are given as a single dose (probably a high potency) when the homeopath may wait a number of weeks to assess fully the response. A remedy can also be given in a lower potency, singly, or repeated daily or more frequently. The homeopath will choose the method to suit the client and the nature of the condition. Individuals respond better to some methods than others and understanding this is part of the skill of the homeopath. It also explains why self-prescribing may prove ineffective, as it is more difficult to be objective. The medicines are most commonly dispensed as drops, tablets, pills, powders and granules. For babies, powders, granules or crushed soft tablets are useful.

In acute situations such as birth, the remedy stimulus is used up quickly and may need to be repeated a number of times, possibly every 5–30 minutes. This is because the condition calling for it is likely to recur. The prescriber must observe the reaction to the remedy and reduce the number of doses when there is improvement, and then stop. It may need to be resumed if the condition worsens again. If after four doses it has not acted, or the picture of what is happening and felt by the mother and baby has changed significantly, then another remedy is chosen. This remedy must be selected on the totality of symptoms as before (Moskowitz, 1992). In the main the general and emotional state of the mother is used to select a remedy. Only one remedy should be given at one time.

The carefully selected and indicated remedy can stimulate reaction and therefore 'act' very fast—30 seconds to 1 minute in serious situations. Professional homeopaths have successfully treated women and babies in life-threatening situations such as uterine haemorrhage and respiratory distress, respectively.

Correct prescribing during the antenatal period or the labour can redress an obvious imbalance. This can be a preventative prescription.

Having acquired the necessary skills of the art and science of homeopathy, the midwife may safely and accurately prescribe. She will, of course, remain primarily in attendance as a midwife and is professionally accountable to her UKCC registration (see Chapter 1).

Substances to avoid when under homeopathic treatment

To avoid the possibility of antidoting the beneficial effect of the remedy, some commonly used substances must be avoided. Coffee, peppermint, menthol, eucalyptus and camphor, and anything containing very strong smells, including essential oils, or flavours, should be avoided. This is because homeopaths have noticed that the remedy action has been interfered with or been arrested in some clients where such substances have been used. It varies from person to person and remedy substance to substance, so it is worth noting this, if the results of treatment are not as good as expected.

It is also worth considering the fact that aromatherapists are treated by homeopaths with success! To avoid confusion, individualising this for each client will help, but coffee (in any form), menthol, peppermint, eucalyptus and camphor seem to antidote remedies—no one is sure why. It could be that as the homeopathic remedy is of a dynamic immaterial nature, which stimulates us on an energy level (or vital force), so too is it very sensitive to strong smells. We all know how the aroma of peppermint can make us 'feel fresh' or the smell of coffee can make us 'feel good' and can be uplifting on an energy level. Hence, in some people, there is an effect from these substances that can antidote or overpower the dynamic stimulus of a remedy, because it is a stronger stimulus.

It is perfectly safe to use homeopathic medication whilst being treated by orthodox drugs (NAHG, 1992). A homeopathic remedy will not interact with orthodox drugs. However, orthodox drugs sometimes affect the remedy's action and, in order to overcome this, the remedy may need to be repeated more often. Where possible, it is preferable that other medication is avoided.

The expectations of homeopathy

Homeopathy cannot repair irreversible damage, structural or mechanical, and is not a substitute for emergency surgery or suturing. It can be considered before opting for conventional obstetric treatment, for instance, or when orthodox methods have failed. After taking a remedy, responses vary from person to person. Some feel an immediate surge of well-being, others may feel tired at first and need to rest before improvement is noticed (Society of Homeopaths, undated). This is notable in pregnancy where energy levels vary during the different trimesters and the mother is very aware of the changes.

Sometimes the original symptoms temporarily worsen, or the mother is made aware of previously felt symptoms from which she has not fully recovered. This indicates that the remedy has stimulated the self-healing or regulating process. These reactions may be subtle and pass unnoticed, or in contrast may be quite marked.

Introduction to therapeutics

The midwife will perceive when her client needs more skilled help than she is able to give and so will refer to another practitioner when necessary.

Arnica (*Arnica montana*, 'Leopard's bane') *Arnica* is the most commonly referred-to homeopathic remedy at birth. C.V. Pink, with over 30 years' experience of obstetrics, recognises *arnica* 30 c or 200 c to be effective in the recovery from birth trauma for mother and baby (Foubister, 1989). Other testimonials to its importance in healing soft tissue bruising include Moskowitz (1992) and Gibson and Gibson (1987).

It is an extremely important first aid remedy and pertains to birth because of the commonly felt sensation of bruising and soreness postnatally. It is excellent where there is trauma from overexertion, tissue damage, bruising, swelling, injury, fear of touch, and shock (mental and physical). *Arnica* has an affinity for blood vessels and muscles.

After labour, *arnica* can be given for bruising of the labia or vagina or where the perineum is traumatised after much pushing, an episiotomy or a mechanical delivery. *Arnica* helps prevent bleeding, retained placenta, sepsis and after-pains. *Arnica* 30 c can be given during a labour as is needed and two to four hourly after birth for a few days, reducing and then stopping when there is improvement.

The midwife is ideally positioned to recognise when *arnica* is indicated, and could safely give this on her own accountability. In hospitals, standing orders could be implemented where there is support from the consultants and the pharmacist.

The baby can benefit from *arnica* also, where there is shock, trauma, bruising or cephal haematoma. Here, *arnica* can be given as a crushed tablet or in liquid form one to two hourly to reduce bruising, or in an emergency, repeatedly 15–30 seconds apart.

Sarah was a primigravida, admitted to hospital for induction of labour for postmaturity, and accompanied by her homeopath. An amniotomy was performed which led to regular painful uterine contractions. Sarah took arnica *at this time in preparation for labour and delivery.*

The fetal position was found to be occipito-posterior and Sarah experienced long, painful contractions and backache, which started in the sacral area. Kali carb. *200 c was given as it is renowned for relieving backache.*

Progress was slow and the obstetrician suggested an oxytocic infusion, which Sarah declined, but she did accept intramuscular pethidine for pain relief. Sarah suffered leg cramps and was given mag phos *6 x, and* kali phos. *30 c to combat tiredness. The* kali carb. *was repeated as the backache increased.*

Eventually, as Sarah went into the transition stage, she became frenzied, biting the pillow, thrashing about and swearing, and chamomilla *200 c was given with good effect. The* arnica *was repeated for overexertion, and shortly afterwards Sarah delivered a baby girl, without trauma to either herself or her daughter.*

Caulophyllum (blue cohosh) This remedy has an affinity for the female organs. It is often prescribed for erratic contractions; labour that does not progress; sharp, crampy, spasmodic pains that fly from one place to another; unbearable 'after-pains' across lower abdomen extending to groins; and also for rheumatism of the small joints with gynaecological ailments.

The value of *caulophyllum* in labour has been confirmed in research on animals. In a British study of over 200 births, it was shown that *caulophyllum* reduced significantly the numbers of stillbirths in a herd of pigs with a high stillbirth rate (Day, 1984).

Douglas Borland prescribed *caulophyllum* 200 c hourly in a labour where progress was slow, the mother was having erratic contractions and was getting exhausted. He considers that it stimulates uterine muscle and brings on the labour. Also it can be used, if there are no individualising symptoms at all, in 'false labours' where the mother is becoming exhausted (Borland, 1982). A later trial by Eid et al. (1993) indicated the value of *caulophyllum* in reducing the duration of labour, although Wood (1991) stresses the need for appropriate prescribing of the remedy by a qualified homeopath.

Chamomilla (German chamomile) This remedy has an affinity for the nerves and emotions. There may be excessive irritability and oversensitivity to pain and external influences. In labour the mother may scream, 'I can't bear it!' and be very uncivil. There will be a capricious attitude and the mother will be averse to being spoken to or touched. Everything will become worse after anger or vexation. *Chamomilla* prescribed in such a situation will bring calm to the room and the mother will no longer complain of the pain but be able to cope and give birth freely. Here, the potency is of less importance. For instance if 6 c is all there is available then this is used. It may need repeating. A 30 c may have the desired effect also, after one dose or three. A 200 c may be the most similar and so need no repetition.

Chamomilla 6 c is used successfully in irritable babies, whether from pain or anger, and is found in 'teething granules'.

MaryAnne, in her forties, was having her third baby at home. She had had influenza for a week before the birth. She felt very tired and congested, when there was spontaneous rupture of the membranes with stale meconium at 6 a.m.

By 11.30 a.m. she was having fair contractions, with slow progress, until the pain increased to 'unbearable'. MaryAnne became irritable and cross, having tried various methods of pain relief. She called out, 'I can't bear it'. This was the key to the remedy needed, as the pain appeared to be extreme but the contractions were fair and short. Chamomilla 200 c was given and there were no complaints after that.

MaryAnne had moderate, regular contractions throughout the afternoon but eventually she became indecisive and craved fresh air and there was an obvious lack of thirst. After pulsatilla *200 c was given, her contractions became stronger and MaryAnne was coping better. A little later* kali-phos. *200 c was given and 'a huge surge of energy' was felt. (This remedy is known to work well where any exertion seems a heavy task.)*

At 5.26 p.m. MaryAnne had a spontaneous vaginal delivery of a baby boy in good condition. The stale meconium was not a problem. There was a natural third stage with blood loss of 50 ml.

Pulsatilla (wind flower) This remedy is most useful in pregnancy. There may be a mild, tearful and apprehensive disposition. In labour there is slow progress and the mother tends to get upset. The emotions affect the labour and can lead to faintness, palpitation and poor contractions. A dose of *pulsatilla* will reduce the apprehensions and tearfulness whilst promoting strong, regular contractions and progress. *Pulsatilla* may be appropriate, in the absence of a clear picture indicating a different remedy, as a treatment for haemorrhoids. Perko (1997) also suggests that, in certain cases, it may be effective in turning a breech presentation to cephalic.

Homeopathic remedies can be used very successfully in pregnancy, labour and the puerperium. However, the diverse range of symptoms between individuals makes it impossible, here, to do more than offer a few examples. Although a limited number of remedies can be used almost universally, such as *arnica*, most conditions require the homeopath or the midwife using homeopathic preparations to identify the full symptom picture of the individual. Midwives should therefore be cautious in advising specific homeopathic remedies unless they have received some training in the subject and must always adhere to the parameters for safe *midwifery* practice.

It must also be noted however that women have the right to administer homeopathic substances to themselves and indeed may present in labour with a variety of tablets supplied by a homeopath for use in specific situations that may occur during the labour.

Conditions of pregnancy which may respond to homeopathy

Carpal tunnel syndrome If the mother finds that this is worse in the morning and is accompanied by wrist and finger oedema and, emotionally, a feeling of fear and anxiety, *lycopodium* may be appropriate. If the syndrome is worse at night but improved by movement and exercise of the wrists, *sepia* may be effective. *Arsenicum* may be prescribed if the condition is worse in the fingertips of the hand on which the mother has been lying but the pain is reduced if the area is warm.

Haemorrhoids *Sepia* may be used for external haemorrhoids accompanied by constipation, whereas *nux vomica* may ease itching internal haemorrhoids which cause backache and constipation but which feel better if the mother bathes in cold water. If the woman feels debilitated, restless, anxious, fearful of being alone and sensitive to cold, *arsenicum* may help; bathing in warm water to ease the discomfort may be stated as a positive factor in the symptom picture. As mentioned previously, *pulsatilla* may be suggested if there is no clear picture to prescribe another remedy.

Nausea and vomiting If the nausea is constant and the mother is vomiting frequently especially in association with the smell of food, *ipecacuanha* may be effective. *Nux vomica* may treat sickness occurring in the morning whilst *pulsatilla* is appropriate where the problem is worst in the evenings but better at night. If the mother constantly feels hungry but eating meat aggravates the symptoms, *petroleum* may be tried. Sickness associated with burning epigastric pain and diarrhoea may be treated with *arsenicum*.

Heartburn Accompanied by bloating and flatulence, with the mother feeling faint and weak, this should be treated with *china*. If there is spasm and reflux acidity, *nux vomica* is prescribed whilst *pulsatilla* may be effective for the woman whose heartburn is worse if she eats fatty foods, who is not thirsty and who emotionally needs sympathy.

Backache *Arnica* is best if the backache is due to strain or injury, and as a universal remedy can be tried if all else fails. Lumbosacral pain with the mother feeling tired and weepy may respond to *Kali-carb.*, while *Rhus tox.* may be the correct remedy if the back initially feels stiff and worse on moving but then gradually improves.

Insomnia Inability to sleep due to an overactive mind will usually respond to *coffea* (where the symptoms are similar to drinking too much coffee late at night). The woman unable to sleep due to a fear of labour and what might happen can be treated with *aconite*.

Homeopathy for labour Induction, acceleration and failure to progress, for a variety of reasons, can be treated homeopathically. *Caulophyllum* may be useful where the mother is exhausted, the cervix is rigid and there are spasmodic contractions. *Chamomilla* is appropriate when the woman is emotionally distressed and 'can't bear it any more', the cervix fails to ripen and the os is rigid. *Cimicifuga* may help the mother who is extremely distressed and hysterical and who talks incessantly even during the contractions, which may cease entirely. The mother who does not want to go through the labour, who desires privacy, is weak, exhausted and who experiences contractive cervical pain, spasmodic back pain and headache, may need *natrum. mur*. *Pulsatilla* can be used where there is uterine inertia, the cervix fails to dilate, the mother feels sick, distressed, has a dry mouth and a changeable mood, laughing, weeping and apologetic.

Following operative procedures such as Caesarean section, forceps delivery or episiotomy, the mother should be given *arnica* to combat the shock, trauma and bruising, and *hypericum* to help wound healing. Following Caesarean section the mother could take one of each tablet hourly on day 1, one of each two-hourly on day 2 and one of each three-hourly on day 3. After normal delivery with some perineal trauma, one tablet of each three- to four-hourly for three days should suffice. Arnica cream can also be used but should not be applied over an open wound. Other remedies which may be of use to relieve specific symptoms after operative delivery include *bellis perennis, calendula, chamomilla, phosphorus, secale* and *staphysagria*.

Homeopathy for mother and baby

Breastfeeding problems such as mastitis may require *belladonna, bryonia, chamomilla, phytolacca* or *silica*. Inadequate lactation may also respond to one of these. When no other symptoms are present to complicate the picture, simple sore nipples can be treated with *castor equi*.

Neonatal colic especially in the evening, when the baby has green stools and diarrhoea, may respond to *chamomilla*, although *colocynthus* may be needed if, in addition, the colic is worse after drinking, especially cold drinks. *Nux vomica* may ease morning colic, particularly if the cause is due to the breast feeding mother having eaten spicy foods or drunk too much coffee, tea or cola.

These examples give a brief introduction to the benefits of homeopathic remedies for pregnant and childbearing women, although they are by no means a complete picture of each condition.

Conclusions

- Informed choice must be offered to women (House of Commons Health Committee, 1992).
- Women and midwives need information on, and access to, homeopathy, amongst other therapies.
- Homeopathy offers swift correction to many of the common problems for which midwives call medical aid.
- Homeopathy can work for emergency obstetric situations and minimise trauma whilst promoting healing.
- Women and babies would benefit from homeopathic preventative medicine—an area with which orthodoxy is relatively unfamiliar.
- Homeopathy can improve the health of the neediest women efficiently, cheaply and safely.

Most obstetricians have ignored evidence that is at variance with their accepted practice and abstain from trials to test the effectiveness of alternatives (Tew, 1990). Midwives are in a position to meet the needs of a woman using or wanting to use homeopathy. The midwifery profession should look to undertake research into the effectiveness of homeopathy in midwifery care. Midwives are experts at observing the progress of pregnancy and birth and their skills could be invaluable in the application of high quality homeopathic care. Those attending mothers and babies can look to homeopathy as an effective system of medicine without risk.

Training   **Homeopathic practitioners** The Faculty of Homeopathy is authorised by Act of Parliament to train medically qualified doctors (as well as dentists, pharmacists and vets) in homeopathic medicine. The Faculty offers short diploma courses for doctors at educational centres in Britain. The examinations lead to membership of the Faculty of Homeopathy (MFHom). This is recognised in medical circles and appropriately trained general practitioners will have these letters after their name. Names of trained general practitioners can be obtained from the Family Health Service Associations (FHSAs). General practitioners offering such specialisation may now publicise it. The local pharmacy will also know of general practitioners in the area offering homeopathy. The NHS prescription form can be dispensed by those chemists registered in the NHS. Notices will be obvious in the pharmacies, stating that they have homeopathic medicines available.

The term 'lay homeopath' usually means non-professional homeopath, i.e. someone using homeopathy without a qualification. There is no all-encompassing register of professional homeopaths. Those registered with the Society of Homeopaths are professional homeopaths who have been fully examined according to the principles and practice established by Samuel Hahnemann. They have a proper understanding and knowledge of homeopathic *Materia Medica* and *Repertory*. They have been adequately trained in the essential medical sciences and skills and have had suitable clinical training and experience. They abide by the Society's Code of Ethics. Practitioners are issued with a Certificate of Registration and may use the initials RSHom. Some will use FSHom: this denotes Fellowship of the Society of Homeopaths, awarded for contribution to homeopathy or the work of the Society. Members include midwives, doctors, nurses, pharmacists, physiotherapists and health visitors.

The Society has a Professional Conduct Director and a complaints procedure. Litigation against homeopathic practitioners is virtually unheard of.

The Society has a list of recognised Colleges of Homeopathy, each of which will have their own awards for graduates to receive a diploma or licence, after completion of a 3–4 year course. The Society also has a list of graduates gaining experience prior to registration or who have chosen not to register with the Society of Homeopaths.

Insurance cover is obtainable from other sources outside the Society. Members of the Royal College of Midwives using homeopathy in their midwifery care have insurance cover for this, but only this, type of practice.

References

Choudhury A C 1988 *Indications of Miasm*. B. Jain Publishers, Put Ltd, New Delhi

Close S (reprinted 1981) *The Genius of Homeopathy*, p. 213. B. Jain Publishers, New Delhi

Coulter H L 1981 *Homeopathic Science and Modern Medicine*, pp. 88, 97. North Atlantic Books, Berkeley, California

Cullen W 1789 *A Treatise of the Materia Medica*. Edinburgh

Day C E I 1984 Control of stillbirth in pigs using homeopathy. *British Homeopathic Journal* 73: 142–143

Dhunny J 1993 Professional issues relating to the use of homeopathy within midwifery practice. Unpublished professional development assignment

Dudgeon R E 1921 *Samuel Hahnemann: Organon of Medicine*, 6th edn, 1842, pp. 31, 40–41, 139. B. Jain Publishers (P) Ltd, New Delhi

Eid P, Felisi E, Sideri M 1993 Applicability of homoeopathic caulophyllum thalictroides during labour. *British Homoeopathic Journal* 82(4): 245–8

Enkin M, Keirse M and Chalmers I 1990 *A Guide to Effective Care in Pregnancy and Childbirth*. Oxford University Press, Oxford

Foubister D 1989 *Tutorials on Homeopathy*, pp. 5, 68. Beaconsfield Press, Beaconsfield, UK

Gibson S, Gibson R 1987 *Homeopathy for Everyone*. Penguin, London

Hahnemann S [1821], reprinted 1987 *The Chronic Diseases*, p. 17. B. Jain Publishers (P) Ltd, New Delhi

Handley R 1990 *A Homeopathic Love Story*. North Atlantic Books, Berkeley, California

House of Commons Health Committee 1992 *Second Report: Maternity Services, Vol. 1*. HMSO, London

Kleijnan J, Knipschild P, Riet G 1991 Clinical trials of homeopathy. *British Medical Journal* 302: 316–323

Koehler G 1986 *The Handbook of Homeopathy. Its Principles and Practices*. Thorsons, London

Moskowitz R 1992 *Homeopathic Medicines for Pregnancy and Childbirth*, pp. 12, 13, 19, 60. North Atlantic Books, Berkeley, California

National Association of Homeopathic Groups (NAHG) (Summer 1992) *National Health Service Homeopathy Newsletter*

Patel M S 1987a Evaluation of holistic medicine. *Social Science in Medicine* 24(2): 169–175

Patel M S 1987b Problems in the evaluation of alternative medicine. *Social Science in Medicine* 25(6), 669–678

Perko S J (1997) *Homeopathy for the Modern Pregnant Woman and Her Infant*. Benchmark Homeopathic Publications, San Antonio, TX, USA

Society of Homeopaths (undated) *Homeopathy: the past, present and future medicine* (leaflet). Society of Homeopaths, Northampton

Society of Homeopaths (1993) *Register of Homeopaths*. Society of Homeopaths, Northampton

Tew M 1990 *Safer Childbirth?* pp. 35, 209, 294. Chapman & Hall, London

Wood J 1991 The use of caulophyllum in pregnancy. *Midwifery Matters* 49: 10

Further reading

Castro M 1992 *Homeopathy for Mother and Baby*. Macmillan, London

Geraghty B 1997 *Homeopathy for Midwives*. Churchill Livingstone, Edinburgh

Katz T 1995 The management of pregnancy + labour with homeopathy. *Complementary Therapies in Nursing and Midwifery* (6): 159–164

Koehler G 1986 *The Handbook of Homeopathy. Its Principles and Practice*. Thorsons, London

Ullman D 1991 *Discovering Homeopathy: Medicine for the Twenty-first Century*. Thorsons, London

Vithoulkas G 1986 *The Science of Homeopathy*, Ch. 5. Thorsons, London

Penelope L. Conway

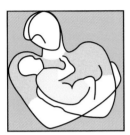

Chapter 3 **Osteopathy during Pregnancy**

The aim of this chapter is to explain how osteopathy can assist midwives to provide optimum care to the women they look after during the various stages of pregnancy, labour and the puerperium.

There is no shortcut to osteopathic diagnosis and treatment, and a four-year full-time course cannot be condensed into one chapter of a book. Because of this, osteopathy is not suitable for the midwife to incorporate in her practice, but rather for her to appreciate when a woman could benefit from referral. Osteopathic treatment is safe, gentle and non-invasive and therefore eminently appropriate for pregnant women.

There are few side-effects and few contraindications to treatment. The main side-effects may be feeling tired after treatment, and a possible increase in symptoms for 24 hours. Contraindications to osteopathic treatment could include:

- any history of or threatened miscarriage;
- active pathology;
- inflammatory conditions;
- some cases of joint hypermobility.

In all these cases the osteopath would discuss the difficulty with the woman concerned, and if necessary with her midwife and general practitioner as well.

Osteopathy is a safe method of treatment even during the early stages of pregnancy. There are no recorded, or even anecdotal, cases of miscarriage or abortion being brought on by osteopathic treatment. However, it is usual practice to avoid strong treatments during the twelfth week and the sixteenth week of pregnancy, when miscarriage is more likely to occur naturally.

This author has not encountered any osteopaths who treat only pregnant women, but naturally there are some practitioners who by virtue of their interest and experience see many more than others. All osteopaths should be willing and able to treat pregnant women.

Historical context

Osteopathy was first conceived over 100 years ago by a physician called Andrew Taylor Still. Still was a country doctor in the Midwest of America who became disenchanted with the medical and surgical knowledge and practice at that time. He spent many years experimenting and developing a new theory of drugless medicine which he called osteopathy. His approach to health care was based on the unity of the body and the proper alignment and function of the musculoskeletal system. He envisaged osteopathy as a complete system of medicine which would employ only manipulative and adjustive techniques which would return to the body the power to heal itself.

Still founded the first School of Osteopathy in Kirksville, Missouri, in 1892. A few American-trained osteopaths came to practise in Britain, and in 1917 the British School of Osteopathy was set up by James Martin Littlejohn who had travelled to America to study. The number of practising osteopaths grew slowly but steadily and in 1934 the profession had progressed sufficiently for a Private Member's Bill to be presented to Parliament calling for state registration for osteopaths. Unfortunately, due to the opposition of the medical establishment, the Bill failed. However at the suggestion of the then Minister of Health, a voluntary Register of Osteopaths was set up to oversee training and provide guarantees of standards and ethics to the public. The Register gave accreditation to osteopathic schools and accepted their graduates as members able to use the designation MRO (Member of the Register of Osteopaths) after their name.

The profession still grew slowly and by 1979 there were only 354 registered osteopaths. Because osteopaths practised under Common Law, anyone could call themselves an osteopath even if they had received little or no training. The Register was therefore vitally important as a safeguard for patients.

Throughout the 1980s public recognition of osteopathy increased, as did acceptance by the medical profession, with many patients being referred by their general practitioner or consultant. State recognition still seemed a long way off, unless as a Profession Supplementary to Medicine, which was not an option many registered osteopaths would consider. Then in 1990 the King's Fund set up a working party to consider the status of osteopathy. Their report incorporated a model bill for statutory registration. A much larger and better organised osteopathic profession was able to find a sponsor for a Private Member's Bill which enjoyed all-party support, and the Osteopaths Act received Royal Assent on 1 July 1993.

Following the passing of the Act the General Osteopathic Council was set up with both Osteopathic and lay members. The process of implementing statutory self-regulation is however taking longer than anticipated. In 1998 all osteopaths, regardless of their previous status, were invited to apply for membership of the first Statutory Register of Osteopaths. This involved completing a lengthy professional profile and portfolio. This method of application will only be available until May 2000. After that date only graduates of institutions with Recognised Qualification (RQ) status will be eligible for registration.

After May 2000 only practitioners on the statutory register will be allowed to call themselves osteopaths.

What is osteopathy?

Osteopathy is concerned with restoring and maintaining balance in the neuro-musculoskeletal systems of the body. This fine balance may have been disturbed by alterations in soft tissues through misuse, or change of use, through trauma to bones or joints, or by modification to the inner-vation of any of these structures. Therefore it is necessary to look at the patient as a whole, not just the area causing symptoms, so that the interaction of the different systems, and the effects they have on each other, can be included in the diagnostic process. Osteopathy is concerned with the biomechanics of the body and the maintenance of appropriate mechanical function.

The osteopath aims to preserve the balance between muscles, joints, liga-mentous structures and nerves which allow the body to function effectively. During pregnancy this balance is constantly under attack from alterations in weight and weight bearing, hormonal changes and fluctuations in fluid balance. In addition there are the 'normal' influences of injury, overuse and physical or mental stress.

The osteopath will attempt to minimise the impact of all these changes by a carefully considered treatment plan formulated for that particular woman. Osteopaths treat people, not conditions.

Osteopathy today

Anyone can self-refer to an osteopath; it is not necessary to have a letter from a medical practitioner, although this is always most welcome. All osteopaths are private practitioners and the cost of treatment varies consi-derably, with most osteopaths operating a sliding scale of fees for those in financial need. Most private health insurance schemes will cover the cost of osteopathic treatment. Fund-holding general practices are now able to employ osteopaths directly, or pay for their patients to have treatment. Several NHS trust hospitals are now purchasing osteopathic treatment for their patients, and with statutory registration this trend is sure to increase.

When people hear the word 'osteopath' most of them immediately think of low back pain, but osteopaths are much more than spinal manipulators. Originally osteopaths treated any and all conditions, but advances in surgery and drug therapies rendered osteopathy obsolete for many complaints. Osteopaths specialised in, and became very proficient at treating, minor orthopaedic disorders. More recently, as people have become disenchanted with drugs and invasive procedures, osteopaths have returned to treating a much wider range of problems. Most now treat asthma, dysmenorrhoea, indigestion and migraine as well as the more common musculoskeletal conditions.

Going to the osteopath

There are registered osteopaths practising in most areas of the British Isles, and a recommendation to a particular Practitioner is often forthcoming from friends or local health professionals. Alternatively the General Osteopathic Council or Osteopathic Information Service will supply the name of a local osteopath. Osteopaths can also be found through Yellow Pages or Thomson local directories. Some osteopaths practise on their own, others in group practices often incorporating several different disciplines.

Most osteopaths will treat pregnant women, but no osteopath will accept a woman for treatment if she is not receiving medical antenatal care as well. During pregnancy osteopathy is truly complementary, not alternative.

Having selected a practitioner and made an appointment, the first part of the initial consultation will involve the osteopath taking a detailed and comprehensive case history. This will include details of occupation and lifestyle as well as information about the problem. For pregnant women obstetric information will also be required, such as estimated date of delivery, home or hospital delivery, any previous pregnancies, and any problems associated with previous deliveries. The next part of the record taking will address past and present medical history including details of diet, genitourinary system, gastrointestinal system and any cardiovascular problems.

Not all pregnant women who consult an osteopath are in pain; some attend just for advice or reassurance, or as part of a 'well woman' approach to pregnancy. They are anxious to be examined for any problems that may arise later so that they can go into labour as well prepared as possible.

The woman would then be asked to undress to her underwear and remove her shoes before the next part of the examination, which is the osteopathic evaluation.

The osteopath will observe the woman standing—checking spinal curves in both antero-posterior and lateral planes, and also areas of weight bearing (Figs. 3.1, 3.2). They would also consider the way in which weight was transferred through the lower extremities, whether this was equally distributed and if the knees were held fully extended and locked, thereby allowing the glutei and hamstrings to relax. They would also check whether the ankles were inverted or everted, and if there was flattening of the medial arch of the foot with associated spreading of the toes to provide a wider base. Medial arch flattening is common in the later stages of pregnancy to accommodate increased weight bearing.

Only by looking at the woman as a whole, not just investigating the area giving symptoms, can the osteopath assess how the body is adapting to the pregnancy.

The osteopath will then palpate the vertebral column and spinal muscles (still with the woman standing) to pick up any areas of increased or reduced tone. They will also be looking for any evidence of localised spinal scoliosis or rotation.

The woman will be asked to perform a range of active spinal movements, which the osteopath will observe for the following:

- range of movement;
- equality of movement throughout the spine;
- any limitation by pain.

The osteopath will ask the woman to sit on the treatment table and her sitting posture and range of movement will be observed. This may also

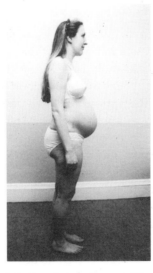

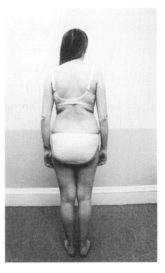

Fig. 3.1. Lateral view of woman, 32 weeks pregnant.

Fig. 3.2. Posterior view of woman, 32 weeks pregnant, to show lateral curves.

Fig. 3.3. Checking mobility of lower ribcage.

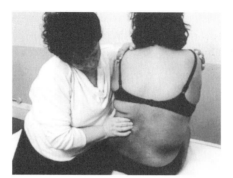

Fig. 3.4. Assessing hip joint mobility.

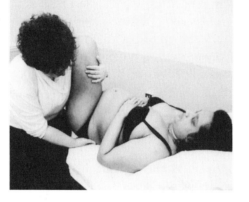

include rib mobility (Fig. 3.3), important for easier breathing, particularly in the later stages of pregnancy when the fundus of the uterus presses on the diaphragm. Active movements of the cervical spine will be checked as a guide to general spinal mobility.

The woman will then be asked to lie supine so that if necessary her reflexes may be checked, and her hip joint mobility tested (Fig. 3.4). Many women with limited spinal mobility overuse their hip joints in order to adapt their posture whilst pregnant, and a good range of movement in the hip joints also increases the options for birth positions. The osteopath will also compare leg lengths and pelvic levels. Most pregnant women are not very comfortable and may become hypotensive lying supine, particularly during the later stages of pregnancy, so other lower extremity joints will only be checked if they are causing problems.

Then the osteopath will make a more detailed assessment of the main area causing symptoms by moving the joints passively and palpating for alterations in local muscle tone and ligamentous stretch (Fig. 3.5). This applies to both spinal and peripheral joints.

If necessary this may be followed by neurological and/or other system examinations. This would usually be carried out if the woman was complaining of any paraesthesia (pins and needles or numbness) or referred pain.

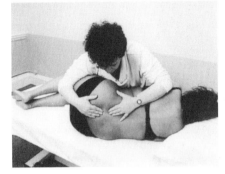

Any unexpected breathlessness or palpitations warrant a cardiovascular system examination.

The osteopath now has all the information from the history and examination and can evaluate the findings in order to reach a diagnosis and formulate a treatment plan. Because pregnancy is a time of so much postural change and adaptation, the diagnosis should be regarded more as an evaluation at that moment in time. There is an immense variation in the rate of growth of every fetus, which necessitates a continuous and continuing reassessment of the woman's stance and mobility. Two weeks later her osteopathic profile could have changed dramatically.

When the diagnosis has been established the osteopath will explain the findings and discuss the aims of treatment. For most people the paramount factor is relief of symptoms, but this may necessitate a change in lifestyle or working practice, as well as osteopathic treatment.

The treatment plan may include:

- Soft tissue techniques to relax and stretch shortened musculature. These are specialised massage techniques which aim to release tension in the muscle fibres which often limit mobility.
- Articulatory techniques to stretch muscles and ligamentous structures rhythmically. These techniques take an area, usually in the spine, through a small range of movement in a repetitive manner, with the osteopath applying a little more force as necessary.
- Friction to improve local circulation. This is usually applied by steady pressure with the thumbs to a particular area of very shortened muscle.
- High velocity thrust (Fig. 3.6)—putting one apophyseal joint through a very specific range of movement. This is the classic osteopathic technique which produces the 'crack' from the joint concerned. Osteopaths limit the movement of surrounding spinal joints by a combination of flexion and rotation so that when a gentle force is applied locally only one joint will separate, causing the sound.

Pregnant women are not comfortable with excessive lumbar spinal

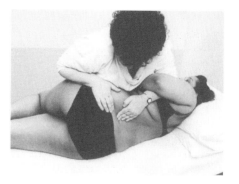

Fig. 3.6. Applying a 'high velocity thrust' technique in the lumbar spine.

rotation, and relax more readily if techniques are adapted to allow for more flexion than is usual. Treatment is usually weekly or biweekly until symptoms improve, and then every 2 weeks. Women are encouraged to attend until delivery if possible, as changes in weight bearing make them vulnerable to recurring problems during pregnancy. They will be advised to return about 6 weeks after delivery so that their posture and mobility can be assessed again. Many women return sooner, particularly if the delivery has been accompanied by backache.

Most of the treatment will be given with the woman lying on her side, with the abdomen supported on a small pillow. This position is often the most comfortable for the mother and all osteopathic techniques can be adapted to take account of this factor. Some of the treatment may be given with the woman sitting. Particularly in the later stages of pregnancy when changing position is difficult, the treatment should be organised to allow the woman to change her position as little as possible. The comfort of the woman is of paramount importance.

At about 34 weeks' gestation, partners or anyone who will be present at the delivery are invited to attend the treatment to be shown some simple pain-relieving techniques that can be used during labour. These are useful for midwives to learn as well and are described in detail later. However, as these techniques are very successful, anyone who starts using them should be prepared to continue until delivery.

Stages of pregnancy

Pre-conception care Pre-conception care is a relatively new area of concern and interest for the medical profession, encouraging women to improve their nutrition and general lifestyle before becoming pregnant. For many years, however, osteopaths have been advising young women to improve their posture and spinal mobility before attempting to become pregnant. This was due to treating so many older women who could trace the onset of their low back symptoms to a pregnancy many years earlier. Low back pain during pregnancy may be common, but that does not make it inevitable.

There is also some anecdotal evidence that osteopathic treatment is helpful in cases of unexplained infertility. To date there has not been any formal research into this subject, but hopefully collaborative endeavours of this type will become easier after statutory registration. The innervation of the reproductive organs arises from the lumbar spine, so it would not seem too unconventional to treat this area in both partners.

The extra weight and changes in weight bearing that occur during pregnancy require good spinal and peripheral joint mobility, so it would seem prudent to deal with any problems in the lumbar or thoracic spine before becoming pregnant. A full range of movement in both hip joints is also important if the woman wishes to have a wide range of options for positions at delivery.

First trimester During the early stages of pregnancy problems often arise in the thoracic spine due to a rapid increase in the size and sensitivity of the breasts. This can lead to flexion of the thoracic spine and internal rotation of the shoulders as a protective mechanism. This can result in muscle shortening and fatigue.

Nausea and vomiting can adversely affect the ribs and thoracic spine as the woman holds on to the basin or lavatory bowl and retches constantly. Gentle osteopathic treatment aimed at releasing the intercostal muscles (Fig. 3.7) and diaphragm is usually very helpful, and work to improve the mobility of the thoracic spine and adjacent soft tissues often relieves the feelings of nausea.

The lumbar spine does not have to undergo much adaptation in the first weeks as the uterus has not risen above the pubic symphysis. However, this author has seen women with severe ligamentous low backache which started at 6 weeks' gestation and could only be hormonally induced, as no other changes were discernible.

Jenny came for advice and treatment after the birth of her second child. She had developed severe backache when only

Fig. 3.7. Technique for stretching intercostal muscles.

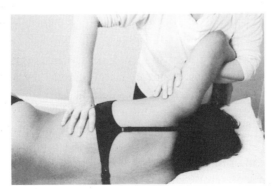

16 weeks pregnant, and had been confined to bed, some of the time in hospital, for the remainder of the pregnancy. A diagnosis was made of ligamentous backache, but no treatment was offered other than bed rest and limiting the size of her family to the two children she had already. Jenny and her husband had planned a much larger family and their religious beliefs did not allow for contraception.

On examination it was found that her lumbar erector spinae and interspinous ligaments were overstretched, causing increased mobility in her lumbar spine and at the thoraco-lumbar junction. During her second pregnancy the increased weight and change in centre of gravity caused further stretch of the spinal muscles and ligaments, leading to early fatigue on any sustained sitting or standing.

Treatment was aimed at encouraging the ligaments to shorten, and increasing the mobility of the underlying lumbar and thoracic spinal joints. Treatment continued for some time, but it was not possible to assess fully a final outcome until Jenny became pregnant again.

After 1 year Jenny was pregnant and continued with treatment. She remained pain free until 36 weeks' gestation and has had two subsequent pain-free pregnancies, only requiring treatment during the pregnancies and not in between.

Second trimester As the pregnancy progresses and the uterus rises out of the pelvic cavity many of the problems encountered are postural—or rather they are caused by the inability of the woman to adapt to her changing centre of gravity. This may be due to an old injury to the lumbar spine several years earlier, perhaps following a fall, or to an immobile thoraco-lumbar area as a consequence of osteochondrosis. The lumbo-sacral and thoraco-lumbar regions of the spine are the main adaptive areas for weight bearing, and therefore bear the impact of the changes taking place.

Whatever the underlying cause, the effect is to prevent the woman from developing a 'pregnant posture'. This normally involves either increasing the lumbar lordosis and tilting the pelvis anteriorly, or flattening the lumbar curve and rotating the pelvis posteriorly (Fig. 3.8). The upper part of the spine adapts accordingly so that a centre of gravity is maintained while standing. The increased weight is thus carried through spinal muscles and apophyseal joints which were not designed for this task. The result is often discomfort and pain. The tone of the abdominal muscles can also affect the way in which the postural changes develop. A woman who has strong abdominal muscles and is a primigravida will develop a very different posture from a multipara with poor abdominal tone.

The other factor which has to be considered is the rising level of

Fig. 3.8. Diagram to show possible changes in weight bearing.

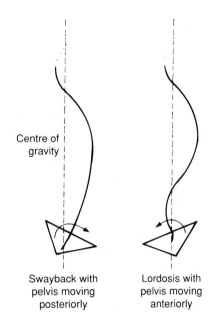

Centre of gravity

Swayback with pelvis moving posteriorly

Lordosis with pelvis moving anteriorly

circulating relaxin, and the effect it has on ligamentous tissue, allowing it to lengthen whilst retaining its stretch.

Adaptation is also occurring at the hip joint, knee and ankle joints, symphysis pubis and abdominal musculature at this time. These are all areas of potential discomfort and pain and all structures which respond well to osteopathic treatment. This may just involve soft tissue relaxation techniques, or articulatory techniques where joints are taken through a range of passive movement in a repetitive manner to encourage ligamentous stretch.

Many women who already have a child carry their toddler on one or other hip. This requires rotation of one side of the pelvis, often resulting in sacro-iliac problems which, as well as causing local pain, often lead to referred pain in the hip or groin and changes in the lateral spinal curves. Any of these problems, which can be both tiring and debilitating for the woman, can be eased with appropriate osteopathic intervention. Symptomatic relief, particularly from sacro-iliac lesions, can be very dramatic and most welcome. However, the woman must also be discouraged from carrying the toddler on her hip in the future, and advised on how to cope with the conflicting demands of her small child and her lumbar spine.

At this stage of pregnancy many women will still be working. This can cause problems if chairs or desks are not adjustable. For anyone working at a keyboard it becomes increasingly difficult to sit really close to the desk. A lower chair may make sitting for long periods more comfortable, and a footrest (it could even be two telephone directories) rotates the pelvis posteriorly so that the lumbar spine is supported by the chair. The osteopath can often suggest such simple alterations to a working environment which make life more comfortable. Allowing the woman to continue working for as long as possible is an important consideration nowadays.

Third trimester In the later stages of pregnancy, as the fundus of the uterus rises and presses on the diaphragm, breathing becomes more difficult, particularly taking a deep breath. The lower ribs are splayed, and upper rib breathing predominates. Gentle rib stretching (Fig. 3.9) and relaxation of the diaphragm can improve this situation.

When contracted, the diaphragm may also constrict the oesophageal opening causing difficulty with swallowing and allowing reflux to occur. Direct treatment to the diaphragm and mid-thoracic spine will ease the discomfort rapidly.

Excessive weight gain at this time will make the simplest everyday tasks difficult to perform. Unfortunately osteopathic treatment does not aid weight loss, but may help the woman to move more easily. Treatment to the feet and knees can assist lymphatic drainage and make walking more comfortable. Advice can be offered on the most suitable positions for sitting and sleeping, and the easiest way of changing position from upright to recumbent.

At this stage of the pregnancy the osteopath may discuss with the woman which birth position would be most suitable for her, taking into consideration her pattern of mobility and any factors which could aggravate a previous injury.

The final pre-delivery treatment should be given as near to the estimated date of delivery with which the woman feels comfortable. Osteopathic treatment is safe at any time during pregnancy and some practitioners have been able to treat women during labour as well.

It must not be overlooked that at any time during her pregnancy a woman may develop a musculoskeletal problem which is totally unrelated to the pregnancy. Pregnant women are more vulnerable to injury because of their increased ligamentous laxity, but any pre-existing condition can continue to be treated.

Fig. 3.9. Sitting technique to separate lower ribs.

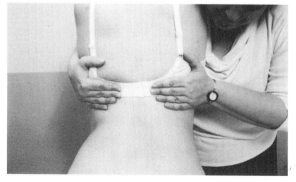

Can osteopathy help?

Sciatica Irritation of the sciatic nerve can occur anywhere along its path, causing pain and or paraesthesia in the lower extremity. The cause of the nerve compression can range from protrusion of an intervertebral disc to spasm in the piriformis muscle. Accurate diagnosis of the level of the nerve root involved and the cause of the irritation is necessary, and most are amenable to osteopathic treatment.

Carpal tunnel syndrome Oedema in the later stages of pregnancy can lead to compression of the median nerve as it passes through the flexor retinaculum at the wrist. The symptoms are tingling and numbness in the hands, particularly in the morning. Osteopathic treatment to the forearm and wrist can help by aiding drainage and improving the mobility of the joints of the wrist. An improvement is seen after only one or two treatments.

Meralgia paraesthetica This is an area of reduced sensation and possibly soreness over the distribution of the lateral cutaneous nerve of the thigh. This corresponds to the antero-lateral portion of the upper half of the thigh. The symptoms often appear at about 20 weeks. Treatment is directed at stretching the nerve root within its fascial sheath, and releasing any compressive tension around the inguinal canal. This involves articulating the hip joint into extension to stretch the tissues of the anterior compartment of the thigh.

Diabetes Diabetes is not usually treated osteopathically, although there are some practitioners who would attempt direct treatment to the pancreas. However, it is important to note that any diabetics who have osteopathic treatment for other problems should always check their insulin levels after treatment. Osteopathic treatment has a similar effect to exercise and can noticeably alter insulin requirements.

Symphysis pubis pain This can be very difficult to treat and does not always respond. This is often the case when excessive separation of the symphysis pubis renders it unstable. Treatment to the sacro-iliac joints may help by encouraging posterior rotation of the pelvis, which takes some of the strain off the anterior structures. Local friction techniques may encourage ligamentous shortening. The woman should be advised to wear some form of support (preferably a maternity panty-girdle) and to sit on a wedge cushion, again to influence posterior rotation. Placing the feet on a box or stool also helps. Pelvic rocking exercises should be suggested.

   If the pain is due to lack of mobility at the symphysis pubis or a shearing movement of the joint, this will usually respond much better to osteopathic treatment.

Coccydynia Localised pain in the region of the coccyx often following a fall or previous difficult delivery can be treated successfully but it may be necessary for the manipulation to be performed per rectum. A chaperone would always be provided if necessary.

Oedematous ankles If the oedema does not require the use of diuretics and is purely gravitational the osteopath may try to improve the lymphatic drainage by releasing any restrictions at the ankle, knee and hip joints and applying longitudinal stretch techniques to the posterior muscle groups. Soft tissue techniques should never be used because of the risk of a deep vein thrombosis.

Indigestion and heartburn These both respond well to relaxation of the diaphragm and techniques to improve the mobility of the ribcage and thoracic spine.

Round ligament pain Pain in the groin is sometimes due to pressure on the round ligament as it passes through the inguinal canal. Local soft tissue and stretching techniques are often helpful in this condition.

Pain relief during labour Simple massage techniques used to relax the erector spinae muscles during the early stages of labour can be very effective for pain relief. They can be performed by the midwife or anyone present at the delivery. The woman can be in any position except supine, but it is easier for the operator if she is lying on her side or sitting astride a chair. The lumbar musculature is then more readily accessible. The lateral border of the thumb and thenar eminence are used to apply pressure with one or both hands. The technique involves cross fibre stretching of the muscles. Baby oil or talcum powder can be applied to the skin to improve contact and lessen friction. The applicator hand is placed on the back in the sulcus (groove) between the spinous processes of the lumbar vertebrae and the muscle belly of the erector spinae (Figs. 3.10, 3.11). By maintaining skin contact and attempting to move the muscle belly away from the centre line the muscle is bowed and stretched.

Fig. 3.10. Stretching lumbar erector spinae muscles.

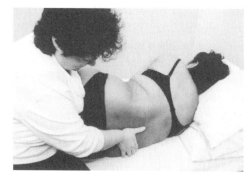

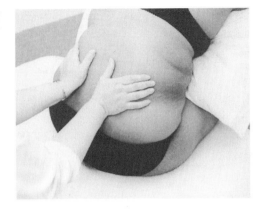

Fig. 3.11. Stretching lumbar erector spinae muscles with woman sitting.

When the limit of the muscle stretch is reached, the pressure is released but not the skin contact. The hand is moved smoothly up or down the spine 2 or 3 cm and the movement is repeated. The pressure should be firm and consistent and the whole manoeuvre slow and rhythmic. The intention is to stretch and relax the muscle belly.

This technique is most effective in the lumbar spine and sacral area, but can be used as far up as the cervico-thoracic junction.

When contractions become more intense, firm pressure can be applied over the sacrum, using the palm of the hand with the fingers pointing downwards (Fig. 3.12). If possible pressure is maintained throughout a contraction, and is applied as if the sacrum formed part of the circumference of a circle, and was being moved round the arc causally. This technique is most useful if the woman is on all fours, as it can be combined with circumduction of the pelvis.

Maintaining firm pressure can be very tiring for the practitioner and she should attempt to use her body weight to apply the force by locking her elbow against her side and leaning on her arm.

During the second stage of labour, between the mother's pushes, it is useful for any of her attendants to massage her neck and shoulders, which take much of the strain along with the accessory muscles of respiration.

Fig. 3.12. Maintaining firm pressure over sacrum.

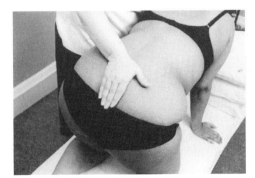

Fig. 3.13. Diagram to show forces acting on lumbar spine in lithotomy position.

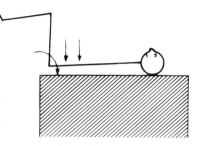

After delivery Women who require an assisted delivery either by forceps or ventouse, or need stitches, are invariably placed in the lithotomy position while these manoeuvres are carried out. At this time their relaxin levels are very high and they are often fatigued. This position results in flattening of the lumbar spine and rotation of the ilia posteriorly (Fig. 3.13). Maintaining this position for any length of time is a source of real concern, due to the excess strain placed on the hip joints and lumbar spine when they are at their most vulnerable.

The situation can be improved by placing a small pillow or even a rolled up towel under the lumbar spine to support the extension curve. This has the effect of balancing some of the downward and rotational forces, thus minimising ligamentous stretch.

Many women experience low backache for the first time in the immediate postpartum period, and this author feels that the lithotomy position is often the cause. Prevention is always preferable to treatment. Some women who have epidural anaesthesia complain of ongoing low back pain. As these are often the same women who require assisted delivery and extensive perineal suturing, with the added disadvantage of loss of proprioceptive control of the lower extremities, the positional factor could be the aetiology in these cases.

Postnatal period Most antenatal education ends with the birth of the baby, and many new mothers are unprepared for the changes that a baby will bring to their lives. These are occurring at a time when the woman is vulnerable both physically and psychologically.

With more home deliveries and 'domino' schemes taking place, and even women who have delivered in hospital being transferred after 24 hours, the transition time from pregnant woman to responsible mother has been considerably shortened. The new mother may not be prepared for the extra bending and lifting involved in caring for a baby, and the fatigue brought on by an altered sleep pattern. This combination can lead to a recurrence of back pain usually at a junctional area. This is the reason for the osteopath asking all pregnant women to return after delivery for an osteopathic examination. This will involve their posture and mobility being reassessed, and the osteopath giving advice on the necessity for further treatment, or possibly just suggestions regarding the height of the changing mat for the baby.

The other major cause of postnatal back problems is the position adopted for feeding, whether breast or bottle. Because of inexperience, and often discomfort from sutures as well, new mothers sit unsatisfactorily when feeding. Breastfeeding mothers bend over the baby rather than raising the baby to the breast. This can lead to mid-thoracic and cervico-thoracic discomfort as well as muscular problems in the shoulder and arm supporting the baby. The woman often fears that if she moves, or even takes a deep breath once feeding is established, the baby will stop sucking and never 'latch on' again. The baby may be being held in an uncomfortable and unsuitable position, which can contribute to sore nipples as well as musculoskeletal problems.

Bottle feeding can also lead to back and shoulder pain, particularly if the baby feeds very slowly and the same unsuitable position is maintained for a long time.

The only alteration required usually involves raising the baby to the breast or bottle by placing pillows on the woman's lap so she no longer has to bend forward. Any treatment to the thoracic spine will have little long-term effect without some adaptation of the causative factors.

Treatment to this area often affects milk production, and many women produce copious amounts of milk during and after treatment.

Aziza developed severe subscapular pain when her first child was 3 weeks old. The pain radiated anteriorly underneath both breasts, and was aggravated by inspiration and rotation. She was given an electrocardiogram and lung function tests and sent to a respiratory consultant because the pain led to panic attacks and hyperventilation. Diolofenac was prescribed and Aziza had to give up breastfeeding. As she could not lift her baby her mother had to take over the care of the baby.

Four years later she became pregnant again and at 26 weeks' gestation the pain returned and Aziza came for treatment. On examination her dorsal spine and ribs had very restricted mobility. Her breathing was mainly upper rib cage and this was aggravated by the fundus of the uterus pressing on the underside of the diaphragm. Treatment was instituted to relax the intercostal muscles and increase the mobility and separation of her ribs and thoracic vertebrae. Over a period of weeks the pains decreased, and with the reduction in symptoms the panic attacks disappeared. It was also recommended that Aziza wore a well-fitting supportive bra as her breasts were very large. She delivered a healthy girl after a 45 minute second stage without any anaesthesia.

The neonate

The postnatal visit is also a useful opportunity to examine the baby osteopathically. This would involve checking the limbs for equal development and full range of mobility, and if the osteopath had specialised training, checking the cranium for equal rhythmic movement. Until recently, cranial osteopathy was not part of the undergraduate course, and had to be studied by choice after qualification. Any osteopath who is not proficient in cranial work will recommend a colleague who is, if this is required.

The difference between osteopathy and chiropractic

Chiropractic also started in America at the turn of the century, but developed from a very different philosophical basis to osteopathy. This however was of little concern to those people receiving treatment. There is only one college of chiropractic in Britain, and until it opened in 1965 all chiropractors trained in America or Europe.

Chiropractors are more concerned with the relative position of joints, particularly vertebral joints, than their relative mobility, and often take X-rays before and after treatment to illustrate the changes brought about by their manipulation. They are also more interested in spinal joints than peripheral joints, and the treatment does not involve much soft tissue or articulation technique.

The main difference noticed by the patient is a different approach to manipulative techniques. Osteopaths usually use long leverage techniques to release a particular joint. This involves locking the joints above and below, using rotation and flexion or extension, so that when a high velocity thrust is applied to the area only one specific apophyseal joint will be released. Chiropractors, being more concerned with positional factors than mobility, apply a very high velocity thrust locally to the joint they wish to move. Many of their techniques require the recipient to be prone during treatment.

The difference between osteopathy and physiotherapy

The practice of physiotherapy has changed considerably during the past 20 years, and many physiotherapists now include massage and manipulation in their treatment regime. However, many people still visit their general practitioner for a diagnosis, with referral to a physiotherapist being just for treatment. While the osteopath is primarily concerned with biomechanical problems, and consideration of the person as a whole, the physiotherapist looks mainly at the area giving symptoms. Osteopaths use just manual treatment, but physiotherapists place significant importance on the use of electrical equipment as well.

Specially trained obstetric physiotherapists are available in some hospitals, but their work is often restricted to ante- and postnatal exercise classes, and advising women after Caesarian section.

Osteopathy in other countries

In most of Europe, which functions under Napoleonic rather than Common Law, osteopathy is technically illegal because it is not state registered. This situation will obviously have to change, at least in the European Community, following the passing of the Osteopaths Act. At the moment osteopaths practising in Europe have to work under the direction of a medical practitioner, or have another qualification themselves such as physiotherapy, which does have state recognition.

There are osteopaths practising in Australia and New Zealand most of whom trained in Britain. Both countries now have their own licensing boards and anyone wanting to practise there may have to take their qualifying examinations.

In America, osteopathy developed in a very different manner from Britain. In the 1960s the American colleges of osteopathy joined the medical establishment, with the result that an American DO is a Doctor of Osteopathy, and in every way the equal of an MD, a Doctor of Medicine. Unfortunately this has had the consequence of American osteopaths doing very little osteopathy as we understand the term. Osteopathic techniques are just one of a whole range of medical and surgical procedures the American DO can employ, and osteopathic hospitals are very similar to general hospitals. Because of the different training in America, and the licensing laws peculiar to each State, it is impossible for a British-trained osteopath to practise in America without undergoing most of their training again.

An American text book, *Osteopathic Obstetrics* by O.P. Grow, DO, published in 1933 contains very little about osteopathic treatment as we recognise it today. However he does recommend direct pressure on the lumbar spine for pain relief, as well as: pressure applied above the symphysis pubis to assist engagement; direct pressure on the clitoris to effect 'osteopathic anaesthesia' before any internal examinations; a sharp tug on the pubic hair to stimulate the uterus to clamp down and prevent excessive haemorrhage; and lumbar extension immediately following delivery to stop haemorrhaging.

Many of Grow's other ideas, such as allowing the woman to walk about during labour, and to put the baby to the breast immediately after delivery, seem very modern, but he also advocated bed rest for 14 days after the birth, which returns the book to its own era.

Research

Research into osteopathy and the outcome of treatment has historically been difficult because of the individuality of the practitioners and their preferred methods of treatment. This renders any trial fraught with complications and inaccuracies. In the past osteopaths attempted to follow the medical model for trials of treatment, but this was always unsuccessful because it proved impossible to treat all volunteers in exactly the same way. The very nature of the treatment made this impractical. Also introducing more than one practitioner into the trial made uniformity of diagnosis and treatment a difficult goal. It is also difficult to quantify the results of a therapy where so much depends on the interaction between practitioner and patient. Obviously some research was carried out, but this was often of a more information-gathering type—what was the most common area for symptoms? or, how far were people prepared to travel to visit an osteopath?, which provided useful statistics but did not add to the body of osteopathic knowledge.

A *Which* report in 1986 suggested that osteopathy was the most widely used complementary therapy, and that 90% of patients claimed to have been cured or improved by treatment. This could not be considered as research, although the findings were most welcome. The dearth of research on pregnant women is even greater, as each practice may have only a few pregnant women attending at any given time, and they could all be at different stages of pregnancy. Even in America virtually no research of a purely osteopathic nature has been carried out on pregnant women. In this country collaborative research has often been hampered by lack of funding or cooperation. Hopefully these problems are all in the past, and several research initiatives are presently under way or in the planning stage. In the interim medical professionals will have to rely on the testimony of thousands of women who have obtained lasting relief from the unnecessary aches and discomforts of pregnancy following osteopathic treatment. There is a large number of small-scale trials which have been carried out by students as part of their degree submissions. While some relate to the increased joint mobility of pregnant women, none so far has resulted in a change to the treatment rationale.

The story so far   The stated aim of this chapter is to inform midwives and other health professionals of the usefulness of osteopathy as an adjunctive treatment for pregnant women. As already stated, osteopathic treatment is safe, non-invasive, usually painless, but primarily effective for pregnant women, and should always be considered a feasible option when offering optimum care. The future of antenatal care must lie in a partnership between allopathic and complementary practitioners working for the better health and well-being of mother and baby.

Training   There are several schools of osteopathy in Britain which together produce about 170 graduates each year. There is also one school which provides a postgraduate course for doctors. The main schools provide a degree course, with either full-time or part-time attendance. One school provides an option with a mixed mode of attendance.

All the schools require 'A' levels or their equivalent for entry by school leavers, but most employ different criteria for mature students to take account of their previous experience. Mature students are welcomed and often make up 50% of a given cohort.

Each institution has its own syllabus but they follow broadly similar lines. The early part of the course will include detailed anatomy and physiology along with sociology, psychology, pathology and osteopathic studies. All the schools have outpatient clinics where students spend hundreds of hours later in the course evaluating and treating patients under supervision.

From May 2000 only schools which have been inspected by the General Osteopathic Council and granted Recognised Qualification status will be allowed to train osteopaths.

At the moment those students on full-time degree courses are eligible to apply for a mandatory award from their local education authority. However, as all the schools are private institutions this only amounts to 15% of the considerable cost of training, and only applies to students who have not had an award before for a previous degree. This is one of the main reasons why there is such a high proportion of mature students—often people who have worked for a few years in order to fund their studies.

References   Consumers' Association 1986 *Which?* (October). Consumers' Association, London

Grow O P 1933 *Osteopathic Obstetrics*. Journal Printing Co., Missouri, USA

King's Fund 1991 *Report of a Working Party on Osteopathy*. King Edward's Hospital Fund for London

Further reading   Hartman 1985 *Handbook of Osteopathic Technique*. Hutchinson, London

Sandler S 1987 *Osteopathy (Alternative Health)*. Macdonald Optima, London

Tone Tellefsen

Chapter 4 **The Chiropractic Approach to Health Care during Pregnancy**

Pregnancy is a time of fundamental change and adjustment for all women. The physical and emotional changes which occur during this short period are among the most profound of any stage of life. Some women pass through these transitions with relative ease but others experience various hurdles along the way: mechanical problems in particular can mar an otherwise trouble-free pregnancy. Recent studies have shown that around 50% of women suffer with low back pain during pregnancy (Fast et al., 1987; Moore, Dumas and Reid, 1990; Ostgaard et al., 1994). Chiropractic offers an effective and gentle way to reduce pain and discomfort during pregnancy without risk to either mother or baby.

What is chiropractic? The science of chiropractic is concerned with the relationship of the nervous system to the mechanical framework of the body. This framework consists of the skeletal system, the joints and attendant muscles and ligaments. In chiropractic special emphasis is put upon the joints of the spine, as these have been shown to have particular significance in movement and posture.

History of chiropractic The word chiropractic stems from Greek *cheir*, meaning hand, and *praktikos*, to do or perform. Indeed the principles of chiropractic can be traced back to the ancient Greeks who were using manipulative techniques to relieve mechanical pains. Hippocrates developed many techniques for the treatment of spinal misalignment and scoliotic curvatures which have been of great influence in the past 2000 years.

Modern chiropractic principles originated in the United States in 1895. Daniel D. Palmer, a student of anatomy and physiology, described the unique relationship between the spine and nervous system and the profound effect of one on the other. He devised chiropractic techniques aimed to improve the function of the musculoskeletal structures and hence the nervous system. Daniel D. Palmer described it like this: 'Chiropractic … done by hand … by one who repairs, one who adjusts'.

Susan had never consulted a Chiropractor before and first considered Chiropractic treatment when she was five months pregnant with her second child. She had experienced quite severe back and neck aches during her first pregnancy two years earlier but had resigned herself to living with it. Like many other pregnant women, she believed that backache was just one of those things that every pregnant woman had to endure. However, suffering with backache the second time was much worse because she now had to keep going for the sake of her toddler.

The chiropractic treatments were focused on improving spinal and pelvic mobility as well as relaxing the soft tissues, especially in the lower back. Susan reported an immediate relief in her symptoms and felt assured that one did not necessarily have to endure backache because of being pregnant! On the last visit prior to birth, Susan also received cranial treatment to relax the nervous system and later reported a feeling of 'floating' out of the clinic. She went into labour less than 6 hours after the visit and gave birth naturally two hours later.

How the physiological changes of pregnancy may alter the musculoskeletal structure

Hormonal changes Progesterone, relaxin and other circulating hormones in pregnancy are known to affect the musculoskeletal system in preparation for labour and delivery (Penna, 1989; Fallon, 1990), although the effects of relaxin are disputed (Petersen et al., 1994; Hansen et al., 1996; Schauberger et al., 1996). Progesterone and oestrogen are said to influence biomechanical structures by changing the structure of connective tissue, and increase mobility of joint capsules and spinal segmental motor units as well as the pelvic joint structures (Fallon, 1986).

Postural changes A chiropractor's primary concern is to diagnose the origin of a complaint rather than chasing symptomatology. It is therefore

Fig. 4.1. Postural changes in pregnant and non-pregnant female.

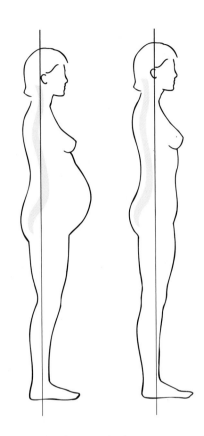

important to understand the postural changes occurring in pregnancy and the possible strains this may cause on the musculoskeletal system and locomotor function.

When examining a non-pregnant woman from the side, the centre of gravity should fall in line with the ear, shoulder joint, hip joint, middle of the knee joint and through the middle of the forefoot. In the pregnant woman the gravity line will fall posterior (Fig. 4.1) to compensate for the increase in weight (Blankenship and Blankenship, 1980; Fligg, 1986).

The pelvis The pelvis (Fig. 4.2) may progressively tilt forward into flexion during pregnancy, which often is due to the growing abdomen and poor postural and muscular strength (Mantero and Crispini, 1982; Fligg, 1986; Bilgrai Cohen, 1989). When the pelvis rotates forward and down it may shorten the ligaments and muscles attached to the posterior and inferior part of the sacrum and iliae (Blankenship and Blankenship, 1980; Chalker, 1993; Harrison, Harrison and Troyanovich, 1997). The sacro-iliac joint is one of the most complicated and disputed joint structures in terms of its shape, function and movement. Its joint motion is complex due to irregularities within the individual joint structures between the sacrum and the iliae. 'The motion involves simultaneous rotations of 3 degrees or less and translations

Fig. 4.2. Normal pelvis with sacro-iliac and symphysis pubis joints.

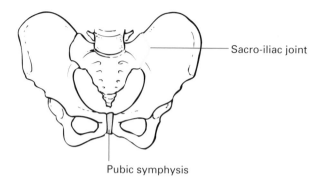

Sacro-iliac joint

Pubic symphysis

of 2 mm or less in three dimensions' (Harrison, Harrison and Troyanovich, 1997). This may explain the multitude of complications that may occur with postural biomechanical stress during pregnancy.

Symptoms associated with the pelvic joints Referred pain from dysfunction of the sacro-iliac joints is usually distributed along the buttocks down the posterior or anterior thigh. There may also be referred pain to the groin and anterior hip (Fligg, 1986; Mens et al., 1996). Muscles involved in sacro-iliac and pelvic conditions are the piriformis, gluteus maximus and medius, iliopsoas, latissimus dorsi, multifidus, obliquus and transversus abdominis, and the leg muscles which attach to the pelvis (Harrison, Harrison and Troyanovich, 1997). Many women will often report a feeling of instability and 'giving way'. This may encourage some women to walk with a waddling gait (Chalker, 1993; Mens et al., 1996).

Symphysis pubis   The symphysis pubis can misalign (Figs 4.3, 4.4) in an upward, downward, lateral or torqued direction. The joint will separate to some degree with

Fig. 4.3. Symphysis pubis misalignment.

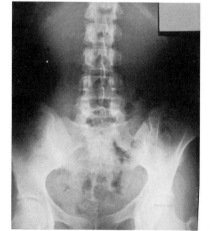

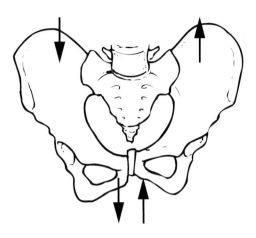

Fig. 4.4. Symphysis pubis misalignment due to pelvic and sacro-iliac asymmetry.

forward flexion of the pelvis such as in the pregnant posture (Chalker, 1993). The normally stable ligaments of the symphysis pubis may elongate or tear during strong abduction of the legs, causing an abnormally large gap in the joint itself. When this gap is more than 10 millimetres it is generally called a diastasis. The separation is most probably affected by the ligamentous laxity during pregnancy. It usually occurs after forceful abduction of the legs in stirrups during labour (Gamble et al., 1983; Walheim et al., 1984; Schwartz et al., 1985; Lindsey et al., 1988).

Symptoms related to the symphysis pubis The pain may be incapacitating and could affect the lives of the whole family. Some women may never be able to carry on a normal life after birth. They may be unable to walk up and down stairs, take care of their child, hold a job or even carry out simple household tasks. Chiropractic care could help to minimise the strain on the symphysis pubis joint by keeping the pelvic ring structure in symmetry and alignment. A support group (see Appendix 2, Useful addresses) has gathered a tremendous amount of information to educate and give support in these cases.

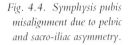

Eva sought chiropractic care in her 33rd week of pregnancy by recommendation from her independent midwife. She had suffered with pelvic joint instability in the first pregnancy which lasted up to 2 years after the birth of her first child. This time the symptoms had started already in the thirteenth week of gestation. The pain was mainly focused in the left symphysis pubis region and both sacro-iliac joints. Her symptoms were aggravated by turning over in bed and pushing the trolley in the supermarket. She had difficulty in walking for any length of time. Eva had had an emergency caesarian the first time but was determined to try for a vaginal

birth this time. The chiropractic examination revealed a pronounced pelvic tilt and asymmetry of the sacro-iliac joints and symphysis pubis articulation. Treatment consisted of gentle manipulative techniques and supine SOT blocking (see treatment section) to realign the pelvic structures. Six weeks later Eva went through a 12-hour vaginal delivery, which was facilitated by the support and persistence of her independent midwife and husband. Treatment was resumed shortly after in correlation with pelvic exercises, and 3–4 months later she reported a full recovery.

Lumbar spine　With the postural changes in the pelvic joints and the added weight distribution of the abdomen, the lumbar lordosis may be accentuated (Fig. 4.5) (Blankenship and Blankenship, 1980; Mantero and Crispini, 1982; Penna, 1989; Fallon, 1990; Chalker, 1993) thus moving the weight-bearing posteriorly from the intervertebral discs to the posterior facet (zygapophyseal) joints (Fig. 4.6). This may stretch the anterior annular fibres of the intervertebral disc itself as well as the anterior ligaments attaching to the vertebral bodies. Mechanically this may cause facet joint irritation and asymmetrical loading of the intervertebral discs (Chalker, 1993).

Interestingly enough, recent research contradicts the previous idea of an increase in lordosis during pregnancy. Moore et al. (1990) and Dumas et al. (1995) found no significant alteration of the lordotic curvature during pregnancy. In fact 56% of the research population showed a flattening of the curvature in comparison to the 16% which displayed an increase in

Fig. 4.5. Increased lumbar lordosis during pregnancy.

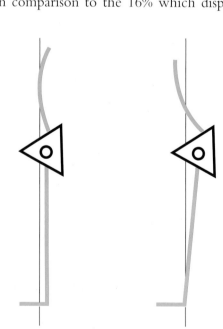

Fig. 4.6. Posterior facet joint of lumbar spine.

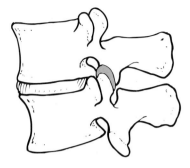

the lordosis. They did however find a positive relationship between pain perception and an increase in the lordosis. It was further postulated that the rectus abdominis muscle, which is attached to the pubic rami, could pull the pelvis posteriorly and superiorly, and in this way reduce the lordosis. This could be further accentuated by a relaxation of the iliopsoas muscle.

Symptoms associated with the lumbar spine It has now been found that as many as 50% of women will suffer various degrees of lower back pain during pregnancy (Fast et al., 1987; Moore et al., 1990; Ostgaard et al., 1994b). The pain associated with lumbar joint subluxation or lesions (such as facet joint syndrome) is either local pain and discomfort from the joint involved and/or referred pain down the posterior thigh, occasionally extending to the foot. When differentiating between a facet joint and nerve root involvement a chiropractor will perform a thorough orthopaedic and neurologic evaluation. Muscle groups involved in lumbo-pelvic complaints are the gluteus maximus, medius and minimus, piriformis, quadratus lumborum and iliopsoas (Bilgrai Cohen, 1989; Hansen et al., 1996).

Thoracic spine and rib-cage With an exaggerated lumbar lordosis, normal spinal coupling will compensate by increasing the thoracic curvature posteriorly. This is called a kyphosis (Fligg, 1986; Moore et al., 1990). The increased size of the breasts may enhance a forward rotation of the shoulders. This may cause an instability of the thoracic spinal joints due to the alteration of the normal mechanical alignment of this area (Chalker, 1993). One of the early changes of the mechanical structure is a change of the rib angles. This may be due to the increased respiratory demand from the growing fetus (Fallon, 1990). The height of the chest cage may be decreased as the uterus enlarges and starts pushing upwards (Fligg, 1986).

Symptoms associated with the thoracic spine Symptoms related to mechanical changes of the chest and rib-cage include joint pain and irritation to the spinal joints and rib articulations (Fallon, 1996). Nerve impingements of the spinal and intercostal nerves are common. These may refer pain anteriorly to the chest. Muscular syndromes include muscle fatigue of the posterior postural muscles, spasm of intercostal musculature and tightness of the diaphragm (Mens et al., 1996). Heartburn is often due to hormonal relaxation of the cardiac sphincter and the fetus pressing up onto the diaphragm.

Katherine sought chiropractic care 4 days after the birth of her second son, on the advice of her midwife. She had suffered with a persistent cough for several weeks and subsequently developed a pain in the right scapular region referring anteriorly to the breast. The pain was aggravated by turning over in bed, breastfeeding and twisting the spine. She had found no relieving factors. After a detailed case history and spinal examination, a working diagnosis was established of costochondral rib subluxations at T9–11. The treatment consisted of gentle spinal manipulation to improve segmental mobility and mobilisation and soft tissue techniques to the surrounding area. Additionally Katherine was given postural advice with regard to breast feeding, and stretching exercises for the shortened musculature. She reported an improvement after the second treatment and was fully recovered after five visits.

Cervical spine In view of the postural changes that take place further down the spine, the neck will compensate for the posterior curvature of the thoracic spine by inclining forward. Lastly the occiput will attempt to regain balance by extending on top of the first cervical vertebra (Fligg, 1986).

Symptoms associated with the cervical spine When these postural changes are exacerbated they may cause tension to the muscles of the back of the neck and base of the occiput (Fligg, 1986; Penna, 1989). This may cause neck and shoulder pain as well as pain referred to the head and skull. Tension headaches are common in pregnancy, although Fallon (1990) reports that approximately 77% of all migraines disappear in pregnancy. This is believed to be due to the hormonal changes of oestrogen and progesterone on the musculoskeletal and vasomotor systems.

Lower extremities Changes of the musculoskeletal function of the lower extremities are often associated with pregnancy alterations in posture. The increased lordosis and forward tilt of the pelvis may influence an external rotation of the hip joints. This is often associated with short piriformis and glutei muscles.

The external rotation of the hips may affect the posture of the feet and cause pronation of the sub-talar joints and flattening of the forefoot (Bilgrai

Cohen, 1989). This may be aggravated by abnormal gait arising from instability at the pelvic joints. The pelvic pattern could also cause an imbalance in the thigh muscles such as the quadriceps and hamstrings (Hansen et al., 1996).

Subluxation theory A subluxation is not merely a 'bone out of place' but a description of the complex relationship between the articulating joint and its adjacent neuro-muscular structure (Chapman Smith, 1997).

Chiropractic treatment during pregnancy

Aims of treatment:

- Improve spinal alignment and stability of the pelvis
- Minimise musculoskeletal and related discomforts
- Optimise neurological function
- Improve posture
- Provide a better space and environment for the baby
- Reduce stress
- Enhance self image and feeling of well-being
- Enable the body to work at its optimum during and after labour
- Accelerate postpartum recovery.

The primary form of care is the specific chiropractic manipulation technique. This is a gentle, specific, high velocity, low amplitude adjustment which is applied to the affected joint, moving it very briefly beyond its normal range of movement. The aim of this is to reduce the subluxation and hence to restore function to the area. Palpation prior to manipulation is shown in Figs 4.7 and 4.8 for the cervical and thoracic spine respectively.

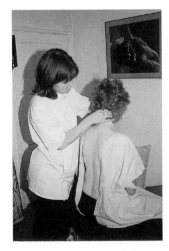

Fig. 4.7. Palpatory technique of the cervical spine to assess subluxation patterns.

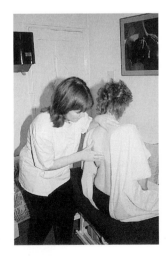

Fig. 4.8. Palpatory technique of the thoracic spine to assess spinal subluxation patterns.

A specific hand contact is applied to a particular part of the involved spinal joint and a short rapid impulse is made in a specific direction. Although the affected area of the spine is often very sensitive, the thrust is usually painless.

The specificity of the thrust is of paramount importance and thus helps to avoid undue stress to any of the surrounding tissues. The adjustments can be carried out sitting, standing, kneeling, lying supine, prone or in side posture. Again these will be adapted and modified to the pregnant woman to ensure comfort and avoid any risk to the fetus.

In addition to the specific chiropractic adjustment, chiropractors will often incorporate other techniques and protocols into everyday practice. This includes various types of mobilisations and traction as well as other more specialised techniques.

Treatment consists of a thorough case history, examination and in non-pregnant women, X-rays to determine the diagnosis. For obvious reasons, X-rays are not used in any woman who is or might be pregnant.

It is essential to take a proper and thorough case history to identify any history of spotting, miscarriage or past trauma. If any suspicion of previous miscarriages arises it is vital to proceed cautiously in the first 3 months (Fligg, 1986). Most women can be treated as normal early on in pregnancy until the fourth to fifth month when the abdomen becomes too large (Fligg, 1986; Esch and Zachman, 1991; Anrig-Howe, 1994).

Later on in pregnancy it is helpful to place a pillow under the abdomen in side-posture to avoid any stretching on either the abdomen or the back (Mantero and Crispini, 1982). Whilst lying supine it is often helpful to use pillows to lift up the upper chest cage and also under the knees to reduce the lumbar lordosis. The nearer to term, the more the adjustment technique is adapted to the laxity of the articulation joints and stabilising structures (Anrig-Howe, 1994). Various soft tissue techniques such as massage, stretching and myofascial trigger point work may be employed.

With regard to hypermobile and unstable sacro-iliac joints, a chiropractor may use special weight bearing wedges in the supine position to realign the pelvic structures (Fig. 4.9). This is a non-force method used in a branch of chiropractic called the sacro-occipital technique (SOT). These wedges will help to realign the pelvic bones in a neutral alignment allowing the muscular and ligamentous structures slowly to relax.

Fig. 4.9. SOT wedges positioned in supine position.

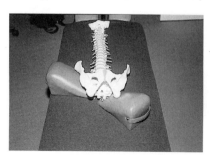

Chiropractic care in pregnancy: some of the conditions that can be treated

Lumbo-pelvic spine

- Lower back pain with or without referred pain
- Lumbar nerve root syndromes such as sciatica or meralgia paraesthesia
- Sacro-iliac and symphysis pubis subluxation and syndromes
- Muscular involvements such as piriformis and gluteus medius syndrome.

Thoracic spine and rib-cage

- Thoracic spinal joint syndromes and costochondral irritation
- Postural strain and muscle imbalance
- Diaphragm spasm and intercostal muscular tension.

Cervical spine

- Tension headaches and migraine of cervicogenic origin
- Neck pain and arm paraesthesia such as pins and needles, numbness and/or muscle weakness
- Carpal tunnel syndrome.

Advice on prevention of back problems in pregnancy

Lumbo-pelvic spine

- It is beneficial to keep an upright posture when gardening, vacuuming and lifting, bending the legs and reducing any twisting avoids strain on the back. Frequent breaks are recommended.
- When lifting a heavy weight, try to hold it close to the body.
- A cushion in the small of the back when sitting can alleviate backache.
- Postnatally, when changing nappies make sure the changing table is at the height of the waist.
- Strength of the transverse abdominal and pelvic floor muscles gives mechanical support, especially later on in pregnancy.

Thoracic spine

- Lifting with outstretched arms may be tiring, especially when lifting children in and out of the car.
- Strength of the posterior back muscles such as trapezius and latissimus dorsi facilitates postural support.
- Pectoralis muscle stretching is helpful for forward rotation of the shoulders.

Cervical spine

- When suffering from neck and shoulder tension an orthopaedic pillow may be of use.

- Bending the neck over a desk for long periods of time can give rise to neck and shoulder tension.
- Lying down with a rolled up towel under the curve of the neck for 10 minutes a day is of benefit and very relaxing.
- Exercises should be focused on strengthening the postural thoracic muscles whilst relaxing and lengthening the neck and anterior shoulder muscles.

Research related to pregnancy

One study by Diakow et al. (1991) involving 400 pregnant women looked at the percentage of women suffering from back pain in pregnancy and whether chiropractic care helped to reduce back pain in labour. Back pain was experienced in 43.5% of pregnancies and 44.7% of the deliveries. Of the 170 pregnancies with reported back pain, 72% also reported back pain in labour. Of the women studied, 37 received manipulation during their pregnancies. It was found that 84% of these women reported relief of back pain during labour.

Treatment was also given during labour in one group, with another group receiving placebo treatment to the thoracic spine. Of the first group, 81% experienced pain relief and 80% felt they required less pain relief or medical intervention. The labour time was decreased in the treated group in 24% of primigravidae and 30% of multigravidae, compared with the control group. Another study by Mantero and Crispini (1982) found as many as 75% of women reported pain relief with chiropractic care.

Joan Fallon has written extensively about pre- and postnatal chiropractic care (1990, 1993, 1996). In one study (1993) she compared her clinical findings of the duration of labour with and without chiropractic care during pregnancy. It was found that primigravidae on average went through a labour time of 14 hours, whereas with chiropractic care the mean labour time was 8 hours. Multiparous women had on average a labour time of 9 hours compared to a 4–5 hour labour in the treated group.

Daly et al. (1991) researched the benefits of manipulation to the sacro-iliac joint in pregnancy. They performed a retrospective study of 100 consecutive pregnancies where 23 of the women reported back pain due to sacro-iliac joint subluxation. Eleven of these women were treated with rotational manipulation, and ten reported relief of pain and no longer exhibited signs of sacro-iliac subluxation after the treatment.

The placebo effect with regard to chiropractic treatment can obviously not be excluded. As far as the author is aware there are unfortunately no research papers available examining this issue in pregnancy; however, it has been shown that the mere fact of being looked after by a caring therapist may give a positive bearing on pregnancy and the outcome of labour. It would be difficult to perform double-blind studies on pregnant women given that they are individually different with different factors such as age, genetic makeup and structural cause of discomfort and pain.

Chiropractic in labour and delivery

The chiropractic approach to facilitating labour and delivery is based on a knowledge of the interaction and interdependence of bones, muscles and nerves. While the peripheral nervous system is responsible for skeletal muscle control and function, it is the autonomic nervous system which is responsible for the control of visceral organs. This is an important factor with regard to labour when the fetus is guided out of the pelvis with the help of maternal uterine muscular contractions. The autonomic and peripheral nerves run down the spine in the spinal cord and exit at each segmental level through the intervertebral foraminae to travel to their specified destination. It is therefore helpful to keep the spinal joints in alignment to reduce any undue pressure or irritation to the passing or local nervous structure. The aim is to provide optimal neurological function to all the structures involved in labour.

The other aspect is related to the mechanical three-dimensional aspect of the pelvis, lumbar spine and diaphragm. The uterus is suspended between the pelvic floor and the pelvic ring structure by strong muscular and ligamentous support. It is then encapsulated by the abdominal wall and spinal structures all the way up to the thoracic diaphragm. If a woman is in a twisted or torsioned posture of the pelvis or lumbar spine, the shape and diameter of the birth canal may be compromised and hence cause obstruction for labour. Figure 4.10. illustrates assessment of pelvic symmetry, and Fig. 4.11 the visual inspection of posture vis-à-vis fetal lie.

Victor Barker (1993) divides the pregnant female posture into the lordotic and kyphotic type. The lordotic pregnant woman will have an increased lumbar curvature which may result in a narrower and more tortuous birth canal. The woman who displays a reduced lumbar curvature and a so-called kyphotic thoracic posture may have an increased space for the birth process. This should allow a larger area for rotation of the fetal head as well as increasing the diameter of the pelvic outlet itself. Figure 4.12

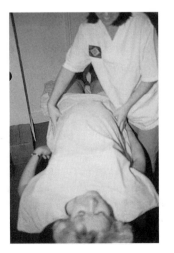

Fig. 4.10. Assessing pelvic symmetry.

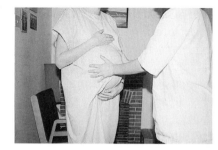

Fig. 4.11. Visual inspection of posture in relationship to fetal lie.

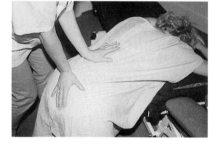

Fig. 4.12. Stretching technique for releasing tension of the lumbo-pelvic spine which can, after instruction, be performed by birth partner or midwife.

shows a stretching technique for release of tension in the lumbo-pelvic spine. The relationship of fetal in utero positioning and the postural alignment of the pelvis has been described by Sutton and Scott (1997) and McMullen (1995). Jean Sutton believes there is an optimal position for the fetus prior to labour, which could facilitate and shorten the birth process.

Maxine McMullen depicts the mechanical forces on the fetal spine, during a transverse lie, breech or brow or face presentation. She advocates chiropractic care to balance the lumbo-pelvic and abdominal relationship and thus try to achieve a better environment for the fetus in utero as well as reducing the possible strain on the neck and cranium during birth.

Sam was already a chiropractic patient when she became pregnant with her first child. She had suffered chronic back pain and symptoms as a result of a whiplash injury in the past. Her symptoms were largely helped by treatments both by the chiropractor and a massage therapist. She was surprised, therefore, not to suffer from back pain during pregnancy, which she had expected due to her history. Unfortunately the fetus was in a posterior position, which caused intense back pain 48 hours prior to labour. This was alleviated however by soft tissue techniques and specific postural positions taught by the chiropractor and carried out by her husband. Sam delivered a healthy boy the following day, after 8 hours' labour, with help only from a TENS machine and gas and oxygen for pain relief.

This is why chiropractic care in pregnancy may appropriately be linked with chiropractic paediatrics, as it is aiming to facilitate a less traumatic birth process for both mother and baby (Anrig-Howe, 1994; Diakow et al., 1991; Esch and Zachman, 1991; Fallon, 1990; McMullen 1995). The midwife or birth partner could learn simple chiropractic techniques aimed to ease discomfort in labour.

Postnatal considerations

It is helpful to have the mother's postural and spinal alignment checked again soon after birth. Contraindications to chiropractic care after delivery would be infection from a caesarean section, severe tissue damage or blood loss. The birth process itself can be tiring and strenuous for the mother and may cause lower, mid back or neck tension, which can easily be helped with chiropractic care. Some women may develop tension headaches after delivery. Many women with pelvic joint dysfunctions find their symptoms aggravated by walking or when lifting their new baby. It can be of help to use specific chiropractic belts to stabilise the sacro-iliac and symphysis pubis articulations during this time.

Training and education

Chiropractic is now the third largest primary health profession in the western world after allopathic medicine and dentistry. It takes five years of full time study to become a chiropractor at the Anglo-European College of Chiropractic (AECC) in Bournemouth, which offers B.Sc., M.Sc. and postgraduate diploma courses. Since 1997 the University of Glamorgan has also offered a four-year full-time B.Sc. (Hons) degree, plus a final vocational year. An M.Sc. course became available at the University of Surrey at the same time. All graduates of these institutions will have been fully trained in anatomy, physiology and biochemistry, leading to an understanding of pathology and diagnosis. Emphasis is placed on neurophysiology and musculoskeletal study, and students are also trained in radiology to nationally accepted standards.

In 1994, the Chiropractors Act received Royal Assent, and set in place the legal framework for the establishment of the General Chiropractic Council (GCC)—the statutory regulator for the profession. The GCC will protect the title 'chiropractor' and will regulate standards of training and safe and competent practice of chiropractic in the UK. The British Chiropractic Association (BCA), established in 1925, is the largest and longest-established association for chiropractors in the UK, and represents 70% of the practitioners working in Great Britain. It runs the most extensive vocational training scheme in Europe as well as a continuing professional development programme and a clinical audit programme.

There are approximately 68 000 chiropractors in the world with 750 members of the British Chiropractic Association practising in Britain, where about 75000 patients consult a chiropractor each week.

References

Anrig-Howe C 1994 Considerations of rendering pre-natal chiropractic care. *American Chiropractor* 34–36

Barker V 1993 *Posture makes perfect*. Japan Publications, New York

Bilgrai Cohen K 1989 Pregnancy and low back pain. *California Chiropractic Journal*: 43–44

Blankenship T, Blankenship V G 1980 Biomechanics of back pain in the gravid female. *American Chiropractic Association Journal of Chiropractic* 1: 113–115

Chalker H M 1993 Spinal compensations of pregnancy. *American Chiropractor* 23–26

Chapman Smith D (ed.) 1997 The role of subluxation in chiropractic. *Chiropractic Report* 11(5): 1–5

Daly J M, Frame S P, Rapoza P A 1991 Sacroiliac subluxation: a common, treatable cause of low-back pain in pregnancy. *Journal of Orthopaedic Medicine* 13(3): 60–65

Diakow R P, Gadsby T A, Gadsby J B, Gleddie J G, Leprich D J, Scales A M 1991 Back pain during pregnancy and labour. *Journal of Manipulative and Physiological Therapeutics* 14(2): 116–118

Dumas G A, Reid J G, Wolfe L A, Griffin M P, McGrath M J 1995 Exercise, posture and back pain in pregnancy. *Clinical Biomechanics* 10(2): 98–103

Esch S, Zachman Z 1991 Adjustive procedures for the pregnant chiropractic patient. *Chiropractic Technique* 3: 66–71

Fallon J 1986 Chiropractic manipulation in the treatment of costovertebral joint dysfunction with resultant intercostal neuralgia during pregnancy. *Journal of Neuromusculo-skeletal System* 4(2): 73–75

Fallon J M 1990 Chiropractic and pregnancy, a partnership for the future. *International Chiropractors Association International Review of Chiropractic* 39–42

Fallon J 1993 Orthopaedic and neurological conditions of pregnancy and chiropractic management of care. *International Chiropractors Association International Review of Chiropractic* 25–30

Fast A, Shapiro D, Ducommun E et al. 1987 Low-back pain in pregnancy. *Spine*, 12(4): 368–376

Fligg B 1986 Biomechanical and treatment considerations for the pregnant patient. *Journal of Canadian Chiropractic Association* 30(3): 145–147

Gamble J G, Simmons S C, Freedman M 1983 The symphysis pubis. Anatomic and pathological considerations. *Clinical Orthopaedics and Related Research* 203: 261–271

Hansen A, Vendelbo Jensen D, Larsen E, Wilken-Jensen C, Kjeld Petersen L 1996 Relaxin is not related to symptomgiving pelvic girdle relaxation in pregnant women. *Acta Obstetrica et Gynecologica Scandinavica* 75: 245–249

Harrison D E, Harrison D D, Troyanovich
S J 1997 The sacroiliac joint; a review of
anatomy and biomechanics with clinical
implications. *Journal of Manipulative and
Physiological Therapeutics* 20(9): 607–617

Lindsey R W, Leggon R E, Wright D G,
Nolasco D R 1988 Separation of symphysis
pubis associated with childbearing. *Journal of
Bone and Joint Surgery* 70-A(2): 289–292

MacLennan A H 1991 The role of the
hormone relaxin in human reproduction and
pelvic girdle relaxation. *Scandinavian Journal
of Rheumatology* 88: 7–15

Mantero E, Crispini L 1982 Static alterations
of the pelvic, sacral, lumbar area due to
pregnancy. Chiropractic treatment.
Chiropractic Inter-professional Research. Minerva
Medica, Torino: 59–68

McMullen M 1995 Physical stresses of
childhood that could lead to need for
chiropractic care. *International Chiropractors
Association International Review of Chiropractic*
24–28

Melzack R, Schaffelberg D 1987 Low back
pain during labour. *American Journal of
Obstetrics and Gynecology* 156(4): 901–905

Melzack R, Belanger E 1989 Labour pain:
correlation with menstrual pain and acute
low-back pain before and after pregnancy.
Pain 36: 225–229

Mens J M A, Vleeming A, Stoeckart R,
Stam H J, Snijders C 1996 Understanding
peripartum pelvic pain. Implications of a
patient survey. *Spine* 21(11): 1363–1370

Moore K, Dumas G A, Reid J G 1990
Postural changes associated with pregnancy
and their relationship with low-back pain.
Clinical Biomechanics 5: 169–174

Ostgaard H C, Zetherstrom G, Roos-
Hansson E 1994a The posterior pelvic pain
provocation test in pregnant women.
European Spine Journal 3: 258–260

Ostgaard H C, Zetherstrom G, Roos-
Hansson E, Svanberg B 1994b Reduction of
back and posterior pelvic pain in pregnancy.
Spine 19(8): 804–900

Penna M 1989 Pregnancy and chiropractic
care. *American Chiropractic Association Journal
of Chiropractic* 31–33

Petersen K L, Hvidman L, Uldbjerg N 1994
Normal serum relaxin in women with
disabling pelvic pain during pregnancy.
Gynecological and Obstetric Investigations
38: 21–23

Schauberger C W, Rooney B L, Goldsmith
L, Shenton D, Silva P D, Schaper A 1996
Peripheral joint laxity increases in pregnancy
but does not correlate with serum relaxin
levels. *American Journal of Obstetric
Gynaecology* 174(2): 667–671

Schwartz Z, Katz Z, Lancet M 1985
Management of puerperal separation of the
symphysis pubis. *International Journal of
Gynaecology and Obstetrics* 23: 125–128

Stern P J, O'Connor S M, Silvano A M
1993 Symphysis pubis diastasis: a
complication of pregnancy. *Journal of Neuromusculo-skeletal System* 1(2): 74–78

Sutton J, Scott P 1997 Understanding and teaching optimal foetal positioning. Lecture notes from seminar in the UK. Birth Concepts, Tauranga, NZ

Walheim G, Olerud S, Ribbe T 1984 Motion of the pubic symphysis in pelvic instability. *Scandinavian Journal of Rehabilitative Medicine* 16: 163–169

Further reading

Chapman Smith D (ed.) 1997 The spine and the nervous system. *The Chiropractic Report* 11(3): 1–6

Fallon J 1994 *Textbook on Chiropractice and Pregnancy*. International Chiropractors Association, Arlington, VA 22201, USA

Haldeman S 1992 *Principles and Practise of Chiropractic*, 2nd edn. Appleton and Lange, Norwalk, CT, USA

Kirkaldy-Willis W H (ed.) 1988 *Managing Low Back Pain*, 2nd edn. Churchill Livingstone, New York

Liebensen C (ed.) 1996 *Rehabilitation of the Spine, a Practitioner's Manual*. Williams and Wilkins, Philadelphia

Schaafer R C, Faye L J 1989 *Motion Palpation and Chiropractic Technique. Principles of Dynamic Chiropractic*. The Motion Palpation Institute, Huntington Beach, CA, USA

Vleeming A, Mooney V, Dorman T, Snijders C, Stoeckart R (eds.) 1997 *Movement, Stability and Low Back Pain. The Essential Role of the Pelvis*. Churchill Livingstone, New York

Sarah Budd

Chapter 5 **Acupuncture**

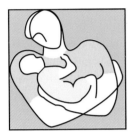

Sarah Budd

Introduction   In presenting acupuncture as it is used today in midwifery, in a Western hospital, it is necessary to review the history of acupuncture. It is also helpful to have an understanding not only of the theory of Traditional Chinese Medicine, but also the underlying philosophical framework of Chinese thought. Modern Western ideas on acupuncture will then be outlined.

The term 'acupuncture' comes from the Latin *acus*, meaning a needle, and *punctura*, punctured. In China, thousands of years ago, it was noted that soldiers wounded by arrows sometimes recovered from illnesses which had affected them for many years. The idea evolved that, by penetrating the skin at certain points, diseases were apparently cured. The Chinese began to copy the effects of the arrow, by puncturing the skin with needles. Acupuncture is an important part of Traditional Chinese Medicine, which includes other techniques such as 'cupping', 'moxibustion', massage ('Tuina'), and Chinese herbal medicine. Over the past 2500 years, medical scholars in every age have contributed to the refinement and development of the art of acupuncture in China. Over the last 20 years acupuncture has dramatically increased in popularity in many parts of the world. There is an increasing interest in the use of it in midwifery practice. The World Health Organization states that there is sufficient evidence supporting the therapeutic effects of acupuncture for it to be considered as an important part of primary health care and that it should be fully integrated with conventional medicine.

Acupuncture is a technique of initiating, controlling or accelerating physiological functions of the body. Acupuncture theory incorporates a complete scientific model that permits the precise calculation of which acupuncture points to use, when and how to combine them, and which points to combine together—all based on observations of the signs and symptoms of the patient (Bensoussan, 1991).

Details of therapy

Needles are inserted into the skin at the acupuncture points. There are over two thousand points on the body, although only approximately two hundred are commonly used in everyday practice. The earliest recorded acupuncture needles were made of stone. In early times, they would also have been made of bone, slivers of bamboo and later bronze, iron, silver and gold. They are now made of stainless steel, are of hair-like thinness, and produce relatively little pain when inserted. The length and gauge refer to the needle body, the part between the handle and the tip. The length ranges from 1.25 centimetres (cm) to 12.5 cm. The gauge ranges from 0.45 cm (26 gauge) to 0.22 cm (34 gauge). In the UK, 30 to 34 gauge would be most commonly used. The length of needle and depth of needling depends on factors such as the location of the point and the size of the person being treated. For example, to treat sciatica, a needle may be inserted into the buttock to a depth of at least 3 cm and the needle would therefore need to be at least 4 cm long, whereas to treat sinusitis, a needle may be inserted alongside the nostril where there is much less flesh; this needle need only be 1.25 cm long and inserted to a depth of 0.5 cm. Figure 5.1 shows acupuncture needles.

Fig. 5.1. Acupuncture needles. (Photo: Nik Screen.)

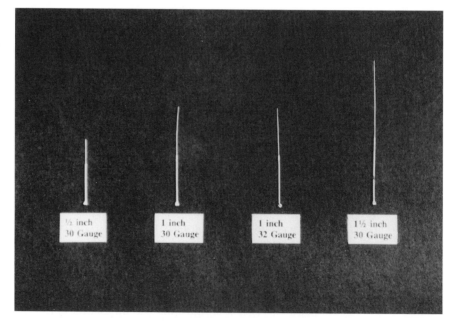

½ inch
30 Gauge

1 inch
30 Gauge

1 inch
32 Gauge

1½ inch
30 Gauge

After insertion, needles are manipulated by rotation according to the condition being treated. This leads to a feeling of warmth and distension around the needle, sometimes also described as a tingling or electric sensation. This is how the practitioner knows that the needle is in the right place. The needles are usually retained for approximately 20 minutes, although this may vary. During treatment, there is often a pleasant feeling of deep relaxation and some people fall asleep. The effect may last for some hours and it is wise to reassure the client that this is normal. In the case of pregnant women, it is often a much needed rest.

Another way of stimulating the needles is by the use of electro-acupuncture. This was first used in China in the 1930s and is now widely employed. Light leads are attached to the handle of the needle by a small clip and a mild electric current passed through the needle. The amount of stimulation can be objectively measured and regulated by adjusting the current, amplitude and frequency. This can produce a higher and more continuous level of stimulation than manual manipulation which is often needed in acupuncture analgesia and anaesthesia. For pain relief in labour, the woman can select the frequency and intensity of the stimulation for maximum analgesic effect. Figure 5.2 shows an electro-acupuncture machine.

Another technique used in Traditional Chinese Medicine alongside acupuncture is 'moxibustion'. This has many applications in general treatment, but in obstetrics, tends to be used for encouraging version in breech presentation. This will be discussed in the section on treatments during pregnancy. A moxa stick is shown in Fig. 5.3.

Acupuncture needles are manufactured in the UK now, as well as being imported from China and Japan. There are several suppliers who provide many different types of equipment which may be used by the acupuncturist. Needles may be disposable or reusable and the choice made by the practitioner may depend on access to safe sterilisation methods. Registered practitioners are required by their local authority to prove they have

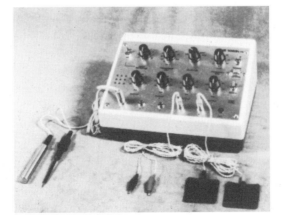

Fig. 5.2. Electro-acupuncture machine.

Fig. 5.3. Moxa stick.
(Photo: Nik Screen.)

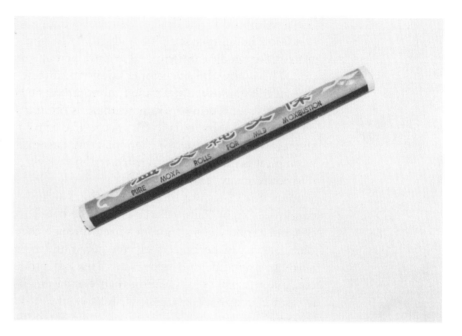

adequate sterilisation equipment, or means of sterilisation at a local hospital, as well as safe facilities for the disposal of both single-use and reusable needles. This is to reassure those coming for treatment that the needles will not be a source of infections such as hepatitis and human immunodeficiency virus (HIV).

Diagnosis   In determining the pattern of disharmony, the acupuncturist needs a detailed understanding of the person's lifestyle, diet, work, medical history, emotional states, etc. The diagnosis is made by questioning, observation, and examination of the pulse and tongue. The practitioner is looking at a whole pattern rather than symptoms in isolation. Tongue and pulse diagnosis are highly refined in Chinese Medicine. The pulse is felt at the wrists on the radial artery and its strength, rhythm and quality indicate the balance of energy and state of the disease. The tongue, through its shape, colour, movement and coating, indicates the progression and degree of the illness.

Just as there are those who do not respond to drugs, so there are those who do not respond to acupuncture. Some diseases are very difficult to cure, particularly if they have progressed to the point where the person is very weak. There are no restrictions on who may have treatment. Babies can be treated, although finger pressure, 'Shiatsu', is usually preferable to needles. Women can be treated for complications of pregnancy without causing harm to the mother or baby, though certain points must be avoided if there is any likelihood of miscarriage. Acupuncture can be combined with

Western drug therapy, or can be used to eliminate dependence on drugs for chronic conditions.

An appointment for acupuncture treatment may be anything from 30 minutes to 1 hour in duration. The first appointment is longer as a detailed case history is taken. The number of treatments needed varies tremendously according to the condition and the person being treated. Women treated for sickness in pregnancy sometimes recover fully after just one treatment, although three or four are usually needed. Some benefit is usually felt after each treatment. Backache in pregnancy tends to take longer, usually needing five or six treatments.

Traditional Chinese Medicine

Traditional Chinese Medicine is a system of medicine which uses not only acupuncture but herbs, diet, massage ('Tuina') and exercise for the prevention and treatment of disease. Acupuncture theory is drawn from an ancient Chinese text, *The Yellow Emperor's Classic of Internal Medicine (The Nei Jing)* compiled between 300 and 100 BC (Kaptchuk, 1983). The theories of medicine it contains are still regarded as the most authoritative guide to Traditional Chinese Medicine.

The Chinese medical system stems from a philosophy very different from that of Western medicine. Acupuncture is a method of using fine needles to stimulate channels of energy running beneath the surface of the skin. This effects a change in the energy balance of the body and works to restore health. The Chinese call this energy or life force 'Qi', pronounced 'chee'. Qi pervades all things, and in humans is derived partly from heredity and partly from the food we eat and air we breathe. It keeps the blood circulating, warms the body and fights disease. Qi flows through channels or meridians which form a network in the body and link all parts and functions together so that they work as one unit. There are 12 main channels, each connected to an internal organ and each named after that organ (Fig. 5.4a). As well as this, there are eight extra channels, which also follow a set pathway in the body. The auricle of the ear has a complete set of acupuncture points corresponding to different parts and systems of the body (Fig. 5.4b). If the ear is likened to the flexed fetus with the lobe representing the fetal head, the acupuncture points correspond approximately with the anatomy of the body. Ear acupuncture originated in China, but was greatly developed in France in the 1950s by Dr Nogier, who added pragmatic points to the traditional ones. It is symptomatic and relatively easy to learn. Short acupuncture needles, usually half an inch in length, may be used at the time of a treatment. Another method is to use stud-like or embedded needles or seeds which may be left *in situ* for several days. The seeds are usually mustard seeds which are very hard, and when pressed, strongly stimulate the point. The advantage of seeds over needles is that they do not break the skin, and therefore are less likely to cause infection when left *in situ* for several days.

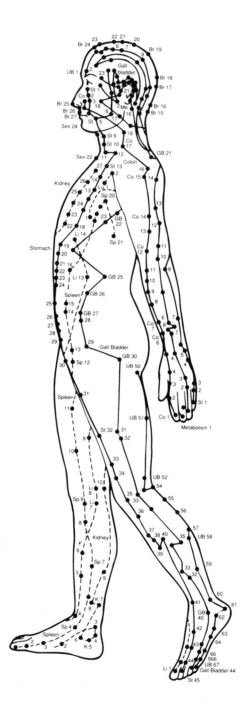

Fig. 5.4a. Illustration of acupuncture channels and points.

In health, the Qi moves smoothly through the channels, but if for some reason it becomes blocked, or too weak or too strong, then illness occurs. The aim of the acupuncturist is to correct the flow of Qi by inserting thin needles into particular points on the channels and so effect a change in a part or function of the body. The logic underlying Chinese medical theory

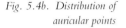

Fig. 5.4b. Distribution of auricular points

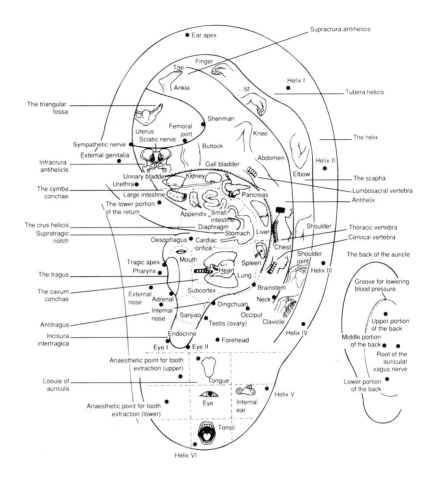

assumes that a part can only be understood in its relation to the whole. The Chinese identify the relationships between phenomena by the theory of Yin and Yang, two opposing forces. Yin, originally signifying the northern side of the mountain, implies coldness, darkness, the interior, passiveness, and the negative. Yang, the southern side, implies warmth, light, activity, expressiveness, and the positive. If either Yin or Yang become out of balance, then health disorders result. An organ that is too Yin is too sluggish, static and accumulates waste. An organ that is too Yang is overactive, out of control, and may generate heat. As well as the principles of Yin and Yang, Traditional Chinese Medicine uses other polarities by which all diseases and disharmonies can be described. Together, they are called the 'eight principles'. They include empty–full, hot–cold, and excessive–deficient, and are used to group symptoms. For example: red face, rapid pulse, fever, dark urine and pain made worse by heat are hot, Yang symptoms, while slow movements, slow pulse, pale tongue, thin clear urine and pain improved by warmth would be symptoms of a cold, Yin condition. This classification of disease suggests suitable methods of treatment; for the patient diagnosed as having a hot condition, the treatment will aim to disperse the heat. If the diagnosis is of weakness and cold it will aim to build strength and warm up by using moxibustion. Traditional Chinese Medicine takes into account not only the disease symptoms, but also the age, habits, physical and emotional traits and all other aspects of the individual, looking at the whole person, as an inextricable part of the environment. Internal causes of disease may be constitutional, of an emotional nature or as a result of habits such as overindulgence. Emotional problems may be traced to a physical origin, and physical symptoms may be emotionally induced. An example would be excess anger, causing the energy to rush up to the head causing a red face, bloodshot eyes, headache, stiff shoulders, etc. Disharmony of the liver may cause irritability, anger, sighing, and depression.

External causes of disease are mostly associated with the environment, especially weather conditions such as cold, damp, heat, etc. and particularly sudden changes in weather; exercise and rest, too much or too little of either can harm the balance of energy; trauma, such as accidents, falls, operations, etc. In China, the emphasis is on prevention of disease. Every morning, one can observe hundreds of ordinary people of all ages practising their Tai Chi or Qi-Gong exercises in the parks or outside their homes, to encourage the free flow of Qi.

Picture a peasant working in the fields in the Han dynasty, 154 BC in northern China. A bitterly cold north wind blows, and in the evening she has an itchy throat, runny nose, cough, severe stiff neck and headache. The local acupuncturist diagnoses 'Exterior invasion of Wind–Cold'. Treatment is given, and after a few hours, there is a marked improvement.

A businessman in the city of London suffers from anxiety, insomnia and headaches. He is under considerable pressure at work, with heavy responsibility and long hours. A friend recommends an acupuncturist, who diagnoses 'Liver Qi stagnation' caused by the pressure at work. After a few weekly treatments, there is much improvement.

Such is the awesome power of Chinese Medicine, that although it originated thousands of years ago, it can still successfully diagnose and treat twentieth century health problems brought about by a lifestyle very different from that of the peasant.

Traditional Chinese Medicine theory and obstetrics

Several of the eight extra meridians referred to in the previous section are very much concerned with women's physiology and with childbirth, particularly the 'Ren' and 'Chong' channels (Fig. 5.5). The Chinese character for Ren means 'pregnancy and nourishment'. If the Ren channel is working well, then one is able to conceive and nourish the fetus. The channel starts in the uterus, emerges at the perineum and ascends the anterior midline of the body. The Chong channel is known as the 'Sea of Blood'. It also starts in the uterus, emerges at the perineum and travels up the trunk bilaterally. It is very much concerned with healthy menstruation and conception.

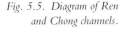

Fig. 5.5. Diagram of Ren and Chong channels.

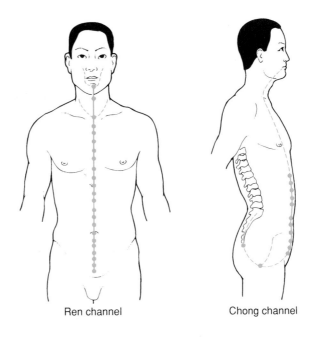

Ren channel   Chong channel

In Traditional Chinese Medicine it is really the ability to conceive that indicates that the *Ren* and *Chong* channels are functioning. Acupuncture has apparently been used successfully in some cases of infertility. Great emphasis is placed on the blood. Nourishment of the fetus during pregnancy via the placenta, and after the baby is born, in the milk, are both considered to make great demands on the woman's blood. In China, great emphasis is placed on the woman's diet during pregnancy as well as observing other lifestyle modifications.

Some of the 12 regular channels are also involved in reproduction, particularly the Kidney, Liver, Spleen and Heart meridians. The Kidney is said to control physical growth, development, maturation, and reproduction. It is also the ultimate control for the other organs and for Qi and blood. The Chinese include the adrenal glands when talking about the kidney, and in Western terms, this importance of the kidney can be understood in terms of steroidal and hormone production. Certain acupuncture points should be avoided during pregnancy as they may cause miscarriage: in particular, points 'Sanyinjiao or Spleen 6' located on the lower leg and 'Hegu or Large Intestine 4' located on the hand (Fig. 5.6). Of course these points may be advantageous in the post-mature woman who is heading for induction of labour.

There are a number of studies on induction of labour with acupuncture (see 'Application to midwifery practice', p. 90).

As the *Nei Jing* is compiled from numerous texts with many revisions and refinements, it will be easy to understand that further details of Traditional Chinese Medicine theory are beyond the scope of this chapter.

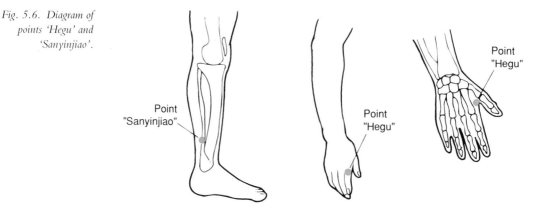

Fig. 5.6. Diagram of points 'Hegu' and 'Sanyinjiao'.

The Western explanation ... and research

There are now both theories and experimental evidence to explain some aspects of acupuncture, particularly its effect in pain relief. A tremendous amount of research has been carried out which attempts to legitimise its use in terms of Western science. To researchers, acupuncture presents a specific problem in that it is a different scientific model from Western medicine and adopts distinct terminology such as 'energy' and 'channels'. The methodology used is extremely variable, and has resulted in many papers which are of poor quality and of little value. It is important that an agreed and satisfactory methodology be established for the evaluation of acupuncture.

The popularisation of acupuncture in the West came about through observation of operations under acupuncture analgesia in China. This led to more research both in the West and in China, where it was recognised that further evidence would promote the use of acupuncture analgesia by Western doctors.

A number of physiological changes have been reported following acupuncture treatment. Functional changes include:

- controlling peristaltic activity in the digestive process, smooth muscle influence in the control of urination and childbirth;
- altering haemodynamics, such as blood pressure, cardiac output and microcirculation;
- the modification of body or blood chemistry as evidenced by production of enzymes and hormones, changes in cellular and humoral immunity, and alterations of blood cell counts, e.g. white blood cells and platelets.

The following trials illustrate some of the above findings. They are not at this stage directly concerned with obstetrics, such trials being included in a separate section, but as pregnancy involves so many physiological changes and a number of patients develop medical complications, they are of some relevance.

Takishima et al. (1982) and Yu and Lee (1976) demonstrated that acupuncture generally improved bronchoconstriction and pulmonary function during clinical attacks of asthma. Altering haemodynamics, Omura (1975) demonstrated that acupuncture had a prolonged effect on microcirculation in the brain and peripheral tissue. Wu (1982) and several other researchers monitored changes in electrocardiograms (ECGs) and cardiac echoes after needling the point 'Neiguan' (or Pericardium 6).

Biochemical alterations include for example restoring levels of stomach acidity, free stomach acids, pepsin and gastric lipase from needling three specific points (Shanghai College of Traditional Chinese Medicine, 1983).

Numerous clinical surveys illustrate that viral, bacterial and protozoal infections may be effectively treated with acupuncture. Qiu (1985) discusses the effect of acupuncture on raising the immunity of the body. The possible changes in the immune system brought about by acupuncture include:

- changes in the cellular immune ability of the body—white blood cells, sensitised T-lymphocytes and their phagocytic activity;
- changes in the humoral immune ability—production of immuno-globulins by B-lymphocytes;
- changes in the reticuloendothelial system—macrophages in the liver, lymph nodes, spleen, and bone marrow;
- the anti-allergic effect of needling (suppressing hypersensitivity).

Bresler and Kroening (1976) comment that 'When an area of the skin anywhere on the body is stimulated, the immune/inflammatory system is mobilised. This reaction to acupuncture may involve histamine, bradykinin, cyclic AMP, serotonin, prostaglandins, and a variety of substances yet to be discovered.'

Trials carried out on patients with a whole range of psychological and emotional disorders show mixed results. Some concluded that it was a cheaper and safer method of treatment than others currently in use (Schaub and Fazal Haq, 1977). Others were more disappointed with their results (Fischer et al., 1984), but it has been pointed out by Bensoussan (1991) that no attempt was made at a differential diagnosis in Chinese terms, which augured badly for their experimental outcome.

In summary, research into what mediates the acupuncture effect focuses on three main areas:

- Neural mediation, which incorporates the concept that nerve fibres transmit and carry the acupuncture effect, and this is confirmed by experiments which test the acupuncture influence after denervation in the region of needling, interference with neural transmission of the acupuncture impulse, or following nerve section.
- Humoral mediation, which includes communication of the acupuncture effect via the circulation of neurotransmitters and other hormones in the bloodstream and cerebrospinal fluid.
- Bioelectric mediation, which maintains that the meridians are electrically

distinct and that changes in them act as precursors to humoral and neurological responses.

Acupuncture today in Britain

The recent British Medical Association report on complementary medicine (BMA, 1993) states that one in four of the 28 000 members surveyed by the Consumers Association in 1991 had consulted a practitioner of complementary medicine in the preceding 12 months. They included the practices of acupuncture, chiropractic, herbalism, homeopathy, osteopathy, aromatherapy and reflexology. The register of acupuncturists published by the Council for Acupuncture at the time of writing has 1114 members. Most are in private practice, but there are a growing number of practitioners working in the National Health Service, some in pain clinics, working alongside anaesthetists, some in general practitioners' surgeries, some in maternity units. Physiotherapists with an interest in acupuncture often combine it with their routine work. There is also a growing number of general practitioners who incorporate acupuncture into their practice.

Application to midwifery practice

Acupuncture is ideal for childbirth. It offers a safe, easy to administer, inexpensive treatment to women during the antenatal, intrapartum, and postpartum period. Women have always been cautious about taking drugs in pregnancy, and since the thalidomide disaster so have their doctors. The so-called 'minor disorders' of pregnancy are anything but minor if you are the one suffering from them, and for years midwives and general practitioners have felt the frustration of not being able to offer much in the way of remedies for these problems. Now there is an answer. It has been around for 2000 years, but has not been readily available to us here in the West until recently.

More midwives around the country are becoming interested in acupuncture as the mothers under their care report the great relief it has given them. There has also been a vast amount of media interest with many articles in journals such as the *Midwives Chronicle* and *Nursing Times*. Several maternity units in England have one or more midwives who offer acupuncture to their patients. Others have shown an interest, and are encouraging midwives to train, in some cases with funding as well. One maternity unit in Plymouth has two midwives trained in acupuncture, and together they have treated over 2000 women with pregnancy-related problems. The service has been available since 1988 and has had tremendous support from both management and medical staff (Budd, 1992).

Uses in pregnancy

There are many conditions which may be helped by acupuncture during pregnancy. In the Plymouth maternity unit, the most common are backache, sciatica and sickness/nausea. The success rate for these is very high. Women are referred for treatment with all sorts of conditions, as illustrated in the table below, but we will look at some of the more common in detail.

Sickness. Hyperemesis	Nausea. Heartburn
Carpal tunnel syndrome	Headaches. Migraines
Varicose veins	Constipation
Vulval varices	Haemorrhoids
Abdominal pain	Backache. Sciatica
Drug addiction	Smoking
Breech presentation	Induction of labour
Skin rashes	Sinusitis.

It is not the purpose of this chapter to discuss all the different treatments for various disorders, but a few examples will be given for the most common of these, illustrated by some case histories. There will be reference made to research where available, although the majority of papers are on the use of acupuncture for analgesia in labour or the induction of labour.

Sickness, nausea and hypermesis gravidarum These can cause absolute misery in early pregnancy, and in the unfortunate few can last the whole duration! Women who have severe hyperemesis needing hospitalisation may be separated from other children, causing much heartache and inconvenience in the home, with partners taking time off work, etc. They can be treated with acupuncture as inpatients, and when well enough to go home again, may continue treatment on an outpatient basis if necessary. The number of treatments needed varies greatly according to the individual and severity. Some women notice an immediate improvement and even cancel their second appointment! This is unusual though, and three treatments is the average. Needles are inserted into the wrists at the point 'Neiguan' (Pericardium 6) and 'Zhongwan' (Ren 12) in most cases, with other points being added if indicated. As mentioned previously, each treatment is adapted according to the individual. Research into the actions of the point 'Neiguan' has been carried out by Professor Dundee, amongst others (Dundee et al., 1988). See also Dundee and Ghaly, 1989; Dundee et al., 1989; Dundee and Yang, 1990; Dundee and McMillan, 1991; Evans et al., 1993; McMillan, 1994; Vickers, 1996; Al-Sadi et al., 1997.

Helen had a history of vomiting until term in her first pregnancy. She presented in her second pregnancy at 12 weeks' gestation, having been referred by her general practitioner. She had nausea and vomiting every day, which was worse in the evenings. She worked full time as a teacher. She was also constipated, having her bowels open only once per week. Otherwise she was well. After the first acupuncture treatment, she noticed less nausea, and a reduction in the frequency of vomiting, which was just beginning to return when she came for her second treatment. She had had her bowels open twice in 5 days. After three more treatments, the nausea had gone completely, and she had not been sick. By mutual agreement, she stopped treatment, with the understanding that she could return if necessary.

Tina B. had suffered from sickness in her first pregnancy until the 17th week. She presented in her second pregnancy at 10 weeks' gestation having been referred by her community midwife. She worked 4 days per week as a midwife (and was also studying for a degree). She complained of constant nausea, and was sick several times per day, morning and evening. She had no appetite or energy. When a full history had been taken, a Traditional Chinese Medicine diagnosis of Stomach/Spleen deficiency was made. After one treatment, she improved immediately, the nausea had gone, and she had only vomited once in 4 days. Treatment was repeated once, and she decided she did not need to continue. She admitted to having felt sceptical before she started treatment. She was delighted with the results, having expected the pattern to be repeated from last time.

Backache and sciatica   This is another common complaint in pregnancy. In many women, it is fortunately just a problem during pregnancy, but there are also those who have had back trouble for a long time, which is often exacerbated by the hormonal influences as well as the postural changes which come about as the pregnancy advances. Physiotherapy is sometimes more appropriate, and with a good relationship between the two departments, referrals may go back and forth. Some women do not have any relief from physiotherapy, and try acupuncture, and vice versa.

In the early stages, it may be possible to carry out the treatment with the woman lying prone, but as the 'bump' grows, she needs to lie on her side with a pillow between her knees. Needles are inserted locally around the area of pain as well as lower down the legs. Points are used which tonify the Kidney Qi, responsible for the health of the lower back area and for bones in general in Traditional Chinese Medicine. The first treatment may well aggravate the situation as the 'stagnant Qi' starts moving, and it is important to warn her of this. After the second treatment, there usually follows a progressive improvement. Again, the number of treatments needed varies from person to person, but is usually around five or six.

Victoria presented at 25 weeks' gestation in her first pregnancy, having been referred by her general practitioner.

She worked full time as a state registered nurse. Five years previously, she had suffered from sciatic nerve entrapment from lifting a patient at work. She had been treated with physiotherapy and three epidurals. She now had low back pain, radiating down her right leg. The first acupuncture treatment stirred up her backache, as she had been warned, but then it eased. After four visits, it had improved enough for her to stop treatment. She needed one 'top-up' treatment 2 months later, but was otherwise delighted with the results.

Constipation Most women notice a change in bowel habit during pregnancy, and again we can probably blame the hormones for this, particularly the relaxation of plain muscle by progesterone. In those who have a problem anyway, it can become a major discomfort and cause great distress. Acupuncture points are chosen according to the individual case, but are usually in the arm, just above the wrist, and in the leg, just below the knee. Results are usually quite dramatic, as illustrated in the following case history.

Tania had a history of irritable bowel syndrome and constipation, with painful bowel movements every 2 or 3 days. She was taking isphaghula husk (Fybogel), senna and lactulose (20 ml three times daily). Like most women, she was keen to stop her medication during pregnancy. Her general practitioner referred her for acupuncture at 19 weeks' gestation in her first pregnancy. Her constipation had started 4 years previously after having glandular fever, with an enlarged spleen. At this time, she had been bedridden for 3 months. After a full case history and examination of her pulse and tongue, the Traditional Chinese Medicine picture was one of 'heat retention', probably due to the glandular fever. After the first acupuncture treatment, she opened her bowels 1 hour later. At her second treatment 10 days later, her bowel movements were noticeably easier, with no bleeding. She had stopped the lactulose. After the second treatment, she was having daily bowel movements, and had stopped all medication.

Breech presentation This area of Traditional Chinese Medicine application to midwifery practice has attracted much attention. The technique used to encourage version of the fetus is called 'moxibustion', which means the burning of the herb 'moxa', the Chinese name for mugwort (*Artemisia vulgaris* or St John's Herb). The technique involves heating an acupuncture point on both feet for 15 minutes, up to 10 times, on a daily basis. This seems to increase fetal activity, hopefully enough to turn the fetus from breech to cephalic presentation. Studies conducted in China on this technique report varying success rates ranging from 80.9% to 90.3% (Wei Wen, 1979; Co-operative Research Group of Moxibustion Version of Jangxi Province, 1984). A study conducted in Italy in 1990 (Cardini et al., 1991) reported 66.6% success rate on a group of 33 women of gestational ages ranging from 30 to 38 weeks. Most research papers on moxibustion show that the 34th week of gestation is the optimum time to carry out the technique, giving a higher success rate. A trial conducted by the author is in progress, which hopes to demonstrate further the effect of this technique on the mother and fetus. Regarding the mechanism of action, a trial carried out by the Co-operative Research Group of Moxibustion Version of Jangxi Province (1984) postulates that the increase in corticoadrenal secretion, through the resulting increase in placental oestrogens and changes in prostaglandin levels which they measured, raises basal tone and enhances uterine contractility, stimulating fetal motility, and thus making version more likely. This increase in fetal motility is one of the more striking features of moxibustion, perceived by almost all the women during the second half of the 15 minute treatment, and persisting even after the end of stimulation.

Figure 5.7 shows the hypothetical mechanism of action of moxa stimulation of the 'Zhiyin' point (Co-operative Research Group of Moxibustion Version, 1984). A second study by the same authors presents the results of 1 week's treatment with moxa in 241 pregnant women of gestational age ranging from 28 to 34 weeks, in comparison with 264 control subjects. In the moxa-treated women, there were 195 versions (81%) as against 130 (49%) in the control group, the difference being statistically significant ($P<0.05$). When moxa treatment was continued for a further 7 days, the overall success rate was 87%.

Cardini's trial confirmed findings in the Chinese trials that the success

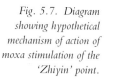

Fig. 5.7. Diagram showing hypothetical mechanism of action of moxa stimulation of the 'Zhiyin' point.

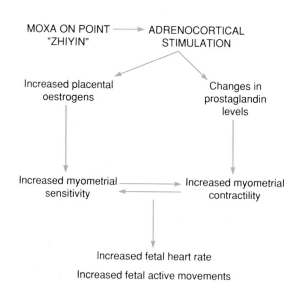

rate is higher in multigravidae, as would probably be expected owing to the reduced tone of the abdominal muscles.

As this technique does not involve any needles, and needs daily application for up to 10 days, the woman's partner or a friend can be instructed in its application, and they can continue treatment at home. This has the advantage not only of convenience, but also gives them a sense of control over the situation, and when successful, a tremendous feeling of having sorted out the problem for themselves.

With further research to prove the efficacy of this technique, it may be possible for it to become a routine treatment in the management of breech presentation. Midwives could easily be trained in its application. The obvious advantages are a decrease in the number of breech births and their complications, as well as a potential reduction in the caesarean section rate in primigravid breech presentation (routine in many units). It is also extremely cheap, with moxa sticks currently costing 50 pence each! Most mothers only need two sticks per course of treatment, with some needing four. (See also Cardini & Weixin, 1998.)

Induction of labour This application of acupuncture in obstetrics has stimulated a number of clinical studies in various countries. In the *Jia Yi Jing* (dated AD 282), a Chinese Jin dynasty classic, it is stated: 'In prolonged labour and retained placenta use *Kunlun*', an acupuncture point behind the medial malleolus. Studies have explored acupuncture's ability to initiate contractions prior to rupture of the membranes, and prior to the woman experiencing any labour pains (Kubista et al., 1975; Ying et al., 1985; Dunn et al., 1989). Other investigators noted that with acupuncture, 'the relation between the force of contraction and the degree of dilation of the cervix differed from that in spontaneous and oxytocin induced labours' (Tsuei and Lai, 1974). The implication here is that different physiological pathways are possibly involved in acupuncture-induced labour. The accumulated results of hundreds of studies have shown that virtually any hormone or neurotransmitter may be affected by appropriate acupuncture stimulation (Bensoussan, 1991). This may explain the difference between the two methods of induction of labour.

In approximately 12 separate clinical studies on the induction of labour with acupuncture, negative side-effects have still to be reported or identified. This is in contrast to the possible side-effects of Syntocinon, such as abnormally strong or prolonged contractions or rupture of the uterus, as well as other responses (Wren, 1985). However, some researchers found a disadvantage in that the strength and frequency of contractions cannot be controlled, although the contractions stimulated by acupuncture resembled those of spontaneous labour (Kubista et al., 1975; Yip et al., 1976). Another disadvantage may be that the period of acupuncture necessary to stimulate contractions can be as long as 5 hours in some cases, which may not be practical or acceptable to the woman. It is the experience of this author that when attempting induction around term, often by maternal request, several treatments are needed, each lasting 1 hour, on a daily basis. However, in the case of a typical para two, whose third labour is slow to establish, or in cases where the membranes have already ruptured, acupuncture stimulation is far easier and has a much higher success rate. This can often negate the need for augmentation with Syntocinon, and the accompanying monitoring by fetal scalp electrode and lack of mobility that go with it.

The acupuncture points most commonly used to stimulate contractions are 'Hegu' or Large Intestine 4, and 'Sanyinjiao' or Spleen 6, needled together, bilaterally. They are often stimulated by an electro-acupuncture unit for maximum effect. They are located on the hand, between the thumb and index finger, and on the leg, just above the medial malleolus. In traditional Chinese medicine terms, they have a very strong effect on the energy of the uterus, causing it to descend, and it is for this reason that both these points are amongst those listed as being forbidden for use earlier in the pregnancy. In some cases, firm pressure to these points may be enough when needles are unavailable, to bring back contractions that have weakened during an established labour.

Analgesia in labour Again, this application of acupuncture in obstetrics has aroused much interest, and a certain amount of research. In some cases, it has been the reason for the introduction of acupuncture into maternity units by midwives (Skelton, 1988; Budd, 1992).

The results of studies on acupuncture analgesia in labour vary tremendously. One of the main problems in assessing analgesia is the subjectivity of pain perception. The methods of assessing this also vary tremendously, making comparisons between trials difficult.

The first reported acupuncture deliveries in Europe were done by Dr Christman Ehrstroem in Stockholm, Sweden, in 1972. In 1974, Darras, in France, reported 20 electro-acupuncture deliveries. They were primiparae and multiparae, all non-operative deliveries without episiotomy or forceps. He reported 16 successful, three partially successful, and one failure.

More recently, Martoudis and Christofides (1990) conducted a trial in Cyprus using an interesting combination of an auricular point with a point on the hand, on 186 parturients. The time of acupuncture stimulation varied from 20 to 30 minutes, and the analgesic effect began to be effective at a mean time of 40 minutes. The duration of the analgesic effect was a mean time of 6 hours. In all the parturients who delivered during this period of time, no analgesic drugs were necessary. In 24 cases, electro-acupuncture had no effect, and these received analgesic drugs. The average Apgar score was 9.60 at 1 minute, a very high average which speaks well for the safety of the method. In order to evaluate the results of the treatment as objectively as possible, questionnaires were given to the parturients themselves, as well as to the midwife in charge of the delivery room and to the delivering doctor.

The recordings taken before the insertion of needles show clearly that pain was felt at the beginning of the contraction, and went at the end of the contraction (Fig. 5.8). Recordings taken when the effect of the electro-acupuncture was maximal show that pain was felt at a much later stage of the contraction, and ended much earlier than the end of the contraction. The authors concluded that their method produced slight to very good results in 87.5% of the cases.

The methods used in other trials on acupuncture analgesia in labour were quite different from the above, and produced just as variable results. One contrasting report is that of Wallis et al. (1974), who studied 21 women in labour with acupuncture analgesia. They concluded that 19 of the 21 re-garded the acupuncture treatment as unsuccessful in providing analgesia

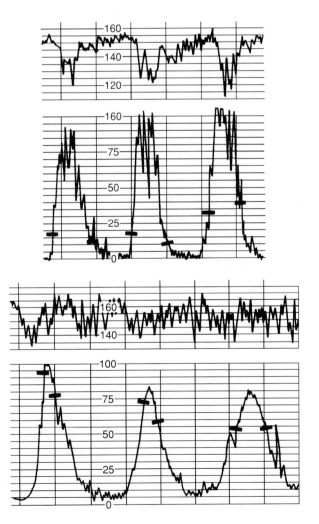

Fig. 5.8. 'CTG' recording from trial. Top: before acupuncture; bottom: after/with acupuncture.

for labour and delivery. The points used were selected on an individual basis, and were taken from a selection of 17! These points were located on the abdomen, back, legs and ear. It is the opinion of this author that the restriction in the mobility of the woman during acupuncture may have had a very negative influence on the effect of the treatment. However, other studies which also used 'body points', such as Perera (1979), showed much higher success rates, so other factors must be involved.

Irene Skelton was the first midwife in Britain to carry out a study on acupuncture and labour, reported in 1988. It was a 2-year study involving 170 births in Glasgow, investigating the comparative effectiveness of conventional analgesics and acupuncture. She concluded that 'Acupuncture has a significant part to play in the control of labour pain ... Women who received acupuncture felt more in control of their labour and delivery and were generally more satisfied with the "birth experience" than the control group.'

In the Plymouth unit, acupuncture analgesia for labour has been offered since 1988. The women hear about it from their community midwives, during parentcraft talks, from the hospital tours, their general practitioners, hospital midwives and doctors, and of course, by the powerful 'word of mouth'. They are then advised to contact the midwife/acupuncturist during the third trimester and then to meet them and see the equipment. A demonstration is often given of the needling of an ear point so they know what to expect, as many have never had acupuncture treatment before. It is pointed out that there are only two midwives trained to provide acupuncture at the moment and it is therefore not a 24-hour service, so they should not rely on it totally. It is made as available as possible within the limitations of running a busy outpatient clinic. There is often the flexibility to stay with the woman in labour and hopefully deliver her, as well as providing the acupuncture. This is extremely satisfying for both parties, and ties in well with the 'Know your midwife' scheme.

The method of application of ear acupuncture for labour has been altered with experience. In the early days, points on the hand and leg were chosen, according to the ancient texts and to methods used more recently by researchers, but these were found to restrict mobility too much. Ear points are now used, usually with electro-stimulation (Fig. 5.9). Half-inch needles are inserted into the chosen points and taped down. The cartilage of the ear is tough enough to hold the needles in place quite firmly. Light leads from the electro-acupuncture machine are attached to two of the needles and the woman is instructed in the use of the stimulator. She is in control of the intensity of the stimulation, but the frequency is determined and pre-set by the practitioner. Once in place, the woman is free to mobilise or assume any position she finds comfortable. If she decides she would like a bath, the electricity is discontinued, but the needles may be left in place. The effect usually takes around 10–20 minutes to build up, and the

Fig. 5.9. Diagram of ear points used for analgesia in labour.

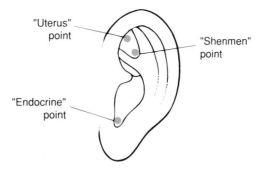

"Uterus" point

"Shenmen" point

"Endocrine" point

labouring woman becomes noticeably more calm and relaxed—able to cope with the contractions, even though she can still feel them. Some start to fall asleep in between contractions and wake up half way through the next one. This sleepy, very relaxed state may well be due to the stimulation of serotonin. The degree of analgesia obtained varies tremendously, as it does with other methods, and is of course subjective. In some cases, the acupuncture is not enough, especially when nearing transition into the second stage of labour. This is when Entonox can be a great help, and is usually enough to see her through until pushing commences. Of course in a very long and tiring labour, possibly with complications, epidural anaesthesia may become necessary and it is important that the woman feels able to ask for this without feeling she has failed by not coping with acupuncture alone. This is pointed out to her when she comes to discuss acupuncture analgesia during the antenatal period.

The points used for analgesia are 'Uterus', 'Shenmen' and 'Endocrine'. The first is chosen for obvious reasons as the organ being targeted. The second point is used for general analgesia and relaxation in the whole body, and the third to stimulate contractions. There is no research available at the time of writing which looks at the use of ear points alone in labour. The clinical trials conducted so far have mainly used body points, although Martoudis and Christofides (1990) used a combination of ear and body points.

In a review of eight clinical trials on acupuncture analgesia for labour, six showed favourable or successful results (Darras, 1974; Ledergerber, 1976; Hyodo and Gega, 1977; Perera, 1979; Skelton, 1988; Martoudis and Christofides, 1990) and two were negative (Wallis, 1974; Abouleish, 1975). Most of these studies were carried out on small numbers of women. They were of differing design, only some using controls, and using varying methods of assessment. As is often the case, further research needs to be carried out in a standardised manner on large numbers of women. One of the problems with this is of course the funding for such research. Another is the availability of suitably trained practitioners to carry it out. As a majority of medical research is funded by pharmaceutical companies, finding money for research into a complementary therapy which may negate the need for medication can be a problem.

Haemorrhoids Haemorrhoids are an extremely common complaint in pregnancy and the immediate postnatal period, causing much discomfort and distress, and may often lead to problems with breast feeding due to poor positioning. There is an 'empirical' point for haemorrhoids called 'Chengshan' or UB 57, which is located on the back of the calf. It is on the urinary bladder meridian which passes around the anus, and even when used on its own, this point can give tremendous relief within hours, reducing the swelling, pain and discomfort in the area. Often one treatment is enough, but if not, and the mother and baby are still in hospital, it can be repeated on a daily basis, which is convenient before the busy times start at home. If necessary, she may return as an outpatient.

Retention of urine This is fortunately not very common, but when it happens can have serious implications, and apart from the distress of repeated catheterisation it causes great unhappiness from being kept in hospital when looking forward, and having planned, to go home soon after the birth. It is often associated with traumatic forceps deliveries, oedematous perinei and sometimes epidural anaesthesia. In Traditional Chinese Medicine terms, the acupuncture can tonify the bladder and draw energy to the area, causing the sensation of needing to pass urine, which is often absent in these cases. Needles are usually inserted into points on the lower leg as well as locally, above the symphysis pubis, and strong stimulation is used. Even when she has already tried for several days without success to begin to empty her bladder, one treatment may well be enough to stimulate the urge to pass a good volume of urine within an hour. Repeated treatments may be necessary.

Insufficient lactation Acupuncture can be particularly useful in the situation where a mother is under a lot of stress, and despite a strong desire to breastfeed her baby, finds that her milk production is reducing. This is often the case with premature births, where the baby is still being cared for in the special care baby unit, and particularly when he or she is unwell and struggling. Part of the physiology of lactation involves the neurohormonal reflex set up by stimulation of the nipple leading to the release of oxytocin from the posterior pituitary. This reflex can be suppressed by the higher centres in the brain, causing stress and anxiety to affect the 'let down' reflex.

Acupuncture treatment can be aimed at strong relaxation as well as providing a 'tonic' to build the mother up, and increase the flow of energy or 'Qi' to the breast. It is known that acupuncture has a strong influence on hormone levels, and there are suggestions of its influence on the higher centres, so it is reasonable to speculate that its success in promoting lactation is due to an increase in levels of oxytocin and prolactin.

The use of acupuncture by midwives

Training, registers, how to find an acupuncturist There are several acupuncture training schools in this country which are listed below. These are all recognised by the Council for Acupuncture, the governing body for the acupuncture profession. Training in some of these schools leads to automatic admission to one of the acupuncture registers. Admission to a register for those who have trained elsewhere is by interview and occasionally examination. The Council for Acupuncture publishes an annual directory of practitioners in the country which is a recommended method of choosing a practitioner. The Royal College of Midwives is aware of midwives who are also trained acupuncturists, especially those practising in the NHS.

Acupuncture training The minimum training period in this country is 3 years (full/part-time) and the British College of Acupuncture is the only one to require students to have some medical, paramedic or other practising qualification prior to entry. Prospectuses and full details of courses can be obtained from the colleges by sending a stamped addressed envelope.

An alternative and quicker training can be found in China! There are many international training colleges in China, a list of which can be found with the above. My colleague trained in Nanjing on their 3-month course, which can be followed by another 3-month advanced course. It is an extremely intensive course, and some knowledge of basic theory and acupuncture point location before departure is highly recommended. Interpreters are provided! Funding may be available, but it takes much patience and many application forms to find it. There are several midwives who have been successful in this, however, and have had their whole training paid for by awards or charitable means. The author has been contacted (for advice) by several midwives in different parts of the country whose health authorities have encouraged them to train as acupuncturists, with sponsorship offered.

References

Abouleish E B 1975 Acupuncture in Obstetrics. *Anaesthesia and Analgesia* 54(1): 83

Al-Sadi M, Newman B, Julious S A 1997 Acupuncture in the prevention of postoperative nausea and vomiting. *Anaesthesia* 52: 658–661

Bensoussan A 1991 *The Vital Meridian*. Churchill Livingstone, Edinburgh

Bresler D, Kroening R 1976 Three essential factors in effective acupuncture therapy. *American Journal of Chinese Medicine* 4(1): 81

British Medical Association (BMA) 1993 *Complementary Medicine, New Approaches to Good Practice*. Oxford University Press, Oxford

Budd S 1992 Traditional Chinese medicine in obstetrics. *Midwives Chronicle and Nursing Notes*, 105: 140

Cardini F, Basevi V, Valentini A, Martellato A 1991 Moxibustion and breech presentation: preliminary results. *American Journal of Chinese Medicine* XIX(2): 105

Cardini F, Weixin H 1998 Moxibustion for correction of breech presentation: a randomized controlled trial. *JAMA* 280(18): 1580–1584

Co-operative Research Group of Moxibustion Version of Jangxi Province 1984 Clinical observation on the effects of version by moxibustion. *Abstracts from the Second National Symposium on Acupuncture and Moxibustion and Acupuncture Anaesthesia, Beijing, China*, p. 150. All China Society of Acupuncture and Moxibustion

Darras J C 1974 Acupuncture update. Symposium, held in New York, by National Acupuncture Research Society, October

Dundee J, Sourial F, Ghaly R, Bell P. 1988 Acupressure reduces morning sickness. *Journal of the Royal Society of Medicine*, 81: 456

Dundee J, Ghaly R, Fitzpatrick K et al. 1989 Acupuncture prophylaxis of cancer chemotherapy-induced sickness. *Journal of the Royal Society of Medicine*, 82: 268

Dundee J W, Yang J 1990 Prolongation of the anti-emetic action of P6 acupuncture by acupressure in patients having cancer chemotherapy. *Journal of the Royal Society of Medicine* 83: 360–362

Dundee J W, Ghaly R G 1991 Local anaesthesia blocks the anti-emetic action of P6 acupuncture. *Clinical Pharmacology and Therapeutics* 50: 78–80

Dundee J W, McMillan C M 1991 Positive evidence of P6 acupuncture antiemesis. *Postgraduate Medical Journal* 67: 417–422

Dunn P, Rogers D, Halford K 1989 Transcutaneous electric nerve stimulation at acupuncture points in the induction of uterine contractions. *Obstetrics and Gynaecology*, 73: 286

Evans A T et al. 1993 Suppression of pregnancy-induced nausea and vomiting with sensory afferent stimulation. *Journal of Reproductive Medicine* 38(8): 603–606

Fischer M, Behr A, v. Reumont J 1984 Acupuncture—a therapeutic concept in the treatment of painful conditions and functional disorders. *Acupuncture and Electrotherapeutics Research* 9: 11

Hyodo M, Gega O 1977 The use of acupuncture analgesia for normal delivery. *American Journal of Chinese Medicine*, 5(1): 63

Kaptchuk T 1983 *Chinese Medicine, the Web that has no Weaver*. Rider, London

Kubista E, Kucera H, Muller-Tyl 1975 Initiating contractions of the gravid uterus through electroacupuncture. *American Journal of Chinese Medicine* 3(4): 343

Ledergerber C P 1976 Electroacupuncture in obstetrics. *Acupuncture and Electrotherapeutics Research* 2: 105

Martoudis S, Christofides K 1990 Electroacupuncture for pain relief in labour. *Acupuncture in Medicine* 8(2): 51

McMillan C 1994 Transcutaneous electrical nerve stimulation of Neiguan anti-emetic acupuncture point in controlling sickness following opioid analgesia in major orthopaedic surgery. *Physiotherapy* 80(1): 5–9

Omura Y 1975 Pathophysiology of acupuncture treatment; effects of acupuncture on cardiovascular and nervous systems. *Acupuncture and Electrotherapeutics Research* 1: 511

Perera W 1979 Acupuncture in childbirth. *British Journal of Acupuncture* 2(1): 12

Qiu M 1985 Lecture Presented on the Occasion of the Fourth International Advanced Studies Program in Acupuncture, Nanjing

Schaub M, Fazal Haq M 1977 Electro-acupuncture treatment in psychiatry. *American Journal of Chinese Medicine*, 5(1): 85

Shanghai College of Traditional Chinese Medicine 1983 *Acupuncture: A Comprehensive Text* (eds O'Connor and Bensky). Eastland Press

Skelton I 1988 Acupuncture and labour—a summary of results. *Midwives Chronicle and Nursing Notes* May: 134

Takishima T, Suetsugu M, Gen T, Ishihara T, Watanabe K 1982 The bronchodilating effect of acupuncture in patients with acute asthma. *Annals of Allergy* 48(1): 44

Tsuei J, Lai Y 1974 Induction of labour by acupuncture and electrical stimulation. *Obstetrics and Gynaecology* 43(3): 337

Vickers A 1996 Can acupuncture have specific effects on health? A systematic review of acupuncture antiemesis trials. *Journal of the Royal Society of Health* 89: 303–311

Wallis L, Shnider S, Palahniuk R, Spivey H 1974 An evaluation of acupuncture analgesia in obstetrics. *Anesthesiology* 41(6): 596

Wei Wen 1979 Correcting abnormal fetal positions with moxibustion. *Midwives Chronicle and Nursing Notes* 92(1): 103, 432

Wren B G (ed.) 1985 *Handbook of Obstetrics and Gynaecology*, 2nd edn. Chapman and Hall, London

Wu Y 1982 Therapeutic effect and mechanism of acupuncture at Neiguan (Per 6) in chronic rheumatic heart disease. *Journal of Traditional Chinese Medicine* 2(1): 51

Ying Y, Lin J, Robins J 1985 Acupuncture for the induction of cervical dilatation in preparation for first trimester abortion and its influence on HCG. *Journal of Reproductive Medicine* 30(7): 530

Yip S, Pang J, Sung M 1976 Induction of labour by acupuncture electro-stimulation. *American Journal of Chinese Medicine* 4(3): 257

Yu D Y, Lee S P 1976 Effect of acupuncture on bronchial asthma. *Clinical Science and Molecular Medicine*, 51(5): 503

Further reading

Bensoussan A 1991 *The Vital Meridian.* Churchill Livingstone, Edinburgh *This book explores the biomedical and scientific aspects of acupuncture. It presents a thorough, easily accessible review of research conducted in China and in the West.*

Kaptchuk T 1985 *Chinese Medicine. The Web that has no Weaver.* Rider, London *An interesting approach to the principles of Chinese medical thought, which develops an interaction between modern Western medicine and traditional Chinese medicine.*

Lewith G, Aldridge D (eds.) 1993 *Clinical Research Methodology for Complementary Therapies.* Hodder and Stoughton, London *This book lays out the fundamentals required for clinical research within a range of complementary therapies and brings together some innovative ideas.*

Low R 1990 *Acupuncture in Gynaecology and Obstetrics.* Thorsons, London *A textbook for practitioners and students of Chinese medicine on the application of acupuncture in this important area.*

Maciocia G 1989 *The Foundations of Chinese Medicine.* Churchill Livingstone, Edinburgh *An excellent textbook on the theory of Chinese Medicine which draws on modern and ancient classical Chinese texts. It explains the application of the theory of Chinese medicine to a Western medical practice, emphasising Western types of diseases and patients.*

Helen Stapleton, Denise Tiran

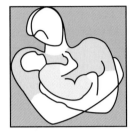

Chapter 6 **Herbal Medicine**

Healing with the use of herbs is undoubtedly the earliest form of medicine, practised primarily amongst women everywhere since human existence has been recorded. For the most part, these ordinary, unremarkable women continued a timeless tradition of 'women's work' in attending labouring women, the sick and the dying. These were the 'wyse wimmin'; the un-licensed doctors, pharmacists, abortionists and midwives who travelled from place to place, collecting and cultivating herbs, learning from each other and passing on their wisdom, experience and knowledge as nameless keepers of an oral tradition.

One such historical figure whose life and practice during the Middle Ages has been well researched was Trotula, a distinguished teacher and physician at the famous Medical School of Salerno, Italy. Amongst remaining writings attributed to her is a treatise on gynaecology and obstetrics: 'Passionibus Mulierum Curandorum' (*The Diseases of Women*), also known as *Trotula Major* (Brookes, 1993). Trotula (the same Dame Trot of Chaucer and children's tales) was a skilled diagnostician in a time when actual knowledge of the inner workings of the body was largely left to the imagination as dissection was rarely, if ever, performed. Her reliance on the skills of urine and pulse diagnosis, in conjunction with careful consideration of the patient's features and choice of words, remain integral to the practice of many non-European systems of medicine in current use today. She wrote on a variety of topics directly related to women, and subsequently made her writings available to them at a time when such activities would have been considered highly subversive by the Establishment. The diversity of her subject matter reflected her understanding of the complexity of women's situations and difficulties, as is expressed when she makes suggestions in a herbal recipe for counterfeiting virginity. Trotula personified the balance so critical but yet so rarely visible in contemporary health workers; a knowledge and appreciation of the importance of science, attention to the 'magical' aspects of healing embedded in the mind, an empathy with the suffering and distress of illness and a willingness to engage compassionately with those who sought her advice.

Herbal medicine continued to be practised throughout the countryside and even up to the 1800s most people, when sick, still consulted herbalists. As women healers were further decimated or their position usurped, the developing fields of chemistry and physiology were subtly supplanting herbal traditions by subsuming them into a 'science'. Only with the rise of the pharmaceutical industries in the late nineteenth century did the intimate alliance between botany and medicine begin to falter. We still owe a considerable debt of gratitude to women persecuted as witches for their accumulated empirical knowledge, as many of the herbal remedies tried and tested by them continue to hold their place in modern pharmacology. Significantly, witches were also known as 'herberia', meaning 'one who gathers herbs' (Walker, 1983).

Contemporary herbal medicine

Since the publication of the British Medical Association's Report into complementary medicine (BMA 1993), herbal medicine is included as one of the five main therapies recognised as 'discrete clinical disciplines' most amenable to statutory regulation and thereby greater accessibility for the interested public. Seriously undermining this increased freedom of choice is EC legislation which has already removed a number of herbal medicines from the UK market and which also threatens the availability of vitamins, minerals and dietary products. At the heart of this conundrum is whether herbs and many other commodities presently classified as foods should be reclassified as medicines, with the associated requirement to show acceptable, 'scientific' proof of efficacy and safety.

Included on the list of herbs banned as medicines in one or other European Community country are those which have been used for centuries throughout Europe to great benefit and with no recorded ill-effects. In many cases, there is no demonstrable evidence that they pose serious health risks, but merely that they contain minute amounts of a toxic substance. This is also true, however, of many of the plants which constitute our daily diet including potatoes, bananas, almonds, lettuce, beans, peas and parsnips, not to mention beer, tobacco, coffee and tea.

Herbalists are seriously challenging the list prepared by the Committee for Proprietary Medicinal Products (CPMP; the European Union equivalent to the Department of Health). When paracetamol, a drug well known to be liver toxic, is freely available to the public, why should herbal medicines such as coltsfoot, angelica, comfrey, borage, parsley seed and pulsatilla be banned for use by the qualified medical herbalist? There are parallels between midwives and herbalists in this situation, in what may be seen as an erosion into the sphere of clinical practice being dictated by an outside agency. Midwifery is only just beginning to show signs of recovery from this, as once limitations have been enforced, practitioners seem to incorporate rather than continue to challenge these changes.

In 1976 the World Health Organization calculated that traditional medicine was the main health source for approximately 75% of the world's population, and across cultures in most areas of the world, herbs are used as antiseptics, coagulants, analgesics, diuretics and emetics. They aid digestion, lower fevers and are used to ease the transitional moments of dying and of being born. Through frequently updated directives the World Health Organization continues to recommend the use of local health measures rather than encourage a dependence on expensive and often inappropriate biomedicine. With many of our clients using herbs as an integral part of their health care, it behoves us as professionals to respect intelligently this different knowledge. As with orthodox medicines, many herbs which have potent but beneficial effects also hold the capacity to exert unwanted or toxic effects if consumed at inappropriate dosages, if prepared incorrectly or if taken at vulnerable times, e.g. pregnancy.

Herbs as everyday foods or medicinal meals

The availability and restorative properties of everyday basic foods such as porridge (oats), barley, horseradish, mustard, garlic, onions, alfalfa sprouts, celery, seaweeds, asparagus, chicory, endive, potatoes, carrots, artichokes, walnuts, almonds, pumpkin and sesame seeds (tahini), watercress, honey, fresh leaves of dandelions, parsley, coriander, dill, chickweed or young nettle tops all offer even the most reluctant an opportunity to begin to think herbally. It may be a useful and normalising process to begin the exploration of using herbs by regarding them essentially as food items at one end of the same continuum which also holds the potential for their transformation into medicines. This approach embraces a period in history which preceded the Cartesian dualism so fundamental to Western biomedicine. It was a time when many classifications were more holistic; where food was medicine and this common knowledge was a legacy enjoyed by people untroubled by the specialisms so divisive in orthodox medicine today. Herbs can be seen as the 'original food' containing all the essential vitamins, minerals and trace elements required by the body. This has great relevance as an ever-increasing range of our food is denatured more and more through the widespread use of fertilisers, pesticides and irradiation. Although herbs suffer in a similar way from environmental degradation, there are sources available for the purchase of organically grown herbs and the amounts required for regular consumption are relatively small. As many herbs are amenable to grow in tubs or windowsill containers, it requires comparatively little effort for even city dwellers to enjoy a year-round supply of many culinary staples such as sage, thyme, chives or mint, all of which also incorporate useful medicinal properties.

How do herbs work? Like other areas of complementary medicine, herbal medicine is health rather than disease orientated, with the aim of enhancing constitutional strengths rather than concentrating on the disruptive effects of illness. As individual needs are distinctive and reflective of a unique physiology, the highly personal experience of suffering is paramount in formulating a prescription which focuses on this person rather than on their complaint. Plants used for both nutritional and medicinal purposes are more in harmony with the natural, physiological rhythms of the body than the orientation of pills, vaccines or other synthetic substances promising instant relief of symptoms. In this way, consideration is given to the overall process rather than the discrete, mechanical functioning of isolated (bodily) parts.

This philosophical concept of holism is further mirrored in the way herbalists use the whole plant for its total medicinal value, rather than the fragmented approach of biomedicine which concentrates on isolating only the active constituent for administration. The lower concentration and more dilute solutions of the complex mixtures of chemicals present in the whole plant also greatly reduces the risk of side-effects. Using all parts of the plant in this way tends to ameliorate the effects of the more potent constituents, thus facilitating better tolerance. Another feature of herbal medicine which helps to keep effective doses low and hence reduces the likelihood of side-effects is illustrated by the concept of synergism. This can be seen where the different ingredients of a single herb or prescription might otherwise interact, thereby increasing the effective response beyond what would be expected from the sum total of the individual constituents. For example, tiny amounts of cayenne (*Capsicum minimum*) will enhance the effectiveness of any other herb included in the prescription by increasing their rate of distribution through the blood vessels. Similarly, the flavanoids found in hawthorn (*Crataegus* spp.) can be isolated, extracted and will still have beneficial effects on the heart, but use of the whole plant in its natural form allows smaller doses, which are even more effective, to be given (National Institute of Medical Herbalists, 1991).

A knowledge of pharmacology, or the effect of drugs on the body, is integral to the study of herbal medicine. Within biomedicine, this fascinating exploration has been narrowed down to an artificial examination of the effects of isolated chemical constituents on isolated cells, structures or functions of the body. An attempt is then made to reassemble these fragmented observations and extrapolate from this the likely effects upon 'real' people with demonstrable illnesses. This approach favoured the development of synthetic drugs from the templates provided by plants and resulted in the extraction of ergotamine from ergot of rye, morphine and codeine from opium poppies, atropine from deadly nightshade, pilocarpine from jaborandi, reserpine from rauwolfia, digoxin from foxgloves, aspirin from willow bark, quinine from cinchona bark, anti-ulcer drugs from liquorice, anti-cancer drugs from periwinkle and yew, and so on.

Offering a sharp contrast to the explicitly material and physical application of orthodox pharmacology, a traditional pharmacology 'must start with the human experience of an agent, a well charted catalogue of effects on mind and body as well as spirit' (Mills, 1993). This view never loses sight of the 'whole' nor of the axiom that not only is this whole greater than the sum of its parts, but actually plays a decisive role in determining them. Carol MacCormack refers to this 'one' as all things; as incomplete without the least of them and yet with all the parts retaining their full identity. She goes on to urge that 'once this concept, so congruent with Bohm's theory of wholeness and the implicate order is grasped, it frees us from Cartesian dualism' (MacCormack, 1991; see also Bohm, 1980).

The medicinal property ascribed to a particular herb, then, is not that of a single, active constituent, but rather an entire orchestra of ingredients working synergistically and thereby reinforcing the overall positive effect of the herb. The incredible complexity of this vast array of chemical components, all possibly interacting with one another in a (mostly) unknown and infinitely variable manner, has posed something of a dilemma for the needs of orthodox medicine regarding standardisation, predictability of action and the need for replication. Yet, as clinical pharmacology knows full well, this state of affairs is illusory, as is demonstrated by the administration of digoxin or insulin with its variable results on different patients, with the acknowledgement that tailoring the dose to the individual's real life situation will inevitably be necessary. The herbalist, in common with most alternative practitioners, begins from accepting the premise that although life is infinitely variable, it does follow a distinct pattern. It is also acknowledged that although fluctuations exist, they are within workable limits.

Herbal pharmacy —including the buying, storing and the making of infusions

Herbs should look fresh and smell lively, so wherever possible, gather them fresh or buy them dried from a reputable supplier with a good turnover of stock. Label and store in a dark glass jar or brown paper bag out of direct sunlight. Use the aerial parts (leaves, stems and flowers) within 6–12 months and the hard, woody parts, (seeds, berries, barks and roots) within 2–5 years. Freshly picked herbs such as lemon balm and basil will freeze well.

Herbs are amenable to administration in a wide variety of ways such as poultices, baths, douches, inhalants, gargles, ear/eye drops, capsules, pills, vinegars, syrups or even wines. Nowadays, the most common techniques include infusions (teas), decoctions, tinctures and infused oils.

Infusion (tea) The standard measure uses 1 oz (30 grams) of dried plant material to 1 pint (500 ml) of water. For freshly picked herbs, use 2 oz to the same quantity of water. This method is appropriate for the softer parts of the herb—flowers, soft stems, leaves and small seeds whose active constituents are readily soluble in water. Pour the boiling water over the herb, cover and leave to steep for 10 or 15 minutes. Strain, press out the herb to obtain maximum fluid and drink with enjoyment, preferably without sweetening.

Some herbs (notably the 'mint' family) have different actions when consumed hot or cold; sage tea prevents sweats if consumed cold but if drunk hot, it acts as a diaphoretic (encouraging sweating).

Decoction This method is used for hard, woody parts of plants where the active constituents are only released at the higher temperatures achieved by boiling.

Use the same measurements as for an infusion but bring cold water to the boil and simmer for 15–20 minutes before straining and drinking.

All water-based preparations of herbs should be drunk within 24 hours. If making more than is required for immediate use, keep warm in a thermos flask or refrigerate and reheat.

Tincture This is the most common form in which herbal practitioners currently administer herbs. They are prepared from either dried or fresh plant material carefully weighed out and left to macerate in varying strengths of alcohol or glycerine for 2 or 3 weeks before pressing out.

Infused oil Not to be confused with essential oils, suitable plants such as marigold, St John's wort, comfrey or chickweed are covered with a cold pressed oil such as sunflower, almond, or olive and either left in strong sunlight for 3–4 weeks or heated over a bain marie for a couple of hours. They can then be directly applied to the skin or used as a base for creams, ointments, pessaries or suppositories.

The use of herbal preparations in pregnancy

The routine use of herbal medicine in pregnancy is generally not advocated unless treatment for an existing complaint has been instigated prior to conception, in which case the advice of the practitioner should be sought. Although most health problems are self-limiting, the appropriate use of herbal remedies during pregnancy ensures that acute episodes of illness do not become established as chronic and debilitating patterns of ill health. Whilst it is an established and commendable principle that pregnant women (and those still in the planning and breast-feeding stages) abstain from taking medicine of any variety, there are notable exceptions to this. In women whose constitutions may be weakened by previous childbirth, poor nutrition, unhappy relationships, unemployment, homelessness, chronic ill health or other stresses associated with the overcrowding and poverty of modern living, pregnancy may be perceived by the body as an intolerable stress. In such cases herbal support from a qualified practitioner may be warranted throughout pregnancy. Herbal remedies can also be used effectively for preconception care and extended well into the period of breastfeeding and early parenthood.

Preconception care

If a conception is planned for late spring/early summer, fortuitous use may be made of the greedy spring herbs, all of which draw up huge quantities of nutrients from the soil to fuel their dramatic growth rate. Examples might include chickweed, comfrey leaves, ground ivy, purslane, samphire, sorrel, nettles, cleavers, lambs' lettuce, wild asparagus, watercress and dandelion leaves. All of these plants, storehouses of essential vitamins and minerals, are powerful cleansing agents in the body, and the leaves when picked young can be used raw in salads or soups. Sorrel and samphire are traditional ingredients in the French 'soupe aux herbes' and the attention this culture gives to the liver in particular, and to eating in general, is well recognised! Spring tonics are not just nutritious foods; they are tonics in the true sense of the word in that they stimulate the liver, invigorate the digestion and thereby increase the body's vitality by promoting more effective assimilation and elimination. Like most tonics, they need to be used regularly for maximum benefit, i.e. three to five times weekly. A reminder might be in order here that this is not the time to 'diet' but rather to use to full advantage the impulse of change conferred by pregnancy to review (unhealthy) eating patterns.

Mandy, a 35-year-old woman, asked for help in conceiving following a 2-year period of infertility.

Her menarche occurred at 13 years of age with a 'regularly irregular' cycle established by her mid teens and which had remained unchanged. One pregnancy had been terminated 8 years previously and was currently a source of great emotional pain and grief. A referral by her GP to her local hospital for blood tests and an ultrasound scan had been inconclusive. She was now awaiting laparoscopy. Assessment of her partner's sperm for motility and volume showed that it was normal.

There had been many episodes of pelvic inflammatory disease during her early twenties following use of an IUD. Current complaints included both occupational stress and that directly related to the consequences of her infertility, skin rashes and osteoarthritis in both feet from years of classical ballet since her teens. There was no other relevant medical or family history. She was not taking any medication apart from vitamin B complex which had been found helpful for dysmenorrhoea. Anticipating pregnancy, I suggested she commence Folic Acid—400 mcg daily—and to continue until 12 weeks pregnancy (Department of Health Expert Advisory Group, 1992).

Dietary advice focused on her patterns of binge eating, particularly fatty and sugary foods, and her high caffeine intake of four cups of tea and six cups of coffee daily. Treatment over the following 3 months focused on balancing her cycle with the use of tinctures of chasteberry and other herbs such as capsicum, cleavers, liquorice, valerian, St John's wort and helionas root to improve circulation, nourish and soothe the organs of the reproductive system and activate the lymphatic system whilst gently repairing a rather frayed nervous system. A tea made from equal parts of lime blossom, catnip, borage and lemon balm was consumed concurrently.

She conceived at the beginning of the fourth month and was advised to stop the main mixture but to carry on with the tea and chasteberry tincture. Two episodes of spotting with fresh blood at 8 and 10 weeks were remedied with an increased dose of chasteberry, which was discontinued in week 15. A pregnancy tea comprising equal parts of lemon balm, nettles and raspberry leaves was enjoyed from about 30 weeks of pregnancy until 2 months postpartum.

A beautiful baby boy was born at home as planned; an ecstatic event in water following a 5-hour labour. The puerperium was uneventful with breastfeeding continuing for 7 months. She is now pregnant again and has achieved this spontaneously, 12 months after weaning.

Herbs to avoid in the first trimester, but where possible during the entire time from planning to the cessation of breastfeeding a baby

Although there is no definitive list of contraindicated herbs, the following herbs, some of which are known emmenagogues, should be avoided. The term emmenagogue refers to herbs likely to induce a period; thus these may also be referred to as abortifacients. Some herbs such as squaw vine, blue and black cohosh, are commonly referred to as 'partus preparators' and may be indicated in the last few weeks of pregnancy, in a stalled labour or in anticipation of postmaturity. Senna, cascara and other purging laxatives should also be avoided. Included are some herbs which may be prescribed by a qualified herbalist for specific problems and for a limited time.

Common name	Latin name
arbor vitae	*Thuja occidentalis*
barberry	*Berberis vulgaris*
beth root	*Trillium erectum*
black cohosh	*Cimicifuga racemosa*
blue cohosh	*Caulophyllum thalictroides*
cinchona	*Cinchona* spp.
cotton root bark	*Gossypium hebaceum*
golden seal	*Hydrastis canadensis*
greater celandine	*Chelidonium majus*
juniper	*Juniperus communis*
marjoram	*Origanum vulgare*
meadow saffron	*Crocus sativus*
motherwort	*Leonorus cardiaca*
mugwort	*Artemisia vulgaris*
pennyroyal	*Mentha pulegium*
poke root	*Phytolacca decandra*
rue	*Ruta graveolens*
sage	*Salvia officinalis*
squaw vine	*Mitchella repens*
tansy	*Tanacetum vulgare*
wormwood	*Artemisia absinthum*

The use of herbal remedies in pregnancy

Gestational sickness There is a connection between nausea in early pregnancy and low blood sugar. Maintain blood sugar levels by frequent snacking, two to three hourly, on high protein/unprocessed carbohydrate foods such as oatcakes with tahini, miso soup with wholemeal bread, peanut butter on rice cakes, etc. Regular exercise will encourage the body to eliminate toxins which may contribute to headaches and nausea. Increase the intake of dietary iron and vitamin B complex. Avoid foods which are spicy or greasy; even the smell may be nauseating. Tea and coffee should be avoided as the tannins in the former inhibit the absorption of iron and the stimulating effect of caffeine contained in both may provoke nausea and headaches.

Herbal remedies Drink a cup of anise, fennel, meadowsweet, spearmint or peppermint tea with a dry cracker on waking. Keep a thermos of hot water or the electric kettle and a choice of teas by the bed to avoid having to get out of bed on an empty stomach.

Before sleeping, enjoy an infusion of chamomile, hops or lemon balm with a small carbohydrate snack. Sip infusions made from grated fresh ginger root or Iceland moss when nausea is particularly bothersome or if compounded by travel sickness. If available, powdered ginger root may be taken in capsule form. A cup or so of raspberry leaf tea daily, besides being a pregnancy tonic recommended from the second trimester onwards, is also effective. All of these infusions may be frozen and sucked as ice cubes if preferred. Some also 'marry' well in combination, for example ginger and chamomile. Chew or suck slippery elm tablets, available from most health food shops.

It is not uncommon to find the beneficial effects of remedies quite short-lived for this particular problem. What often works is drinking the herbs in rotation over a cycle of a few days in order to avoid incurring the tolerance which temporarily renders the herb ineffective. In persistent cases, a visit to a qualified herbalist may be necessary for more specific herbs such as wild yam or gentian roots. Many of these more powerful herbs are restricted from over-the-counter use and are administered in the form of tinctures. Very small doses in the form of drops are often all that is required.

Threatened miscarriage The outcome for women with a history of repeated miscarriage will be greatly improved if treatment has been given for varying lengths of time before pregnancy is attempted. This will enable nutritional deficiencies to be corrected, lifestyle habits to be addressed and any specific problems to be diagnosed. Both partners may require treatment.

Once bright red blood loss occurs, especially if accompanied by cramping, it is generally acknowledged that the pregnancy cannot be conserved. It is recommended that a scan be performed on any woman reporting fresh blood loss at any stage of the pregnancy, particularly in the second and third trimester.

Folklore has it that if the miscarriage results from a fetal abnormality or misplacement of the placenta, herbal remedies will not impede this natural process.

Herbal remedies Crampbark, as the name suggests, is specific for the relief of muscular tension and is a useful remedy where there is no suggestion of an underlying hormonal dysfunction. As a preventative, it may be taken in the form of a cup of the decoction daily throughout pregnancy or as drops: 10–20 drops at 30–60 minute intervals until symptoms subside.

Black haw bark, closely related to crampbark, is specific as a sedative and relaxant to the uterine muscle and may be taken in the same way.

Helonias root is a powerful tonic particularly where women report a history of repeated miscarriage and the suggestion emerges of irritability of the uterus or poor tone in the cervix. A decoction of the root is prepared and a half teacup consumed twice daily, or five drops of the tincture twice to three times daily is recommended.

Chasteberry has a balancing action on the activity on the female sex hormones, making it a herb of choice where miscarriage threatens around the time when placental functioning begins. It is generally administered in the form of a tincture, 10–20 drops at 15–60 minute intervals until symptoms have subsided.

Raspberry leaf tea may be consumed throughout pregnancy in the form of one to two teacups daily when miscarriage has threatened or where a previous pattern exists. As a 'partus preparator', the astringent, tightening properties of this herb suggest its application be reserved for the last trimester in primiparous women or from the middle of the second trimester in multiparous women. As the toning action lends itself to the process of involution, infusions can be enjoyed for 1–2 months after childbirth.

Wherever possible, encourage women to rest in bed and spend a little time doing pelvic floor and appropriate visualisation or relaxation exercises. Support this process with soothing infusions of lime blossom, skullcap, orange blossom or lemon balm. In cases of severe anxiety, a herbalist might recommend the addition of valerian root.

If it seems apparent that a miscarriage has occurred and the woman would prefer to allow the process to complete itself naturally without recourse to an evacuation of the retained products of conception, in the absence of infection or haemorrhage the following herbal support may be advised:

- To control bleeding drink infusions of raspberry leaf, Lady's mantle, plantain or freshly picked shepherd's purse. Tincture of golden seal may also be administered at a dose of 10 drops four to six times daily.
- Recommend that the diet contain plenty of iron rich foods and a clove of raw garlic daily as a protective measure against infection. Crushing and mixing the latter with yoghurt, tahini or peanut butter before spreading on bread or a cracker will reduce any tendency toward digestive upset. The superlative antiseptic effects of garlic are nullified by heat; cooked garlic has negligible medicinal effects.

Varicose veins, haemorrhoids and constipation Varicosities may occur in the legs, vulva or at the anus as haemorrhoids. A tendency towards them is often inherited but much can be achieved through implementing lifestyle and dietary changes. Leg cramps or spasms may be an accompanying feature which may indicate a deficiency of calcium in the diet.

Yoga positions which hold gentle, inverted postures such as lying in the dorsal position with the feet and legs raised above the hips are recommended. Relax in this position for 10 or 15 minutes and repeat twice daily. Fully inverted poses such as the plough, shoulder and head stands should not be attempted without expert guidance.

Regular swimming or a daily brisk walk stimulates the circulation, aids digestion and encourages regular bowel function.

Constipation, if a feature, may be lessened or eliminated by ensuring that the diet comprises a wide variety of fresh fruits, vegetables, unrefined carbohydrates, grains, nuts and pulses with a minimum of 2 litres of water daily.

Ordinary tea and coffee should be avoided, as should bran. The latter absorbs fluid from the colon, hardens the stool, and aggravates constipation. Linseed, acting as a gentle aperient, may be used as an alternative to bran and sprinkled over food or mixed with water.

The inclusion of raw garlic and onions is strongly recommended as powerful circulation tonics with the former having marked antihypertensive properties (Foushee et al., 1982). The addition of both fresh parsley and nettles in the diet, whether directly in salads or soups or enjoyed as herbal infusions, will gradually improve the elasticity of the veins.

Herbal remedies Lotions, compresses or creams made from comfrey, marshmallow, marigold, plantain, yarrow or hawthorn berries can be used.

If staining of the skin is not worrisome, use a decoction of oak and witch-hazel barks combined with any of the above herbs as a local wash or sitz bath for particularly painful veins or haemorrhoids. Grated raw potato may be applied directly to haemorrhoids to ease swelling and pain. For longer term treatment and particularly following defecation, use pilewort cream combined with an equal quantity of comfrey cream. Add 10 drops of essential oil of Cypress to 30 grams of cream where rectal bleeding is an accompanying feature.

Decoctions of dandelion root have a gently laxative effect, thereby counteracting any tendency toward constipation. Regular infusions of lime blossom or fresh ginger root soothe and strengthen the tone of the venous system with overall improvement in the entire circulatory system.

Anaemia In the majority of cases where an uncomplicated iron deficiency anaemia presents, concerted dietary efforts may be all that is required:

- Ensure the diet is wholefood-based with an abundance of fresh, green leafy vegetables including seaweeds, watercress, dandelion leaves, nettle tops, lamb's lettuce, parsley, chicory, sprouted grains and seeds, spring onions and chives.
- Include plenty of dried, dark fruits such as hunza (or other unsulphured) apricots, figs, raisins, currants and of course, prunes. Soak overnight in plenty of water and eat as a breakfast compôte. Add blackcurrants, black-berries, loganberries, etc. as seasonally available.
- Incorporate wholegrains present in bread, chapattis and oatcakes; also nuts (almonds), fish (shellfish, pilchards, kippers, salmon), legumes (pea and bean families) and include vecon concentrate in soup stock.
- Use cane molasses as a sweetening agent in place of honey or sugar.
- Offal, particularly liver, although rich in stored iron may also contain residues of waste toxins. Locate an organic source if possible.

Iron absorption is seriously compromised by the ingestion of bran, which forms insoluble phytates in the digestive system, thereby inhibiting the uptake of available dietary iron. The drinking of tea and coffee worsens the situation especially if these are consumed with meals.

Vitamin C facilitates iron absorption and is found in most fresh fruits and vegetables but particularly in the following: kiwifruits, potatoes, fresh oranges, rosehips freshly gathered in the autumn, parsley leaves, broccoli, Brussels sprouts and cauliflower.

Floradix, a concentrated iron preparation from vegetable sources, is a useful alternative to ferrous sulphate. Unfortunately, its tendency to fermentation makes it unsuitable for women with a history of thrush (*Candida albicans*), for whom a better recommendation would be chelated iron, generally available from wholefood shops.

Herbal remedies Decoctions of yellow dock root combined with infusions of leaves from nettles, parsley, comfrey and peppermint are useful.

Heartburn Employ the usual measures such as eating small, regular, frequent meals which are well chewed and enjoyed in a calm, unhurried atmosphere. Avoid drinking whilst eating but do ensure an adequate fluid intake between meals. Eliminate any foods which aggravate (e.g. spicy, greasy or unfamiliar) and be mindful that common culprits include coffee, alcohol and cigarettes.

Herbal remedies Add carminative seeds of anise, caraway, dill or fennel to cooked food. These can also be chewed or enjoyed as decoctions after a meal. Infusions of Iceland moss, lemon balm, chamomile or meadowsweet may be consumed throughout the day. In severe cases, a teaspoon of powdered slippery elm bark mixed with water and honey, or flavoured with a little cinnamon or ginger, soothes the oesophageal and gastric mucosa whilst also neutralising gastric acid. Slippery elm is commonly available from wholefoods shops in the form of tablets or lozenges which should be slowly sucked or chewed before swallowing. Follow with a small glass of fluid.

Infections Where a history of any urogenital infection exists, employ the usual measures such as wearing loose, cotton underwear which is changed daily; avoid all refined sugars (and in the case of *Candida*, all yeast-containing products), tea, coffee and alcohol; drink at least 2 litres of water daily; gently wash the genital area after urinating, defecating or sexual intercourse.

As with any infections, these are more likely to occur when the body defences are not functioning to full capacity. Lowered resistance may be due to a number of things such as chronic tiredness, emotional shock, poor diet or chronic constipation, all of which need to be remedied if recurrence of infection is to be prevented.

Partners of sexually active women require concurrent treatment even in the absence of symptoms. The use of condoms is advisable for male partners until laboratory investigations return negative cultures.

If antibiotics are required, concurrently take a course of yeast-free acidophilus with bifidus capsules and vitamin C (1 gram daily for a week) in conjunction with liberal helpings of live yoghurt to rebalance the intestinal/vaginal flora and reduce the likelihood of initiating the common cycle of cystitis–antibiotic treatment–*Candida* infection.

Herbal sitz baths or washes can be used instead of soaps or body shampoo. Use clean hands for washing yourself, rather than damp flannels which simply encourage the spread of infection. Vaginal deodorants have no place in women's hygiene but especially where the genital area is troubled.

As acute infections of the urinary and genital tracts may be implicated in the onset of premature labour, the expertise of a qualified herbalist should be sought if symptoms persist.

Herbal remedies The ubiquitous garlic holds pride of place in treatment: ingest at least a clove daily in the manner previously described. Any partners of sexually active women should indulge in a similar fashion.

Cystitis Cook pearl barley with double the usual quantity of water; strain off and drink the remaining fluid as barley water to which may be added a little lemon juice. Where this has been a recurring problem, alternate infusions of nettle and marigold and drink one or two teacups daily throughout pregnancy. Consume a minimum of 1 pint of tea (infusion) brewed from equal quantities of thyme and marshmallow with either cornsilk, couchgrass or horsetail. A decoction of liquorice root may be added to the mixture for its soothing and aromatic qualities. Where fever or haematuria are present, use equal parts of yarrow, agrimony, plantain and uva ursi, two to three cups daily for no longer than 7 days. Where kidney pain is present or there is a past history of pyelonephritis, refer early to a qualified herbalist.

Jill was a 29-year-old mother of two, who came at 16 weeks' gestation for herbal treatment of recurrent urinary tract infections. In her first pregnancy this had led to hospitalisation for pyelonephritis. Her second pregnancy followed a similar pattern, although hospitalisation was avoided by the continuous use of antibiotics from 24 weeks through until her mid-stream urine returned clear at 8 days postpartum.

Her second son, a healthy term baby, was born at home as planned. After discussion with the midwives she and her partner decided against the administration of vitamin K. Unfortunately at 5 weeks, this baby became seriously ill and required a blood transfusion because of vitamin K deficiency. It was eventually postulated that this had been caused by the prolonged use of antibiotics affecting the intestinal mucosa and interfering with the production of intrinsic factor. She had not been warned that her baby was at any greater risk from not receiving vitamin K.

Jill's past medical history included bladder problems as a child manifesting in bed wetting and incontinence until 12 years of age. All investigations at the time were negative and symptoms ceased spontaneously until her first pregnancy. Family history also revealed that her father underwent a unilateral nephrectomy for kidney stones, and recent ultrasound indicated the presence of stones in his remaining kidney.

A recent mid-stream urine showed positive growth, for which antibiotics had been advised but which Jill had refused to take. The usual measures outlined later in the chapter for the management of cystitis were instigated, as was ingestion of a clove of garlic daily, which the whole family enjoyed rather than suffer the secondhand effects. Herbal treatment included using herbs such as golden rod, lemon balm, roses, plantain and thyme in the form of a tea with additional support from a tincture including horsetail, agrimony, uva ursi and marshmallow. The aim was to strengthen the mucous membrane of the urinary tract and gently stimulate the immune system whilst reducing the irritation in the genitourinary system with soothing demulcents. A base oil containing essential oils of hyssop, pine and lavender was prepared and massaged over the kidney area four or five times weekly from 30 weeks onwards.

Two acute episodes of cystitis were treated using tincture of purple cone flower with parsley piert. One further episode at 32 weeks, precipitated by Jill omitting her medicine for a whole week as she had felt so well, required a course of antibiotics. These were taken in conjunction with vitamin C and acidophilus with bifidus capsules.

Jill went on to deliver her third baby boy at home after a quick labour in her 43rd week of pregnancy and was subsequently transferred to the care of the health visitor for non-herbal care, with the advice to continue the tea for a further 6–8 weeks.

Herpes The use of nerve tonics such as oats, St John's wort, vervain, damiana and lavender are indicated and taken as an infusion, two or three teacups daily. Decoctions prepared from roots of dandelion and burdock will support this action by acting as internal cleansers and restoratives. Sitz baths of herbs such as lavender, thyme, marshmallow, marigold and witch-hazel will all provide local relief. Ointments from marigold or St John's wort, combined with either comfrey (where the skin is friable) or chick-weed (when itching is present), may be liberally applied. Infused oils of any of these herbs may be used instead of ointments. Essential oils of Ti tree, melissa or geranium may be added directly to the sitz bath, or 5–15 drops per 30 gram base cream or per 30 ml base oil. Diluted tincture of myrrh, if applied to the blisters, will sting but will encourage them to dry up quickly.

Candida Most commonly isolated from the vagina, mouth or nipples, but may be systemic or may first appear as a red, angry 'nappy rash' in a new born infant. Many of the recommendations for cystitis and herpes above are applicable and may be tried. In a breastfeeding mother, anticipate an infective 'loop' between her and baby. Both will need treatment.

Immune system restorative herbs such as purple cone flower, marigold, thyme or wild indigo are indicated in persistent cases. Use these in combination with mucous membrane restorative herbs such as golden rod, ground ivy or plantain. A clove of peeled, raw garlic wrapped in muslin, well oiled and placed in the vagina will act as an effective local antiseptic. Change once or twice daily, being careful not to nick the flesh of the clove when peeling as the juices will sting the inflamed mucous membrane.

Mood changes or fatigue Pregnancy is a time when the sensitivities of both mother and baby are very powerful. Herb baths using the flowers of roses, lavender, borage, daisies or chamomile all nurture this aspect.

Women and midwives often need encouragement to take their 'soul' needs seriously; to make space for music, art and contact with nature, all of which are too often considered an irrelevant indulgence in the mainstream of antenatal 'care'.

Given the influence that food has on emotions and moods, concentrate on high protein snacks and eliminate all refined carbohydrates, especially anything containing white sugar.

Herbal remedies Infusions of raspberry leaf in combination with equal quantities of either peppermint or spearmint will calm and lift the spirits. The addition of the bitter tonics such as burdock, blessed thistle or orange peel help to maintain emotional balance. Where sleep is of poor quality, an infusion of hops or skullcap before bedtime will facilitate a more restful night. In addition, a qualified herbalist might prescribe a little tincture of rosemary or motherwort for overwhelming symptoms.

Uses in labour **Exhaustion in labour** This is relatively uncommon when women have been encouraged to follow their natural rhythms in eating, drinking and taking short naps.

Herbal remedies Infusions of fresh ginger root either alone or added to raspberry leaf tea with a little honey will enhance stamina and mental focus. As ginger stimulates local circulation, do not use when birth is imminent or within an hour afterwards. An infusion of rosemary, either added to the bath water or sipped as a tea, acts as a stimulating tonic where fatigue and a sense of hopelessness threaten. It may be combined with vervain. Ginseng, either as a decoction, the root chewed whole or in tincture form, increases vitality and physical performance during long, arduous labours. A substantial body of research supports many of the traditional claims for this herb, including its effective use in supporting the body to better withstand stress (Fulder, 1987). Ginseng should not be taken in conjunction with caffeine or other stimulants or where there is a history of hypertension or headaches.

Perineal care Massaging the perineum from 37 weeks of pregnancy onwards invites women and their partners to give some attention to an often neglected, but very important, part of the body. As with so many aspects of pregnancy care, there is a dearth of research on this subject, although it seems plausible that regular applications of nourishing oils such as wheatgerm or avocado combined with sweet almond oil encourages suppleness, elasticity and a sense of familiarity and deepening trust.

Encouraging a hopeful, optimistic attitude is particularly important where a woman's previous experience of childbirth has left her feeling miserable and anxious after months or years of pain or infection and the inevitable build-up of scar tissue in the perineal area.

A perineal tear where the edges approximate well does not need suturing if the mother can rest in bed for a few days, eat well and use the perineal soaks suggested below. Low haemoglobin and zinc status compromise tissue healing. To raise haemoglobin levels, employ the dietary and other recommendations for anaemia. Dietary sources of zinc include ginger root, parsley, potatoes, garlic, turnips, carrots, beans, muscle meats (lamb chops and steak), split peas, corn, nuts, egg yolk, wholewheat, rye, oats, buckwheat and fresh oysters.

Herbal remedies Following birth, where the perineum is swollen, torn or bruised, use a warm decoction of oak and comfrey barks, to which is added an infusion of marigold and lavender flowers. Where damage to the deeper muscle layers is evident, or where there is a risk of infection developing, add a tablespoon of slippery elm and golden seal powders mixed in equal quantities. Strain off the liquid, add sufficient water to a large washing-up bowl or bidet, and soak the perineum for 20 or 30 minutes twice daily. Where sutures have been inserted, limit the soaks to once daily. Encourage pelvic floor exercises during the soaking time to draw a little of the healing fluid into the vagina.

Pain   When women are supported and encouraged to labour in a familiar environment where they feel safe and secure, pain is generally within the expectations of a normal labour. Within this context, it serves as an early warning signal that all is not well.

Herbal remedies   Motherwort is a useful herb for allaying anxiety and tension, particularly in early labour or for 'false' labour pains. As it is very bitter, it is best taken in tincture form: five to ten drops in a small glass of water, repeated once or twice hourly.

The sedative effect of skullcap makes it a useful herb throughout labour, acting by generally easing and dispersing the tension accompanying and accumulating with pain. It may be drunk as an infusion or sipped from a glass of water to which has been added one teaspoon of the tincture.

St John's wort is a useful remedy for relieving the crampy, spasmodic pains which are a specific feature of some labours. Use in the form of an infusion or add 20 to 30 drops to a glass of water. It combines well with skullcap.

Infusions of catnip leaves are an effective remedy for afterpains, helping to relieve cramping uterine spasm and facilitating the flow of lochia.

Herbal remedies for postpartum use

Engorgement and mastitis   Anticipate mastitis at the engorgement stage and act accordingly, as herbal treatment is sure but slow-acting.

Herbal remedies   In cases of uncomplicated engorgement, use the leaves of a green or white cabbage as a lining inside the bra. This will draw heat from the breast, cooking the cabbage as it does so. Change when limp. Cold poultices from grated raw potato or carrot have a similar effect.

Hot compresses of parsley or comfrey, prepared by tying a handful of the leaves into an old piece of cotton material and immersing in simmering water for 10 minutes, are also effective. Allow to cool until just tolerable before applying to the breast(s).

Immersing the breast(s) in an infusion of marshmallow root and fennel seeds (prepared and left to stand overnight before reheating and leaving to cool) makes a delightfully soothing, slippery soak for tender, inflamed breasts.

In stubborn cases, give 20–40 drops of purple cone flower tincture at hourly intervals until symptoms subside.

The ingestion of garlic in breastfeeding mothers significantly improves suckling time, with the obvious effect of improved drainage and reduction in engorgement. Research into the sensory qualities of human milk found that babies sucked more efficiently and for longer periods when the milk was flavoured with garlic (Mennella and Beauchamp, 1991). Garlic also has the antiseptic effect described earlier, an important consideration in avoiding the unnecessary use of antibiotics.

Sore nipples   If thrush is suspected, employ the measures suggested earlier.

Herbal remedies   As it is difficult to remove all traces of creams and ointments from the nipple/areola, treat conservatively where possible by washing the nipples well with infusions of marigold or comfrey and expose to the air or sunlight. The application of crushed ice made from either of the above herbs and applied just before feeding is an effective local painkiller and also draws out soft, small or partially inverted nipples. Ointments from comfrey or yarrow are particularly effective in healing cracked nipples and relieving pain. The clear gel of a fresh aloe vera leaf will soothe and heal sore nipples but care must be taken to wash it off properly before nursing as the bitter taste will prevent the baby latching on correctly. The underside of geranium leaves soothes and heals cracks if placed in direct contact with the nipple inside the bra.

Heavy bleeding   Once the initial emergency has been effectively dealt with, employ the measures suggested above for threatened miscarriage.

Herbal remedies   Two to three teacups daily of infusions of Lady's mantle or freshly gathered shepherd's purse, combined with raspberry leaf and nettles, is recommended for 3–4 days following birth where heavy blood loss has been sustained. Continue infusions of raspberry leaf and nettles for a further 4–6 weeks.

Lactation   Establishing lactation in a first-time mother requires enormous amounts of patience and time for midwives and mothers.

Herbal remedies   Supporting herbs for this process include infusions of comfrey, milk thistle, red clover, alfalfa, nettles, fenugreek and hops. Borage, blessed thistle, wood betony and oats (as porridge) all act as antidepressant herbs, lifting the spirits as well as ensuring an abundant milk supply. Fennel seeds make a delicious tea to be sipped throughout the day before chewing and swallowing the seeds. Besides improving milk flow, fennel has the added bonus of relieving infant colic.

Neonatal care   Although it is possible to use herbal preparations for babies, more appears to have been written regarding the potentially harmful effects of inappropriately used herbal remedies than on the application of herbal principles to neonatal care (Rosti et al., 1994; Yeung et al., 1993). Herbal tonics used in the East have been cited as possible causes of fetal alcohol syndrome (Pradeepkumar et al., 1996) and other neonatal problems (Utter, 1990). Mothers may wish to administer herbal remedies to their infants and some, such as camomile tea, widely available in health shops and supermarkets are unlikely to cause harm if used in moderation. The antispasmodic and anti-inflammatory chemicals in camomile tea make it a useful remedy for neonatal colic (orally) and non-infective moist eyes (as an irrigation fluid). However, in general it would be wise for midwives to be cautious in advising mothers about herbal remedies for neonatal use unless they are qualified herbalists.

Training

Training for membership of the National Institute of Medical Herbalists may currently be undertaken either as a full-time course attending 3 days per week over 4 years or as a part-time correspondence course to accommodate those with occupational or family commitments. A B.Sc. degree in Herbal Medicine in conjunction with the National Institute of Medical Herbalists is available at Middlesex University in North London. Besides the usual academic pre-entry requirements, students are required to pass examinations in key subjects throughout the course. Five hundred hours of clinical attendance must be certified before the final exams may be taken. The letters MINIH or FNIMH indicate an accredited member of the institute.

References

Bohm D 1980 *Wholeness and the Implicate Order*. Ark, USA

British Medical Association (1993) *Complementary Medicine, New Approaches to Good Practice*. Oxford University Press, Oxford

Brookes E 1993 *Women Healers Through History*, pp. 36–39. The Women's Press, London

Carper J 1992 *The Food Pharmacy*. Positive Paperbacks, USA

Davies S, Stewart A 1987 *Nutritional Medicine*. Pan Books, London

Ehrenreich B, English D 1973 *Witches, Midwives and Nurses, A History of Women Healers*, p. 13. The Feminist Press, USA

Ernest E 1987 Cardiovascular effects of garlic: a review. *Pharmatherapeutica* 5: 83–89

Department of Health Expert Advisory Group 1992 *Folic Acid and The Prevention of Neural Tube Defects*. Department of Health, London

Foushee D B et al. 1982 Garlic as a natural agent for the treatment of hypertension. *Cytobios* 34: 145–152

Fulder S 1987 *The Root of Being* Hutchinson, London

Lau B H et al. 1983 *Allium sativum* and atherosclerosis: a review. *Nutritional Research* 3: 119–128

MacCormack C P 1991 *Holistic Health and a Changing Western World View*. In: Pfleiderer B, Bibeau G *Anthropologies of Medicine*, vol. 7

Mennella J A, Beauchamp G K 1991 Maternal diet alters the sensory qualities of human milk and the nursling's behaviour. *Pediatrics* 88(4): 737–743

Mills S 1993 *The Essential Book Of Herbal Medicine*, p. 261. Arkana Penguin, London

National Institute of Medical Herbalists 1991 *What is medical herbalism?* Draft paper.

Pradeepkumar V K, Tan K W, Med M, Ivy N G 1996 Is 'Herbal Health Tonic' safe in pregnancy; fetal alcohol syndrome revisited. *Australia and New Zealand Journal of Obstetrics and Gynaecology* 36(4): 420–423

Rosti L, Nardini A, Bettinelli M E et al. 1994 Toxic effects of a herbal tea mixture in two newborns. *Acta Paediatrica* 83(6): 683

Utter A R 1990 Gentian violet treatment for thrush: can it cause breastfeeding problems? *Journal of Human Lactation* 6(4): 178–180

Walker B 1983 *The Encyclopedia of Myths and Secrets*, p. 1076. Harper and Row, USA

Yeung C Y, Leung C S, Chen Y Z 1993 An old traditional herbal remedy for neonatal jaundice with a newly identified risk. *Journal Paediatrics and Child Health* 29(4): 292–294

Further reading

Bairacli Levy J de 1982 The natural rearing of children. In: *The Illustrated Herbal Handbook*. Faber and Faber, London

Brooke E 1992 *A Woman's Book of Herbs*. The Women's Press, London

Grieve M 1980 *A Modern Herbal*. Penguin, London

Griggs B 1981 *Green Pharmacy, A History of Herbal Medicine*. Jill Norman and Hobhouse Ltd., London

Hoffman D 1991 *The New Holistic. Herbal*. Findhorn Press, Findhorn, Scotland

Mills S 1993 *The Essential Book Of Herbal Medicine*. Arkana Penguin, London

McIntyre A 1992 *The Herbal for Mother and Child*. Element Books, Shaftesbury, UK

Ody P 1993 *The Herb Society's Complete Medicinal Herbal*. Dorling Kindersley, London

Parvati J 1977 *Hygeia, A Woman's Herbal*. Freestone, USA

Weed S 1986 *Wise Woman. Herbal for the Childbearing Year*. Ash Tree Publishing

Botanical names of herbs referred to by common names

Common name	Latin name
aloe vera	*Aloe vera*
agrimony	*Agrimonia euphatoria*
anise	*Pimpinella anisum*
black haw bark	*Viburnum prunifolium*
blessed thistle	*Cnicus benedictus*
borage	*Borago officialis*
burdock	*Arctium lappa*

Common name	Latin name
capsicum	*Capsicum minimum*
caraway	*Carum carvi*
catnip	*Nepeta cataria*
chamomile, German	*Matricara recutita*
chasteberry	*Vitex agnus-castus*
chickweed	*Stellaria media*
cinnamon	*Cinnamomum zeylanicum*
cleavers	*Galium aparine*
comfrey	*Symphytium officinale*
cornsilk	*Zea mays*
couchgrass	*Agropyron repens*
crampbark	*Viburnum opulus*
damiana	*Turnera diffusa*
dandelion	*Taraxacum officinale*
dill	*Anethum graveolens*
fennel	*Foeniculum vulgare*
fenugreek	*Trigonella foenum-graecum*
garlic	*Allium sativum*
gentian	*Gentiana lutea*
ginger	*Zingiber officinale*
ginseng	*Panax ginseng*
golden rod	*Solidago virgaurea*
golden seal	*Hydrastis canadensis*
ground ivy	*Glechoma hederacea*
hawthorn	*Crataegus* spp.
helionas	*Chamaelirium luteum*
hops	*Humulus lupulus*
horsetail	*Equisetum arvense*
hyssop	*Hyssopus officinale*
Iceland moss	*Cetraria islandica*
Lady's mantle	*Alchemilla vulgaris*
lavender	*Lavandula officinalis*
lemon balm	*Melissa officinalis*
lime blossom	*Tilia europea*
linseed	*Linum usitatissimum*
liquorice	*Glycyrrhiza glabra*
marigold	*Calendula officialis*
marshmallow	*Althea officinalis*

Common name	Latin name
meadowsweet	*Filipendula ulmaria*
milk thistle	*Carduus marianus*
motherwort	*Leonorus cardiaca*
myrrh	*Commiphora molmol*
nettles	*Urtica dioica*
oak bark	*Quercus robur*
oats	*Avena sativa*
orange blossom	*Citrus aurantium*
parsley	*Petroselinum crispum*
parsley piert	*Aphanes arvensis*
peppermint	*Mentha piperata*
plantain	*Plantago lanceolata* or *major*
purple coneflower	*Echinacea angustifolia*
raspberry leaf	*Rubus idaeus*
red clover	*Trifolium pratense*
rosehips	*Rosa canina*
rosemary	*Rosmarinus officinalis*
roses	*Rosa* spp.
St John's wort	*Hypericum perforatum*
shepherd's purse	*Capsella bursa-pastoris*
skullcap	*Scutellaria laterifolia*
slippery elm	*Ulmus fulva*
spearmint	*Mentha* spp.
thyme	*Thymus officinalis*
uva ursi	*Arctostaphylos uva-ursi*
valerian	*Valeriana officinalis*
vervain	*Verbena officinalis*
wild indigo	*Baptisia tinctoria*
wild yam	*Dioscorea villosa*
witch hazel	*Hamamelis virginiana*
wood betony	*Stachys betonica*
yarrow	*Achillea millefolium*
yellow dock	*Rumex crispus*

Denise Tiran

Chapter 7

Massage and Aromatherapy

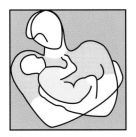

Aromatherapy is the very ancient art and, more recently, the science of using highly concentrated essential oils or essences distilled from plants in order to utilise their therapeutic properties. It is the combination of various chemical compounds which gives each oil its own particular properties and indeed different parts from the same plant may produce several different oils, e.g. the orange tree provides orange oil from the peel, neroli from the orange blossom, and petit grain from the leaves and twigs.

The term 'aromathérapie' was first used in the 1920s by René Maurice Gattefossé, a chemical perfumier. During his laboratory experiments he burnt his hand and plunged it into the nearest available liquid, which happened to be essential oil of lavender. He was astounded to find that his hand healed rapidly with no pain, blistering, infection or scarring, a fact which led him to research extensively into essential oils for medicinal purposes.

However, in Britain aromatherapy has developed not from the medical perspective but from the beauty therapy angle. This has resulted in both public and medical opinions that massage and aromatherapy are merely a luxury with which to pamper oneself and that essential oils are harmless, pleasant-smelling substances to assist in the process. This is not so, and in the last 10–15 years health professionals have begun to take an interest in their uses for treatment.

The history of aromatherapy

Essential oils or the chemical properties of plants have been used since ancient times and have even been found in fossilised pollen from archaeological exploration of primitive burial sites. The Chinese are thought to have used the medicinal properties of plants as early as 4500 BC, including opium, pomegranate and rhubarb; the mummification of the dead incorporating essential oils not only for their fragrances but also for their antibacterial properties is well documented (Worwood, 1990, p. 9; Lawless, 1992, p. 120; Arcier, 1992, p. 8). The Greeks are thought to have used many plants including myrrh for the treatment of wounds sustained in battle, and fennel seeds were chewed to suppress appetite during marches. Even Hippocrates acknowledged the benefits of plant substances.

However, the 'father of aromatherapy' was the Arab physician Avicenna, who documented the effects on the body of over 800 plants and is credited with discovering the method of extraction of essential oils. Sadly the European Dark Ages of the tenth century, during which many written records were destroyed, deprived future generations of much of the abundant contemporary knowledge of plant medicine. By the sixteenth century herbs and other plants were once again being used for their therapeutic characteristics and many herbalists compiled relevant texts—some of which, such as Culpepper's Herbal, are still in use today.

Unfortunately for herbalists, the growing science of chemistry in the seventeenth century elicited new substances for use in medicine and this seems to have coincided with the practice of burning witches at the stake, who were often merely women who had been found collecting plants to treat illnesses.

Although essential oils remained in limited use, synthetic production of drugs, with their attendant side-effects, has increased up to the present day. It is perhaps due to public challenge of these drugs that we are now seeing a return to natural plant remedies and that the medical and allied professions are beginning to examine the scientific basis of the essential oils.

As previously mentioned, Gattefossé was instrumental in reviving interest in essential oils in the early twentieth century, and other French physicians and scientists have continued his research. Doctor Jean Valnet used the oils during the First World War to treat burns and injuries, to good effect. He is still considered one of the world's leading authorities on the therapeutic uses of essential oils, and his book *The Practice of Aromatherapy* (Valnet, 1980) is considered one of the definitive texts on the subject.

How do essential oils work?

Essential oils are highly concentrated substances containing a variety of chemical compounds which give them their therapeutic properties. It is the scientific analysis and the acknowledgement that the compounds have various medical qualities which will convince sceptical doctors, midwives, nurses and others that there truly are clinical benefits to their use. Indeed, essential oils have been used in French medicine for many years and much of the research that has been performed was carried out in France.

All of the constituents in essential oils are organic, their molecular structures being based on carbon atoms bonded to one another and to hydrogen atoms. Some essential oils contain oxygen atoms, sometimes with nitrogen and/or sulphur atoms. Essential oils typically contain several hundred different constituents, although when one sees an analysis of an individual oil it is the major components which have been classified.

The chemical components, grouped into hydrocarbons and oxygenated compounds, have been known since 1818 when the first analysis was carried out. The hydrocarbons contain hydrogen and carbon atoms only, and the oxygenated compounds contain hydrogen, carbon and oxygen atoms in their molecules.

Hydrocarbons Hydrocarbons take the form of terpenes which are broken down into monoterpenes, diterpenes and sesquiterpenes, each of which can be further subdivided. Terpenes are found in all essential oils in varying amounts. Gattefossé stated that the highest proportion of terpenes is found in oils distilled from wood, then those extracted from leaves, with the smallest quantities in oils produced from flowers (Tisserand, 1993, p. 40), although Tisserand himself, a leading contemporary authority, disputes this (p. 141).

Monoterpenes are found in most essential oils and are antibacterial, antiviral and mildly analgesic. They may be a skin irritant so should not be administered neat. Sesquiterpenes are also anti-infective but in addition act to reduce inflammation, are antispasmodic and can lower blood pressure. Diterpenes are mildly anti-infective and expectorant.

Oxygenated compounds Oxygenated compounds are divided into esters, aldehydes, phenols, ketones, alcohols and oxides.

Esters Esters are acidic compounds which Gattefossé states can produce epileptiform fits (Tisserand, 1993, p. 45) and while Tisserand agrees in part, it is generally felt that ketones are more toxic than esters (p. 142) (see below). Massive doses have also been found to produce fatal cardiac failure (Tisserand, 1993, p. 45). Linalyl acetate (in lavender, clary sage and bergamot) and geranyl acetate (in marjoram) are antifungal and sedative while benzyl benzoate (in ylang ylang) is antispasmodic.

Aldehydes The antiseptic properties of aldehydes are considered to be much safer than those of phenols (Tisserand, 1993, p. 45). All essential oils have some degree of antiseptic property although certain oils are more readily used as such, e.g. lavender, eucalyptus and lemon, while others have antiseptic effects on specific systems of the body, such as bergamot, camomile, sandalwood, and lavender for the urinary tract, eucalyptus, tea tree, basil and myrrh for the respiratory tract, and marjoram, lemon, camomile and juniper for the gastrointestinal system. This is due in the main to the presence of the aldehyde citral, which can be found in the citrus oils such as lemon, lemongrass, verbena and some eucalyptus. Aldehydes are also sedative, particularly camomile, lavender, clary sage, sandalwood and ylang ylang.

Phenols Phenols are extremely effective antibacterial compounds and also act as stimulants. The degree to which they can cause skin irritation is disputed between Gattefossé and Tisserand (Tisserand, 1993, pp. 48 and 143), although Lawless (1992, p. 35) seems to agree with the latter. Thymol found in thyme oil can be an extreme irritant to mucous membrane, yet in small doses can be effective in treating infections of the upper respiratory tract. Thymol is, in addition, a particularly good disinfectant and vermifuge and although Gattefossé (Tisserand, 1993, p. 48) found another phenol, carvacrol, to be equally effective but less toxic than thymol, new research confirms the effectiveness of thymol.

Ketones Ketones are considered to be the most toxic of all substances found in essential oils, especially thujone which is present in sage, mugwort and tansy. Gattefossé's observations that fenchone in fennel oil can 'turn livers brown' (Tisserand, 1993, p. 47) was after 'repeated ingestion' of fennel solution and neither Tisserand (1993, p. 142) nor Lawless (1992, p. 35) considers fenchone to be toxic. Ketones can in fact be useful in respiratory infections, serving to ease congestion and aid the flow of mucus—hyssop and sage are particularly noted for these purposes. Other similarly useful ketones include camphor, menthone and pinocamphone, all of which are present in oils such as eucalyptus, although pinocamphone, also found in hyssop oil, may be neurotoxic and could lead to epileptic fits. The ketone pulegone, found in peppermint and in pennyroyal, the latter being known for its abortifacient properties, is useful for its calming effects on the digestive system.

For midwives therefore one of the most significant toxic effects of ketones is the abortifacient action they may have on the pregnant woman, especially oils such as sage, a powerful emmenagogue.

Alcohols Alcohols comprise the greatest quantity and strength of any of the chemical compounds found in essential oils, even more so than terpenes. They are antiseptic and antiviral and are also uplifting. Generally too they are not toxic. Types of alcohols include linalol (in lavender and rosewood), citronellol (in lemon, rose, geranium and eucalyptus), geraniol (in geranium), borneol, menthol and others.

Oxides Oxides such as cineol, a principal constituent of eucalyptus, tea tree, cajeput and rosemary, are those with a noticeably camphorous odour. Trials in France have concluded that eucalyptus is safe to use in pregnancy, contrary to previous thinking (Pages et al., 1990).

Toxicity of essential oils

Many essential oils can cause a variety of adverse effects ranging from skin irritations to death, for example from liver toxicity or cardiac failure. Some, such as sage, rosemary, fennel and hyssop, may initiate epilepsy in someone who has never had a fit before. Certain oils are hypertensive, especially rosemary, sage, hyssop and black pepper; others lower the blood pressure, including lavender, clary sage and ylang ylang. Clary sage can potentiate the effects of alcohol; some oils are stimulating, for example basil, peppermint, black pepper and rosemary. Still more increase photosensitivity and should be avoided if the skin is to be directly exposed to the sun, particularly bergamot. If the therapist wishes to achieve one of these effects, then judicious use of appropriate essential oils can be valuable aids to treatment, but it can be seen that misuse through lack of knowledge could produce disastrous consequences.

There are many oils which should not be used for babies and children. It is important to note that in no case, child or adult, should any one oil be used continuously for more than 3 weeks as skin sensitivity may occur. The safest route of administration for children and babies is via the skin in massages or in the bath water.

Pregnancy and childbirth

Midwives need to consider a variety of safety issues in relation to the use of essential oils in pregnancy and childbirth. Some oils are contraindicated in pregnancy because they are thought to be teratogenic, mutagenic or abortifacient. Some are classified as emmenagoguic, i.e. they may induce uterine bleeding, although Tisserand and Balacs (1995, p. 110) dispute the possibility that emmenagoguic oils are abortifacient. Similarly, where research on animals has elicited a degree of fetotoxicity or mutagenicity, most researchers conclude that the doses needed to demonstrate the same effects in humans would be so large as to be more likely to produce maternal toxicity and death before affecting the fetus. High doses of beta-myrcene, found in nutmeg oil, administered to pregnant rats, were found to cause fetal retardation, skeletal malformations and maternal toxicity (Delgado et al., 1993), and Nogueira et al (1995) found similar effects with citral, an aldehyde found in lemongrass oil (85%) and citrus oils. Pages et al (1996) found that sabinyl acetate, the main component of juniperus sabina oil, was responsible for failure of ovum implantation in mice.

The difficulty for midwives is that essential oils are assumed to be safe to use because there is no real evidence to the contrary. Indeed there are many generalised unproven claims made for aromatherapy generally. However, until more clinical research trials have been undertaken it would be prudent for midwives to work cautiously with essential oils, using the

Table 7.1. Safe use of essential oils in pregnancy

Nature/level of hazard	Essential oils
COMPLETELY CONTRAINDICATED in aromatherapy	Arnica Bitter almond Boldo leaf Broom Buchu Calamus Camphor Cassia Chervil Cinnamon bark Clove Costus Deertongue Dwarf pine Elecampane Exotic basil Fennel (bitter) Horseradish Jaborandi leaf Melilotus Mugwort (armoise) Mustard Origanum Pennyroyal Rue Sassafras Savin Summer Savory Tansy Thuja Tonka Vanilla Wintergreen Wormseed Wormwood
May be **DERMAL IRRITANTS**	Basil (French) Benzoin Bergamot Camomile Cedarwood Cinnamon leaf Citronella Geranium Ginger Jasmine Lavender Lemon Lemongrass Melissa Peppermint Orange (sweet) Tea tree Thyme
May be **PHOTOTOXIC**	Bergamot Ginger? Lemon Lime Mandarin Neroli Orange (bitter and sweet)
May be **EMMENAGOGUIC**	Angelica Aniseed Basil Calendula Camomile Caraway Cedarwood Celery seed Cinnamon leaf Citronella Clary sage Cumin Cypress Fennel Galbanum Hyssop Jasmine Juniper berry Lavender Marjoram Melissa Nutmeg Parsley Peppermint Rose Rosemary Sage Tarragon Thyme
May be **OESTROGEN STIMULATING**	Aniseed Fennel
May be **CARCINOGENIC**	Basil Cinnamon Nutmeg Tarragon
HYPERTENSORS (avoid in pre-eclampsia)	Hyssop Rosemary Sage Thyme
HYPOTENSORS (?avoid with epidural)	Clary sage Garlic Lavender Lemon Marjoram Melissa Ylang ylang
May **INDUCE EPILEPTIFORM FITS**	Fennel Hyssop Rosemary Sage
RUBEFACIENT (avoid if pyrexial)	Basil Black pepper Cajeput Camomile Eucalyptus Fennel Garlic Ginger Hyssop Juniper berry Lavender Melissa Myrrh Peppermint Rosemary Tea tree
DIURETIC (?avoid after PPH)	Benzoin Black pepper Camomile Carrot seed Cedarwood Cypress Eucalyptus Fennel Garlic Geranium Hyssop Juniper berry Lavender Lemon Parsley Patchouli Rose Rosemary Sage Sandalwood
Potential **DRUG INTERACTIONS** (probably ingestion of oils)	Nutmeg potentiates pethidine Geranium has anticoagulant effect—? avoid with anticoagulants, e.g. warfarin Cinnamon interacts with paracetamol and anticoagulants

lowest possible dose and on the least number of occasions. There is much confusion amongst even the most notable of aromatherapy authorities regarding the safety of different oils, and midwives must ensure that they are as up to date as possible with contemporary research.

Lavender, for example, is quoted in many texts as being one of the safest, most versatile oils and which is safe to use in pregnancy, yet if one considers its frequently-mentioned emmenagoguic property, with the uncertainty as to whether this equates to an abortifacient effect, midwives may be wise to err on the side of caution and to refrain from using it at least in earlier pregnancy.

Distinct from the specific knowledge of the chemical actions of essential oils and their potential effects on gestational physiology, pathology and pharmacology, are the health and safety issues pertinent to midwives. The very fact that essential oils are volatile and produce vapours which are inhaled by the client to enhance the therapeutic effect, also means that anyone else in the vicinity will inhale them. Perhaps we should question whether informed consent should be obtained by all other mothers in a four-bedded bay or Nightingale-style postnatal ward where one mother is receiving aromatherapy. Supervisors of midwives may wish to consider the effects on decision-making or driving capabilities of delivery suite or community midwives caring for labouring women using sedative essential oils. Central nervous system effects of cineol, jasmonate and jasminlactone in jasmine oil, one which is useful for reducing pain and enhancing uterine action in labour, have been demonstrated on electroencephalograms by Nakagawa et al. (1992). Effects on therapists of using the essential oils continually have not yet been fully evaluated, although dermal irritation with prolonged use of tea tree oil has been reported (Selvaag et al., 1994; Selvaag et al., 1995; Southwell et al., 1997; De Groot, 1996) and a physiotherapist was found to develop contact dermatitis from the lavender essential oil added to an anti-inflammatory, analgesic gel administered to patients (Rademaker, 1994). Camomile oil has also been shown to cause dermatitis (McGeorge and Steele, 1991; van Ketel, 1982). Volatility of the oils also means that naked flames should not be used to vaporise them in the maternity unit where the fire hazard is increased with the presence of oxygen cylinders.

Essential oils are as potent as pharmacological drugs and are as equally open to misuse or abuse, whether intentional or not. In the maternity unit, the oils should be kept in a locked cupboard, preferably cool and dark to prevent deterioration of the oils due to light and heat. Essential oils should not be stored near homeopathic remedies as the strong odours may antidote the remedies, even when the bottle tops are on. Mothers using them at home should be advised to keep them out of the reach of children. Reports of near fatal ingestion of essential oils by children are not uncommon (Beccara, 1995; Bakerink et al., 1996; Jacobs and Hornfeldt, 1994). Olowe and Ransome-Kuti (1980) reported an increased risk of jaundice in African babies deficient in glucose-6-phosphatedehydrogenase who had a mentholated powder applied to the umbilical cord prior to separation. Weiss (1973) reported that accidental ingestion of camphor oil by a pregnant woman at term resulted in grand mal seizures. She delivered a live healthy baby the following day (although he smelt of camphor!), and the mother recovered fully. The author suggested that delaying the onset of delivery should be advocated in these cases to allow time for maternal detoxification, and mentioned that a previous case had led to severe pregnancy complications and neonatal death. It is interesting to note a trial by Mennella et al. (1995) in which the amniotic fluid samples of women given oral garlic capsules 45 minutes before the procedure smelt significantly of the essential oil. The authors noted that antenatal exposure to different odours affected postnatal preferences for smells in animals but has not yet been determined in humans.

Midwives may be asked by mothers about the use of aromatherapy oils during pregnancy, and should advise them to purchase good quality essential oils from a reputable supplier, and generally to avoid the popular high street shops. Many essential oils are very expensive, due largely to the availability and extraction processes, but oils may be adulterated with similar smelling alternatives which do not have the same chemical constituents and are therefore not able to perform the same therapeutic role. Organically grown essential oils are best but naturally are the most expensive. Midwives are advised to purchase small quantities of a limited number of versatile oils with which they can become totally familiar. The oils should be in dark glass bottles, and many need to be kept in the refrigerator. Light, heat and exposure to other chemicals such as those in plastic bottles, or even water, will cause oxidation and deterioration.

Mothers who use fresh or dried herbs in cooking should be reassured that the amount of essential oil in each plant is very small and they are safe to add to recipes or to drink as herbal teas, although none should be taken to excess. Similarly the mugwort sticks used by acupuncturists to turn a breech to a cephalic presentation (see Chapter 5) will not harm the mother or fetus as it is not the concentrated essential oil which is being used.

It should be stressed that the benefits to be gained from using essential oils for pregnancy and childbirth are enormous if they are used with care. However, midwives wishing to enhance their care of women in this way must be as fully informed about the oils they are using as contemporary knowledge allows. It is not necessary for all midwives to be fully qualified aromatherapists but each individual is accountable for her or his own practice and must therefore be able to justify their actions.

Blending oils   Essential oils should principally be chosen to elicit the desired therapeutic effect in the client, although midwives are advised to use as few oils as possible in order to eliminate any which cause adverse effects on the mother. A maximum of five oils can be blended together and it is in the blending that the art of aromatherapy is seen. Using more than five oils may over-power the person's olfactory sense, and the versatility of many oils makes it unlikely that more than five oils will be needed to obtain the required effects. It is perfectly acceptable to use a single oil for a specific purpose but the combined effects of more than one oil will be greater than if each oil was used separately—this is called the synergistic effect. Additionally the end product needs to have an aroma which is pleasing to the recipient and therapists should always be guided by their client's choice; some aromatherapists believe that clients will automatically choose the oil which is not only the most pleasing but also the most appropriate therapeutically.

There are several different means by which therapists will choose oils to blend. Some aromatherapists use the perfumery system of 'notes' to achieve a balanced blend. The therapeutic oils are usually the middle notes; those which 'fix' the blend and have a long-lasting effect are the base notes; and the presenting aroma of the blend will be the top notes. Oils derived from roots and wood are the base notes, those which are from leaves, particularly the culinary herbs, are the middle notes and oils produced from flowers constitute the top notes. Others select oils according to the botanical family, or simply for the desired therapeutic effects.

Whichever method the therapist uses to decide on a blend, the rules in relation to therapeutic use of essential oils are exactly the same as for conventional medicines, i.e. the blend chosen must be the correct dose of the correct oils given to the correct person by the correct route and at the correct time.

As a general rule a 1–2% blend would be used for massage of an adult, or for inhalations, although in pregnancy this should be reduced to 1%. If using essential oils in the bath a mix of 4% could be used but it is always best to err on the side of caution in pregnancy and use a 3% blend as maximum.

To calculate the correct number of drops of essential oil to be added to the base or carrier oil, the following formula is used:

> To every 5 ml of base oil add the same number of drops as the percentage required
>
> i.e. for a 1% blend—5 ml of base oil + 1 drop of essential oil

If more than one essential oil is used the number of drops is the total amount:

i.e. for a 1% blend using lavender and camomile, one drop of each essential oil would be used but the amount of base oil would be doubled to 10 ml.

Base or carrier oils   The oil used as a base into which essential oils are blended will vary according to the purpose for which it is required, in addition to being merely a lubricant. For example a nourishing oil such as avocado may be used for very dry skin, while wheatgerm is rich in vitamin E and good for scar tissue, but as it is thick it usually needs diluting with another thinner oil. The most commonly used carrier oils in aromatherapy (and the most economical) are grapeseed and sweet almond, although sesame seed oil has the advantage of washing out of towels more easily than the others.

Methods of administration of the oils

Essential oils can be administered either through the skin, by inhalation or orally, although the latter should only be used by medically qualified aroma-therapists as in France.

Massage Massage is perhaps the most usual and certainly the most relaxing means of administration via the skin, and one which provides its own additional benefits, i.e. massage is de-stressing (Field et al., 1993, Fraser and Kerr, 1993), it relaxes muscles, aids circulation, excretion and digestion, reduces pain perception (Ferrell–Torry and Glick, 1993) possibly by the release of endorphins, and facilitates communication between giver and recipient.

Although there are many different forms of massage there is nothing especially difficult about intuitive massage—if it feels right to the recipient it is right! Simple stroking will often suffice in the absence of knowledge or confidence to attempt more specific techniques.

Due to lack of time midwives wishing to administer essential oils to mothers will probably not perform a full body massage, although this can be wonderfully relaxing in cases where the woman is stressed, anxious or depressed. It is far more likely that midwives would choose to massage a particular part of the body for a specific reason, for example, the feet in labour to warm them, an aching back in pregnancy or labour, oedematous ankles, or the scalp to relieve headache.

Midwives occasionally question the cost of the time involved in perform-ing massage on clients, for it is true that it costs more in the short term to massage them, for instance to aid sleep, rather than to give them night sedation, but it is more difficult to count the long-term cost. The very act of touching the women for whom we care has become 'functional' rather than nurturing, perhaps due to excessive workloads and staff shortages, but perhaps also because of the trend towards the promotion of self-help, almost in a 'do it yourself' way. Additionally for some health carers, not touching clients/patients facilitates a professional 'distance' which avoids the need to become too emotionally involved. Obviously these are generalised state-ments and there are many midwives who provide excellent nurturing for the mothers in their care, but often this is related to the personality of the individual midwife as to how close she becomes to them, either physically or emotionally.

Massage, with or without essential oils, is increasingly being used in midwifery and nursing, to enhance care and to regain a sense of nurturing. Baby massage is particularly popular and midwives and health visitors are keen to teach parents how to do this, to help calm their babies, and, indirectly, themselves. (Dellinger-Bavolek, 1996; Porter, 1996; Walker, 1996; Graef and Price-Douglas, 1997). Mothers can be taught to massage their babies following daily hygiene routines, as a means of strengthening their emotional relationship and their manual dexterity; massage can also be used to calm a fractious infant, for example when suffering from colic. Preterm infants have been shown to respond well to tactile stimulation, with improved 'bonding' between babies and parents, and positive behaviour, developmental and prognosis outcomes (Halbardier, 1995; Bond, 1996; Porter, 1996; Appleton, 1997; Harrison, 1997; Young, 1997). Adamson-Macedo et al. (1997) explored the effects of TAC-TIC (Touching and Caressing, Tender in Caring) therapy on oxygen saturations in neonates and found no danger in manual handling of ventilated preterm infants. Physiological effects on blood profiles have also been demonstrated (Harrison et al., 1990; Johanson et al., 1992; Kuhn et al., 1992; Acolet et al., 1993; Adamson-Macedo et al., 1993; Scafidi et al., 1993; de Roiste and Bushnell, 1995).

Performing a massage Before beginning any massage adequate preparation is necessary. Both the mother and the midwife should be comfortable in a warm, quiet room where they will not be disturbed. (Remember to disconnect the telephone if at home, or give ward keys to a colleague if in the maternity unit.) Towels should be used to cover the mother for dignity, and for warmth after the massage has finished; this is particularly important as it is thought that occlusion of the skin may facilitate absorption of the essential oils into the bloodstream. The midwife should remove rings and wrist watch to avoid scratching the mother and should warm her hands before commencing.

The oil is poured into the hands, never directly onto the recipient and, if used without therapeutic essential oils, acts merely as a lubricant to prevent friction of skin to skin rubbing. It is preferable to start with a little oil, about 5 ml, as it is easier to apply more than it is to remove excess. If this occurs, wiping the hands on a towel will leave sufficient oil on the mother to continue the massage. Occasionally women with very dry skin will require more oil to be applied.

Massage should be rhythmical but varied using different pressures, speeds, parts of the hands and techniques. As a general rule slow deep massage will calm and relax whilst brisker movements will stimulate and act as a 'pick me up'. The one exception to performing a deep, slow, soporific massage would be in a woman who is pathologically (clinically) depressed, for this could deepen her sense of introversion and introspection; this woman would benefit from a much more stimulating massage with refreshing oils.

Fig. 7.1. Pregnant mother receiving abdominal massage. (Courtesy of Nursing Times.)

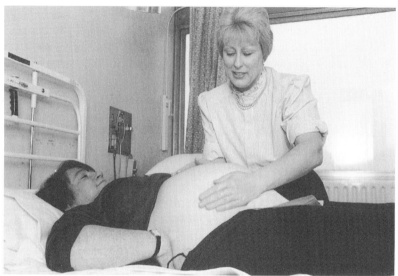

Figure 7.1 shows a pregnant woman receiving abdominal massage.

The movements There are several simple massage movements which can be used in any sequence to make the massage a pleasurable experience.

- Stroking—using the flat of the hands, fingertips or thumbs, enables the oil to be spread over the body surface and creates a flow between other more specific movements. It is important to be creative and imagine you are 'performing a ballet' on the skin, which will enhance the feeling of nurturing. Stroking has the physical effect of relaxing muscles and improving circulation and has a calming effect upon the emotions. The massage is more pleasurable if a variety of strokes are used, with a combination of straight, circular, small, large, deep, light, brisk and slow movements. Stroking should normally be in the direction of venous return, towards the heart, although on the legs, stroking down from the thigh to the feet will give the sensation of removing tension. On the face movements are performed upwards ('in a smile') taking the tension out of the top of the head (Fig. 7.2).
- Kneading—grasping the flesh between thumbs and fingers in a flowing motion alternating from one hand to the other is particularly effective on the shoulders, hips and thighs. Kneading can also be used on other fleshy parts of the body to relax muscles, aid circulation and excretion and to work more directly on certain areas. Where muscles are very tense, for example the shoulders, kneading may be uncomfortable, but by working briefly, moving elsewhere and then returning to the area the desired effect can be obtained (Fig. 7.3).
- Pressure—using fingertips and thumbs to work directly on specific

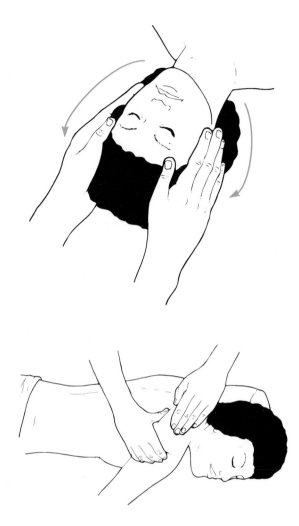

Fig. 7.2. To show direction of stroking movements on the face.

Fig. 7.3. To show kneading movements.

muscles, sometimes with small circular movements, can be very pleasurable, especially either side of the spine during a back massage (Fig. 7.4). The knuckles can also be used to produce a different sensation.

- Percussion—cupping, hacking and pummelling, as in Swedish massage, can be used on fleshy muscular areas for stimulation and to improve circulation, although it may be omitted during a very relaxing massage. This is one of the techniques used by physiotherapists when treating postoperative patients.

Massage in pregnancy Abdominal and sacral massage is to be avoided during the first trimester of pregnancy to avoid any risk of stimulating neural pathways or specific acupuncture points contraindicated in pregnancy.

Regular massage during pregnancy can be extremely beneficial, calming both mother and fetus.

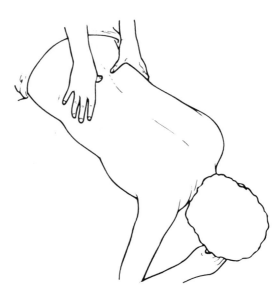

Fig. 7.4. To show pressure movements avoiding direct pressure over the spine.

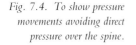

Melanie was a particularly anxious woman for whom weekly massage was performed from about 10 weeks' gestation, commencing initially with just upper back, shoulders, neck, face and head. Back, abdominal and leg massage was added in the second trimester. Melanie always slept exceptionally well following the session, which was usually in the evening at her own home, and the fetus seemed calmer without its usual burst of evening activity. She was so enthusiastic about her weekly 'fix' that on one occasion the massage was continued in total darkness throughout a power cut! In fact the lack of visual stimuli seemed to enhance the effects so much that she felt this was the best massage of any she received during her pregnancy.

This example serves to raise the issue of the environment. Obviously one would not normally perform a massage in total darkness although dimmed lighting can be calming; the masseuse however needs to observe the client for non-verbal signs that she is relaxing or alternatively perhaps uncomfortable or ill at ease.

Auditory stimuli are also questionable. A full body massage will take longer to perform than a foot massage and the degree of relaxation achieved will be greater. Therefore it may be preferable not to initiate conversation with a mother who may opt to be silent. Other women may choose to talk and indeed the sense of being cared for can trigger emotional responses which may otherwise have remained hidden. In a few cases it may be necessary to cease tactile contact and resort to a counselling session if appropriate. Many massage therapists believe that counselling skills are a vital prerequisite for good practice, and midwives using massage in their work must be confident and competent enough to deal with this scenario if it arises.

The use of music is also debatable as some therapists feel it may detract from focusing on the sensations of touch, while others believe that carefully selected music can enhance the relaxation; however only specific relaxation music, of which there is a good selection at most health shops, should be used. With repeated listening the music itself will have a Pavlovian effect and trigger relaxation.

Positioning the mother for massage requires the midwife to be flexible. For example back massage can be performed with the mother lying on her front in early pregnancy if she is comfortable, then on her side, changing to the other side as appropriate, or sitting leaning over a chair as the pregnancy progresses. There are also various aids which can be used to make her more comfortable, including a cushion designed to enable her to lie face downwards to receive back massage.

If the mother has varicose veins of the legs deep localised massage is contraindicated as this may not only be painful but also precipitate release of clots into the circulation. However, simple light stroking over the affected area can be incorporated. Foot massage is an excellent means of offering therapeutic touch to the woman and in reflexology terms she is receiving the equivalent of a full body massage (see Chapter 8). However, in the first trimester it is important to avoid vigorous movements around the heels as these are the reflex zones for the pelvis and this type of massage could potentially disrupt the pregnancy.

The midwife should also be comfortable, paying particular attention to her back through good posture, for there is no point in achieving relaxation for the mother if the midwife ends up needing a massage herself!

Use of essential oils in baths   The addition of a few drops of essential oil to the bath water can be relaxing and therapeutic. Midwives could advocate this method in the postnatal wards as it does not require the midwife's presence and is therefore more cost-effective. (Dispensing by appropriately trained personnel and the usual issues of professional accountability apply—see Chapter 1.) However, as with massage the dose used is important and the essential oils are normally diluted in base oil to disperse them. This is because oil floats on water, and skin contact with undiluted oils can cause dermatitis in women with sensitive skin.

The essential and base oil mix is added to a warm bath under running water and thoroughly blended. A 4% blend is sufficient in pregnancy and this can be increased to a 6% blend postnatally, i.e. 4 or 6 drops of essential oil respectively to 5 ml of base oil. For neonates only a 1% blend should be used, i.e. one drop of essential oil to 5 ml of base oil thoroughly dispersed in the bath water. Doors and windows should be closed to contain the vapours which are inhaled and add to the benefits obtained through skin absorption. If the bath is not enamalled the surface should be cleaned immediately after use to avoid permanent stains from some of the darker oils. For more localised treatment the mother could use a foot bath or a bidet.

Inhalation Inhalation of essential oils is particularly valuable for respiratory tract infections but may be the preferred method of administration for other conditions as the chemical constituents of the oils will be absorbed and act systemically. Facial saunas are also useful. A number of proprietary tools are available to facilitate vaporisation of the volatile essential oils which can then be inhaled, although electrical apparatus will need checking in accordance with health and safety regulations in a maternity unit, and obviously those with candles should not be used as they constitute a fire risk. These are ideal to give a room a pleasant but also therapeutic odour. Indeed, the concept of the 'fragrant hospital' is promoted in some states of America (Steele, 1992), although the ethical issue of administering the oil to everyone in the room should be resolved.

Compresses Compresses act more locally than an all-over massage or bathing and are useful for inflamed or infected areas of the body, for example the perineum following delivery. A cloth soaked in either hot or cold water to which has been added the required essential oil is wrung out to remove excess liquid and then applied direct to the affected area. Compresses containing an appropriate essential oil applied to the sacral and suprapubic area in labour can ease the intensity of pain during contractions.

Ingestion Oral administration of essential oils is recommended by medically qualified doctors in France and is very successful in the treatment of many conditions. However this is only suggested under strict control and it is to be totally avoided by anyone without the relevant knowledge. Inappropriate use may lead to damage to the gastrointestinal tract and other problems. The therapeutic properties of the oils can still be ingested by using the whole plant in cooking or as herbal teas. Certain United Kingdom insurance policies specific to aromatherapy would be invalidated if the therapist was found to have been prescribing essential oils for internal use.

Essential oils for use by midwives   Midwives need to become totally familiar with a few versatile essential oils. Micheline Arcier (1992, p. 86) recommends the use of mandarin (tangerine) as one of the gentlest oils for relaxation in pregnancy, except for anyone who is allergic to citrus fruit. Perhaps the most universal oil is lavender although this is classed as an emmenagogue and is therefore best avoided until the third trimester, and camomile is beneficial in small amounts. Neroli, sandalwood, tea tree, and geranium are also of value for specific conditions. In labour jasmine and clary sage can be added, and of course once the mother is puerperal, any of these and many other oils can be utilised. For babies mandarin and camomile can serve a multitude of purposes.

Let us then examine in detail the characteristics and properties of this small but flexible selection of essential oils.

Mandarin (tangerine)—*Citrus reticulata* (Rutacea family) Essential oil of mandarin is derived from the rind of the fruit and has a light, refreshing aroma reminiscent of the actual fruit. Most authorities are of the opinion that mandarin is safe to use in pregnancy (Arcier, 1992, p. 44; Lawless, 1992, p. 125; Sellar, 1992, p. 100), although the danger of phototoxicity has been questioned but not proved conclusively. Occasionally mandarin may be adulterated with the cheaper oils of orange or lemon. This is important particularly with the latter as lemon is even more phototoxic than mandarin is claimed to be, so it is important to ask specifically for the oil by its Latin name of *Citrus reticulata* or *nobilis*.

Mandarin, in common with other citrus oils, deteriorates quickly so it is best to buy it in small quantities, store it in the refrigerator and only blend the amount required. It blends particularly well with lavender and neroli, but can also be mixed with camomile, sandalwood, geranium and jasmine to produce a pleasant aroma. The oils chosen will of course depend on the desired therapeutic effects.

The chemical constituents include limonene (terpene), methyl methylanthranilate (ester), geraniol (alcohol), citral and citronellal (aldehydes) and other lesser compounds.

Mandarin is antispasmodic, antiseptic, sedative, tonic and digestive. It is useful for constipation, colic and for an uplifting, relaxing massage.

Lavender—*Lavandula augustifolia/officinalis* (Labiatae family) Lavender oil is obtained from the leaves or the flowers and that produced from Alpine lavender is considered to be the best. Inexpensive lavender oil may have been adulterated by lavandin (spike lavender) which has a different balance of chemical constituents and will therefore have different therapeutic properties.

Lavender has a high proportion of phenols which give it a very strong antiseptic and antibacterial action. It contains the alcohols borneol, geraniol, linalool and lavandulol, together with esters (geranyl acetate, lavandulyl acetate, linalyl acetate), terpenes (limonene, pinene, caryophyllene) and the ketone cineole.

Due to its emmenagoguic action lavender should be avoided during the first and probably the second trimester, but is safe to use in small doses towards the end of pregnancy. Many authorities do feel that lavender oil is safe to use throughout pregnancy but as there is no research evidence to demonstrate its safety and as it is classified as an emmenagogue, it is the belief of this author *as a midwife* that its use should be restricted in pregnancy.

Lavender is analgesic, antiseptic, antidepressant, antibacterial, antispasmodic, antiviral, carminative, decongestant, deodorant, diuretic, emmenagoguic, sedative and hypotensive. It should be used prudently for women who have an epidural in situ to avoid exacerbating the hypotensive effects of the bupivicaine. It aids wound healing and is an excellent treatment for burns and scalds, relieving pain and preventing blistering and infection. Lavender is one of the few oils which can be applied neat to the skin in this instance and should be poured liberally over burns. The analgesic property makes it useful for headaches, and in labour.

It can be seen that lavender has many different uses, but as with all other oils it should not be administered for more than 3 weeks without a break. Arcier (1992, p. 32) states that it may overstimulate the nervous system if used in excess; this author personally finds that it can cause irritation of the eyes if inhaled for a prolonged period of time; and dermal toxicity has been reported (Brandao, 1986).

In general healthcare lavender is effective in treating eczema and other skin rashes, is antipyretic and antispasmodic. Holmes (1992) identifies the cardiotonic, cell and biliary stimulant, immunostimulant and antiemetic properties amongst others.

Lavender blends well with most of the oils in the selection outlined but especially with mandarin, camomile, jasmine and geranium.

Neroli (orange blossom)—*Citrus bigaradia/aurantium* (Rutaceae family) Neroli oil is obtained by an intricate process of enfleurage (see Glossary) from the delicate petals of the bitter or Seville orange tree and is therefore one of the most expensive oils and something of a luxury. However the price is worth paying as a very few drops can be extremely effective in a variety of conditions.

The chemical compounds include phenylacetic acid, linalyl acetate, neryl acetate, methyl anthranilate (esters), nerolidol, linalool, geraniol, terpineol (alcohols), camphene and limonene (terpenes) and jasmone, a ketone, in small amounts.

Neroli is an excellent antidepressant and is effective in alleviating nervousness, tension and anxiety. It can be invaluable in times of hormonal upheaval such as premenstrual tension, postnatal depression and again at the menopause. In addition the sedative action of neroli has recently been demonstrated in research on mice (Jaeger et al., 1992) and its relaxing and calming effects were evaluated in research carried out in the intensive care unit at the Middlesex Hospital, London on patients who had had cardiac surgery (Stevenson, 1992).

As with all essential oils it is antiseptic and antibacterial and could be used in a room spray to ward off infections, such as colds in the winter months, whilst also making use of its deodorising effects. It is carminative and regulates the digestive system, being useful for constipation, flatulence, diarrhoea and sickness. Combined with mandarin as an abdominal massage it can be extremely effective for any of these conditions, but in particular for constipation. Neroli also has a toning effect and could be beneficial to aid circulation in the legs with massage or in a foot bath.

Camomile—*Matricaria chamomilla* (German)/*Anthemis nobilis* (Roman) —Compositae family

Camomile essential oil is another oil with many uses and is so gentle that it is sometimes referred to as 'the children's oil'. It is distilled from the flowers of the camomile plant and, depending on its geographic origin and the consequent amount of azulence (see below) within it, may be any colour from a pale to deep blue or yellow to green. The quality will also of course affect the price, with some camomiles being extremely costly.

The most important constituent is not present in the flower but is formed during the process of extracting the oil from the plant. This is a fatty aromatic substance called azulene which has strong anti-inflammatory properties and aids wound healing and other skin problems. German camomile contains a higher proportion of azulene than Roman or Moroccan but otherwise the properties of the different camomiles are very similar to one another.

Other constituents include coumarin, the esters of angelic and tiglic acids, pinene (terpene), farnesol and nerolidol (alcohols) and pinocarvone (ketone), plus others in smaller amounts.

Camomile can be used in any situation where there is inflammation and infection, for its anti-inflammatory and antibacterial characteristics come into their own. Menstrual or labour pain may be eased by the use of camomile in massages, baths or as a tea, and hormonal tensions and depressions can also be alleviated—premenstrually or postnatally. Use in pregnancy should however be delayed until the last trimester as it is thought to have some emmenagoguic properties, particularly Roman camomile (*Anthemis nobilis*) which has a higher proportion of ketones than German camomile (*Matricaria chamomilla*), although Tisserand and Balacs (1995) suggest that it is safe to use camomile oils throughout pregnancy.

The soothing and calming nature of camomile is helpful in promoting rest and sleep, and could be of use throughout the childbearing period and for children and babies. Its action on the digestive tract will ease colic and diarrhoea in children, and a 1% blend rubbed into a teething infant's cheeks reduces fretfulness at these times.

Camomile has an affinity with the urinary tract and can act as a urinary antiseptic. A compress over the kidneys may ease discomfort during an infection. It may also be useful to put camomile tea bags, which have been soaked in boiling water and cooled, over the eyes in cases of conjunctivitis, or on the neck over the Eustachian tube when there is an ear infection. Influenza responds well to an inhalation using camomile oil and this will also relieve blocked sinuses.

Tea/ti tree—*Melaleuca alternifolia* (Myrtaceae family) Tea tree oil is a wonderfully versatile oil derived from the leaves of an Australian bush, and which has been used by the Aborigines for centuries. Indeed its fame grew in the middle of the twentieth century but later declined due to its relative inaccessibility (it grows in snake-infested marshes in New South Wales) and due to new drugs being manufactured. However it is enjoying a resurgence of popularity and the many purported benefits of tea tree oil are now being scientifically investigated.

Tea tree oil contains a massive 60% of terpenes as well as various alcohols and sesquiterpenic alcohols. It is the large proportion of terpenes which make tea tree such a useful oil for it is antiseptic, antibacterial, antiviral, antifungal and immunostimulant, a fact which has led to investigation of its use in HIV and AIDS, and for various infections including *Candida albicans*, *Escherichia coli*, *Staphylococcus aureus* and others (Carson and Riley, 1994; Zarno, 1994; Belaiche, 1995; Raman et al., 1995).

Tea tree products are now widely available from health food stores, including the essential oil, creams and pessaries. It is effective in treating candidal and other vaginal infections, including those in which causative organisms cannot be found, as reported by Blackwell (1991).

Although it has a rather pungent medicinal smell this can be subdued by blending it with other oils such as lavender, which will enhance the therapeutic properties of each oil. Tea tree could be used as a room purifier where there is generalised infection, as an inhalation for respiratory infections, as a douche for infections of the reproductive tract (although this is not to be advised by midwives unless qualified aromatherapists), or applied neat to spots, verrucae or other localised inflammations and infections. Mixed into an appropriate cream in a regulated dose it could be applied to the buttocks of babies who develop infected nappy rash.

A massage with dilute tea tree oil over the kidneys and suprapubic area can also be effective in cases of cystitis. Doses should be kept low for dermal application as there are some reports of skin irritation (De Groot and Weyland, 1993; Southwell et al., 1997).

Sandalwood—*Santalum album* (Santalaceae family) This is a rich exotic-smelling oil which has popularly been known for its aphrodisiac properties. Due to its price, as a result of near-extinction of the trees, sandalwood is another oil subject to adulteration, so it is best to purchase from a reputable supplier, in small quantities.

Sandalwood's chemical constituents include the alcohol santalol, santalene, a sesquiterpene, and various aldehydes (Jirovetz et al., 1992). Therapeutically sandalwood is antiseptic, antispasmodic, aphrodisiac, astringent, carminative, diuretic, expectorant, sedative and tonic. It is beneficial in women with urinary tract or respiratory infections and is generally a relaxing oil. It blends well with lavender, rose, jasmine, geranium, neroli and ylang ylang.

Geranium—*Pelargonium odorantissimum* (Geraniaceae family) The essential oil of geranium is derived from the flowers and leaves of the plant and has a heavy but sweet smell, sometimes thought to be similar to rose, a fact of which unscrupulous suppliers take advantage by adulterating rose oil with geranium.

Geranium contains a high proportion of alcohols such as terpineol, geraniol, citronellol and linalool, plus the phenol eugenol, citral, an aldehyde, sabinene, a terpene and methone, a ketone. It is best avoided in large amounts during pregnancy, particularly around the abdominal and sacral areas, for it is known as a hormone regulator. It can however be used for specific massage such as ankle oedema and is useful for other hormonally related periods such as premenstrually, at the menopause and postnatally. Alternatively the application of geranium leaves to the legs should reduce oedema and applying the leaves to sore nipples may reduce pain and inflammation (Minchin, 1994).

Geranium is analgesic, antidepressant, antiseptic, astringent, diuretic, haemostatic, vasoconstrictive, insecticidal and tonic. It blends well with bergamot, clary sage, jasmine, lavender, neroli, orange, rose and sandalwood.

Rose—*Rosa centifolia/damascena* (Rosaceae family) Rose is one of the most luxurious oils for, like jasmine and neroli, the delicate nature of the petals makes extraction of the essential oil an expensive process. However it has a wonderful aroma which is particularly feminine and lends itself to use in midwifery and gynaecology. The cost can sometimes result in adulteration with cheaper oils so it is important to ask for the oil by its Latin name; *Rosa damascena*, produced mainly in Bulgaria, may be called rose otto or attar of roses, while the French *Rosa centifolia* produces a rose absolute which is by far the most expensive.

The principal constituents include geranic acid, alcohols of citronellol, geraniol, nerol and farnesol, the phenol, eugenol and the terpene, myrcene. These chemicals result in rose being an especially effective antidepressant, but also antiseptic, antispasmodic, diuretic, emmenagogue, haemostatic, laxative, sedative and tonic. Its use is contraindicated in pregnancy as it may initiate uterine bleeding but it can be used with caution in the last 2–3 weeks and is good to use in labour.

Massage with essential oil of rose in labour will not only calm and cheer the mother but enhances uterine contractions; this same property can be harnessed in the premenstrual phase for non-pregnant women, and again postnatally to aid involution and prevent postnatal 'blues'. It is thought to be of use for nausea and vomiting but as it is contraindicated in the first and second trimester it is not appropriate for gestational sickness although Tisserand and Balacs (1995, p. 111) suggest it is safe to use throughout pregnancy.

Rose is also recommended for sexual difficulties including frigidity and impotence and could be helpful in the early weeks of the puerperium to facilitate the resumption of sexual activity.

Rose blends well with mandarin, camomile, neroli, jasmine, lavender, sandalwood, clary sage and geranium; if mixed with tea tree oil it is effective for respiratory tract infections.

Jasmine—*Jasminum officinale* (Oleaceae family) This is another costly oil which has a truly exotic aroma but which can be quite oppressive for some women so care should be taken in the amount used.

There is a variety of alcohols in the oil such as geraniol, terpineol and nerol, as well as esters, linalyl acetate and methyl anthranilate, and the ketone jasmone. It is this latter with its adverse effect on the fetus which makes jasmine contraindicated in pregnancy, but it is perhaps the best essential oil to use in labour. Jasmine can enhance uterine action, accelerating or regulating contractions and easing pain and discomfort, and is useful in cases of retained placenta.

Jasmine is also antidepressant, and is therefore a valuable addition to a massage or the bath in the puerperium and is noted for its beneficial effects in severe depression. Jasmine appears to work as a regulator for lactation, and has been shown to be effective in suppressing milk production (Abraham et al., 1979; Shrivastav et al., 1988). Premenstrual tension and menstrual pain also respond well to jasmine, and it can be valuable in cases of infertility as is it said to increase spermatozoa production.

Jasmine blends well with mandarin, rose, sandalwood, neroli and geranium.

Clary sage—*Salvia sclarea* (Labiatae family) Clary sage is a member of the same family as sage (*Salvia officinalis*) but because it contains a far lower proportion of the ketone thujone it is much safer to use in women of reproductive years. Menstruating women have suffered menorrhagia after using sage oil, and although it can be useful in certain circumstances such as sports injuries, sage oil is best avoided by the novice.

Clary sage contains other ketones such as cineole, as well as the sesquiterpene caryophyllene and various esters and alcohols. It is anticonvulsive, antidepressant, antiseptic, antispasmodic, aphrodisiac, digestive, hypotensive, sedative and tonic. However, overdosing can result in headaches or loss of concentration so clients should be advised not to drive immediately after use. It is also known to potentiate the effects of alcohol—but is not a cheap means of becoming inebriated! Indeed it is thought that clary sage was sometimes added to cheap wines in the eighteenth century as it gave them a taste rather like muscatel.

Clary sage can be very relaxing for women who are stressed and anxious and can be safely used in labour to ease pain and create a sense of euphoria. Its emmenagoguic action precludes its use in pregnancy but it comes into its own in early labour and the postnatal period. Like rose and jasmine oils, clary sage also reduces abdominal and sacral pain during menstruation, labour and involution.

Digestive and kidney problems may respond to the use of clary sage, especially if blended with an oil such as mandarin for constipation.

Clary sage blends well with geranium, grapefruit, orange, mandarin, jasmine, lavender and sandalwood.

Many other essential oils can be used, with caution, throughout the child-bearing period, although some should be restricted in pregnancy. For a more comprehensive discussion of oils relevant to maternity care see *Aromatherapy in Midwifery Practice* (Tiran, 1996).

Utilising essential oils for pregnancy, labour, the puerperium and neonates

Anxiety Periods of anxiety or worry are a common occurrence in pregnancy and essential oils are invaluable in these situations. There are many oils which are safe to use either for massage, in the bath, in room vaporisers or as teas.

For women in the first trimester camomile tea is one of the safest means of providing the effective ingredients, without the potential problems of massage or concentrated oils directly on the skin. Room vaporisers are useful and it is possible to purchase traditional joss sticks of sandalwood, which is one of the most suitable oils. Later in pregnancy, massage (foot, back, face or the luxury of a full body massage) or oils added to the bath can be used, taking into account the correct blending as discussed previously.

Essential oils which can be beneficial in cases of anxiety include bergamot, camomile, lavender, neroli, mandarin, sandalwood and rose. In labour jasmine, clary sage and ylang ylang may also be used.

During her sixth pregnancy Mary was seen in the hospital antenatal clinic for her 32 week examination. The midwife spent a long time with Mary, who seemed particularly anxious. From discussion it transpired that, although all previous labours had been normal, as each had approached Mary had become increasingly agitated and convinced of her own impending mortality. In her mind she knew this was illogical but the feelings had worsened with successive pregnancies so that by now she was emotionally drained and her concerns were affecting the rest of the family.

Mary had no knowledge or experience of complementary therapies but was 'willing to try anything'. At that appointment she was given a simple foot and leg massage, ostensibly to reduce ankle oedema, and she found this very pleasurable and relaxing. No essential oils were available at that time but the effect of the massage was very positive and it was suggested to Mary that someone at home could perform a similar massage for her. Mary was also recommended to drink camomile tea, and to purchase a small bottle of Rescue Remedy to take when the feelings of panic were overwhelming.

About 7 weeks later the same midwife met Mary leaving the clinic after a subsequent appointment. Mary reported that she had followed the suggestions and used the Rescue Remedy in addition to the camomile tea and that this had been the best pregnancy of all. The following day she was to have labour induced due to mild cephalopelvic disproportion but with the help of her 'anti-anxiety remedies' she felt ready for labour and for the process of induction.

Backache The effects of progesterone and relaxin can cause chronic backache throughout pregnancy, labour and the puerperium, which is very wearing for the mother. A gentle massage over the sacral area (except in the first trimester) can ease the discomfort, and if essential oils of lavender and/or camomile are added to the base oil the effects will be even more dramatic. These oils can also be added to a deep warm bath. Some aromatherapy books advise the use of rosemary for relieving backache in pregnancy but this is better avoided because of its tendency to raise the blood pressure.

Backache in labour due to occipitoposterior position of the fetus can best be relieved by sacral massage with lavender, which will also facilitate effective uterine contractions and possibly anterior rotation of the fetal head. The massage can be performed by the midwife or by the birth companion and carried out between contractions. Firm circular movements with the heel of the hand around the sacral area can be very soothing, as can small circular movements with the thumbs up either side of the spine.

In addition a simple shiatsu technique is useful in relieving the intensity of backache during labour and can be performed by the midwife or the mother's partner (Fig. 7.5).

Breastfeeding Lactation can be stimulated by encouraging the mother to drink herbal teas such as fennel, dill or aniseed, or by using one of these plants in cooking, especially fennel. Sore and cracked nipples may be relieved by the use of calendula and there are several proprietary calendula creams available to recommend to mothers.

Relief of milk engorgement can be achieved by using cabbage leaves, and recently geranium leaves have been used with similar but not quite such dramatic effects. Rhubarb leaves can also be used, although the breasts should be wiped before feeding as rhubarb leaves are poisonous if ingested; it is probably advisable, therefore, not to recommend them to mothers for use at home. If the mother uses cabbage it should be very dark green as

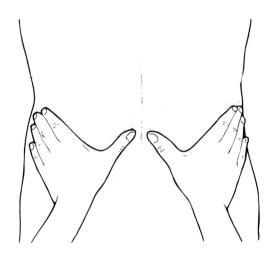

Fig. 7.5. To show shiatsu technique for relief of backache in labour (see also Fig. 9.15).

it is thought to be a substance in the chlorophyll which is the active ingredient. The leaves are wiped clean and cooled in the refrigerator, then applied to the breasts, left in place until wet, and then replaced with two more. This process is repeated until relief is obtained; in some cases the leaves become wet in seconds as the osmotic pressure takes effect.

Essential oil of peppermint can be used in a cold compress for the same reason but this must be wiped off before the baby goes to the breast to avoid ingestion, and for both practical and professional reasons cabbage leaves are the treatment of choice here.

Colic Neonatal colic can be as distressing for the parents as it is for the newborn baby. Simple abdominal massage with a base oil such as sweet almond is all that is required in most cases. If the 'wind' appears to be near the beginning of the intestines, anticlockwise abdominal massage will cause the air bubble to move and be expelled upwards, whereas air lower in the intestines should be encouraged to be expelled via the rectum by performing clockwise massage. If in doubt it is best to carry out clockwise massage, which will stimulate peristalsis in the direction of the rectum.

Community midwives could employ this simple remedy if they are called out by distraught parents in the middle of the night. Not only will the massage calm the baby but the manner in which it is performed, of necessity, will help to relax the parents. It may be even more beneficial if after a few minutes the mother or father is encouraged to carry out the massage themselves.

Figure 7.6 shows a gentle back massage for a baby.

Constipation By far the most effective treatment for constipation in pregnant or postnatal women or their babies is to use abdominal massage in conjunction with essential oils. The massage should be in a clockwise

Fig. 7.6. A baby being massaged. (Courtesy of Nursing Times.)

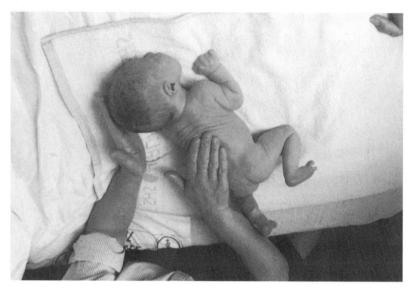

Fig. 7.7. To show abdominal massage for ante- and postnatal constipation and neonatal colic.

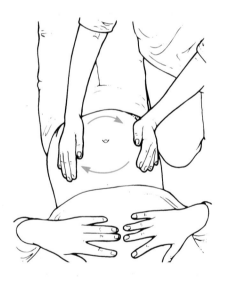

direction across the whole abdomen, following the direction of the large intestine (Fig. 7.7).

The oils most appropriate for constipation are mandarin, orange, bergamot, lime and grapefruit, especially if used in combination.

Ruth was a 30-year-old lady expecting her fifth baby. She had always had a tendency towards constipation, particularly in pregnancy which, on this occasion, was exacerbated by painful haemorrhoids which prolapsed following defecation.

Ruth was seen by the midwife at 30 weeks' gestation

when the problem was causing her great distress. The midwife, an aromatherapist, performed clockwise abdominal massage for about 10 minutes, using a 2% blend of mandarin and orange oils. Normal advice about dietary and fluid requirements was reiterated.

Ruth was given a small amount of the blended oil to take home with her to perform abdominal self-massage. In addition she was given essential oil of lemon and juniper in a 1% blend to use in the bidet or a small bowl for her haemorrhoids. She was visited at home 2 weeks later and reported that she had used the oils as suggested with great relief to both her constipation and her haemorrhoids. She asked her husband to perform the abdominal massage which he normally did just before she went to bed, and the calming effect of the massage had improved her quality of sleep as well.

Postnatally Ruth again had problems, particularly with the haemorrhoids, and she used a combination of cypress and juniper oils in the bidet for local relief and took homeopathic pulsatilla as the appropriate remedy, which eased the haemorrhoids quickly and effectively.

Cystitis   It is obvious that in some women the symptom of cystitis indicates a more serious urinary tract complication which requires medical consultation. However, for those women who experience mild cystitis essential oils may reduce the symptoms, and can be an additional means of treating infection in conjunction with antibiotics.

The essential oils which have a particular affinity for the urinary tract include camomile, sandalwood, bergamot and lavender, all of which could be used for suprapubic massage, in compresses or in the bath, and garlic which could be added to the diet.

Bhupinder had a long history of cystitis. Although she was delighted at being pregnant she was nevertheless worried about the effects it would have on the urinary tract. Bhupinder's mother was instrumental in encouraging her to use complementary therapies, for cultural traditions at home involved the use of essential oils and other plant products.

The first episode of cystitis occurred at 9 weeks' gestation when mild burning sensations were felt during micturition. Bhupinder was advised to drink copious amounts of camomile tea, which acts as a urinary antiseptic. She also increased the amount of garlic in her diet. This can be done by using greater numbers of cloves of garlic but without cutting or crushing them. If used whole in cooking the taste and odour will not be overpowering but the active ingredients will be present in larger quantities.

Sandalwood sticks were used regularly around the home so that Bhupinder would inhale the vapours. This combination of remedies seemed to be effective and the symptoms subsided.

However, the cystitis returned with a vengeance at 34 weeks of pregnancy. The previously used regime was implemented and in addition Bhupinder was advised to wash the vulval area following micturition with a strong solution of warm camomile tea to cleanse the area and reduce stinging. She also prepared compresses to apply suprapubically when the discomfort was at its worst—she soaked a cloth in a solution of warm water (half a litre) to which had been added the essential oils of bergamot and camomile in a 2% blend. She asked her mother to use the same blend as a massage around the sacral area and this combination served to reduce the symptoms considerably.

The general practitioner was amenable to Bhupinder's self-treatment but following laboratory analysis of a mid-stream specimen of urine antibiotics were also prescribed. It poses a difficult ethical dilemma to withhold conventional treatment in order to await the results of 'alternatives' but it would have been interesting to observe the effects of the essential oils alone rather than to pursue the 'just in case' philosophy which can be so much a part of both medicine and midwifery. In Bhupinder's case the use of the essential oils truly was complementary to the orthodox care and caused no problems either for mother or fetus.

Haemorrhoids The pain of severe haemorrhoids, especially when they prolapse, can be relieved as described earlier by sitting in a bowl of warm water to which has been added the essential oil of cypress and/or juniper in a 2% blend (i.e. to 5 ml of base oil add one drop each of cypress and juniper). These are both astringent and will reduce the throbbing sensation which often accompanies 'piles'. In addition lemon has a toning effect on the circulatory system and lavender can be beneficial as it will reduce pain and act as an antiseptic agent to cleanse the area. The mother could be given a bottle of the blended oils to use in the bidet after each bowel action. This would need to be prescribed on 'standing orders' in agreement with medical staff.

Headache The headaches of early pregnancy which are a result of the action of progesterone on the cerebral blood vessels do not normally herald a more serious problem, but those occurring in the third trimester may obviously require further investigation as they may be associated with pre-eclampsia. However, some symptomatic relief can be obtained by using lavender oil. This is one of the few exceptions to the rule of never using essential oils neat on the skin, for two drops on the forefingers of each hand rubbed gently into the temples can work wonders for a mild headache. Alternatively an ice cold compress made by soaking a cloth in iced water with a 2% blend of lavender may be welcomed by some women. Simple head massage, without oils, in a 'hair washing' action can also be effective.

In someone who is not pregnant the synergistic effect of using lavender and peppermint together is even better, but as mentioned previously, peppermint oil is contraindicated in pregnancy.

Hypertension Massage alone can be extremely beneficial for the hypertensive woman, and for those admitted antenatally a simple back or foot massage could be effective in lowering the blood pressure. Its cumulative nature means that its optimum effects are obtained when the massage is repeated regularly, and midwives could teach partners to perform massage, perhaps during visiting hours for inpatients or prior to bedtime in the home.

Lavender and camomile essential oils both have hypotensive and sedative properties and these could be alternated or combined for their synergistic effect (in which the combined effects are greater than the oils used singly).

Mandarin and neroli are also useful for their indirect hypotensive effects through their anxiety-relieving action on the mother.

McArdle describes her care of a woman with impending eclampsia who was not responding to intravenous therapy. Essential oils of rosewood and ylang ylang were massaged into the mother's back and legs for half an hour until the blood pressure decreased to within relatively normal limits. She poses the question, 'Was it due to the continuous infusion of drugs, was it due to the essential oils or was it due to the massage?' (McCardle, 1992)—a question which repeatedly presents problems for those attempting to carry out research.

Indigestion Many women suffer heartburn in later pregnancy to such an extent that it interferes with their appetite, sleep pattern and mood. Camomile and ginger are useful oils, and the mother could prepare a tea from grated ginger root or use one of the proprietary camomile teas. A gentle abdominal massage using camomile oil would be very relaxing, or a compress with camomile placed over the upper abdomen may help.

Insomnia Women nearing the end of pregnancy often experience difficulty in sleeping due to a variety of discomforts. The midwife can advise the ubiquitous camomile tea to be drunk just before retiring. Camomile or lavender oil added to a bath in a 3–4% blend could also be tried by the mother at home or in the antenatal ward. Massage could be even more relaxing, but for women in hospital it may be a less practical suggestion due to lack of time or other resources.

It may be possible in both ante- and postnatal wards to use electric vaporisers to dispense relaxing and calming oils into the air—ylang ylang is perhaps the most effective but as some people find its aroma rather cloying it could be blended with neroli or lavender. Staff would however need to obtain permission from all women in the ward/bay as everyone in the room would be receiving the vaporised oils.

Nausea and vomiting   One of the difficulties in using essential oils to treat nausea and vomiting in pregnancy is that the symptom occurs usually in the first trimester when the woman is seen less often by the midwife, and at a time when many essential oils are contraindicated.

The safest method of utilising the therapeutic properties of appropriate plants is to make a tea, and camomile is the optimum choice. It is a gentle oil which will also relieve the anxiety which can occur and assist in promoting sleep. Women can buy this for themselves and it is acceptable for midwives to recommend it as an adjunct to any other treatment for sickness. Ginger is also very effective in relieving nausea and vomiting, and drinking ginger tea will utilise the therapeutic properties of the plant without too high a proportion of essential oil. Alternatively the mother could chew on crystallised ginger pieces.

Sickness in labour, which sometimes occurs, could also be relieved by sipping camomile tea, either hot, perhaps with the addition of honey, or iced, or encouraging the mother to inhale from a tissue or a piece of gauze to which has been added 2 drops of peppermint oil. Midwives conducting parent education classes could suggest that the women bring in their own flask of camomile tea. If the partner drinks it as well it could serve to calm him down!

For neonates who posset frequently or for those who suffer vomiting caused by swallowing mucus during delivery, an abdominal massage with a 1% mix of camomile would be helpful. Encouraging the mother to perform this massage will have the additional benefit of relieving her anxiety at seeing her baby in distress.

Oedema   Geranium and rosemary work well in reducing ankle and leg oedema if combined with bimanual upwards massage of the legs (Fig. 7.8). Midwives can demonstrate this to mothers in the antenatal clinic or parent education classes and the women could then perform it on themselves or ask their partners to do it, even without the essential oils. However, care should be taken with the use of rosemary oil in pregnancy as it has hypertensive properties. Geranium, too, requires caution as, in a similar way to alcohol, it may exacerbate the mood of the mother, so that if she is depressed it can worsen the condition. Wrapping geranium leaves around

Fig. 7.8. To show leg massage for oedema.

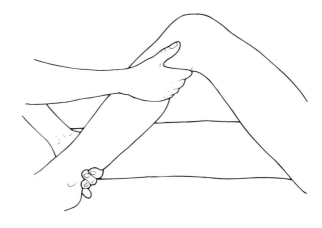

the mother's ankles and legs should have the desired effect without exposing her to excessive quantities of the essential oil.

Pain relief in labour Aromatherapy has a very real part to play in the care of labouring women and can truly be used as an adjunct to any other conventional means of pain relief. It is the time when midwives often feel at a loss to offer sufficient choice to the mothers, particularly as many of the traditional methods have associated side-effects or possible complications.

It is important to recognise that some women do not like to be touched during labour, but in fact if the midwife gently perserveres with a massage the mother often accepts it and then enjoys it. The most effective essential oils in labour include clary sage, lavender, mandarin and jasmine. For women who are coping with contractions but seem anxious, a foot massage with mandarin and rose can be very comforting—women in labour quite literally experience cold feet for their energy is focused elsewhere. Gentle but firm massage of the heel and sole in particular will also stimulate the appropriate reflex zones to enhance uterine action. However, care must be taken with the use of lavender oil if the mother is hypotensive, for example, as a result of epidural anaesthesia, as the hypotensive effects attributed to the oil may exacerbate the condition. Similarly, lavender's alleged contractile effect on the uterus must be borne in mind if the mother is to have labour induced or accelerated. Burns' and Blamey's work at the John Radcliffe Hospital, Oxford, involved the use of a combination of essential oils to ease discomfort and other symptoms in labour in over 500 women (Burns and Blamey, 1994). Reed and Norfolk (1993) also reported their use of aromatherapy in the delivery suite.

Margaret was a 33-year-old primigravida, booked for a home birth with two midwives and a consultant obstetrician, all of whom were personal friends. She had performed nipple massage daily from the 37th week of pregnancy, had been taking raspberry leaf tablets since 30 weeks and went into labour on exactly her due date. During the early hours Margaret used a combination of transcutaneous nerve stimulation alternated with periods in the bath, to which had been added essential oil of clary sage and lavender. It was unfortunate that after the second episode in the bath she returned to using the TENS machine only to find that the batteries were inactive. The delay in obtaining new batteries resulted in labour having progressed too far for the TENS to have any real effect so Margaret turned to the clary sage again. She made a compress from a clean sanitary pad and immersed it in a solution of warm water and clary sage (2% blend)— this was pressed against the suprapubic area with considerable relief.

The fetal position was found to be occipitoposterior and the first stage lasted 23 hours, including what appeared to be a 3-hour transition period between first and second stages. Margaret continued to use the clary sage for most of this time in conjunction with inhalational analgesia, relaxation and distraction techniques and accompanied throughout by one or both of her midwives.

Eventually the obstetrician joined the midwives and after a short period of spontaneous pushing everyone decided that a forceps delivery was needed. Twenty-four hours after the onset of labour (still at home), Margaret was delivered of a healthy baby boy weighing 4.6 kg (10 lb 4 oz)!

Perineal care Some mothers can be advised to perform daily perineal massage in the last 6 weeks of pregnancy to stretch and lubricate the area in preparation for the delivery. Using a few drops of base oil they should massage both outside and inside the perineal area, paying special attention to previous scars, and stretching the tissue by inserting their two thumbs inside the introitus and pressing downwards in the direction of the rectum. This should facilitate stretching of the perineum during delivery and can make the difference between needing an episiotomy or not (Labrecque et al., 1994; Mynaugh, 1991; Avery and Van Arsdale, 1987).

Following delivery, trauma to the perineum, either due to episiotomy or lacerations, can be encouraged to heal more quickly by using lavender oil in the bath or bidet. Research by Cornwell and Dale at Hinchinbrook Hospital in Huntingdon, Cambridgeshire, has shown that, while there was no statistically significant difference in wound healing, the use of lavender oil as a bath additive resulted in less perineal discomfort between the third and fifth days post-delivery (Dale and Cornwell, 1994).

Postmaturity In the absence of any fetal or maternal contraindications, aromatherapy could be used to initiate labour in a mother whose pregnancy is postmature—42 weeks' gestation or more. A daily gentle abdominal massage with a 3% blend of lavender, jasmine and clary sage (i.e. one drop of each in 5 ml of base oil) should stimulate uterine action. This same mix can be used in labour which has commenced spontaneously but in which the contractions are either irregular or ineffective. However, it is important to remember that induction is normally the province of medical staff and midwives must therefore consult with them prior to using essential oils likely to trigger contractions.

Postnatal 'blues' In the early days when many new mothers react tearfully to minor upsets, essential oils can again be of benefit. Room vaporisers with uplifting oils such as orange, mandarin and neroli or bergamot, geranium and rose will help to cheer everyone including the staff, if in hospital, or the rest of the family, if at home. The oils can also be added to the mother's bath in a 6% blend.

For a mother who becomes clinically depressed jasmine, sandalwood and ylang ylang are valuable in the bath or as a massage although the latter should be lighter and brisker than the normal deep, slow, relaxing massage, to avoid the mother becoming even more introspective. On the other hand the woman who has developed puerperal psychosis could benefit from a short but relaxing massage with rose essential oil, together with intermittent oral administration of the Bach Rescue Remedy, in conjunction with medically prescribed treatment.

Retained placenta Delay in separation and delivery of the placenta need not become a medical emergency which may result in a manual removal under anaesthetic. There is an expectation amongst many midwives that the placenta should be delivered within 10–15 minutes of the birth of the baby and that any delay is abnormal. Midwives need to relearn patience in their work, particularly at this stage of labour. However, if after allowing for nature to take its course there still appears to be no separation and descent of the placenta and membranes natural methods to encourage it to do so can be employed.

Nipple stimulation, either by putting the baby to the breast or by manual stimulation will obviously increase the pituitary release of oxytocin. In addition a compress of lavender and jasmine against the suprapubic and fundal areas should initiate further uterine contractions.

This treatment was employed for Prudence, a para three with a history of previous retained placentae. Fifty minutes had elapsed since the baby's birth and the midwife applied a compress of lavender and jasmine to the abdominal area. She also performed reflexology (see Chapter 8) to stimulate contractions. Ten minutes later the placenta was seen at the introitus to the vagina and delivered complete with membranes. One could question whether the outcome was the result of the natural course of events, or due to the aromatherapy or the reflexology—but does it really matter? For the purposes of research it would be important to isolate the causative factors, but on its own merit this case illustrates the virtue of patience.

Striae gravidarum Daily abdominal massage throughout the second and third trimesters of pregnancy with a rich base oil such as jojoba, avocado or peach kernel with added wheatgerm can be enhanced by the addition of a gentle essential oil such as mandarin. Whether this actually prevents stretch marks appearing is questionable, as they might not have manifested in the first place, or if none appear this may be due to the rich base oil rather than the essential oil. However it is certainly pleasurable for an expectant mother to receive a daily massage (she can do this for herself) and many mothers report that their fetuses seem to respond with a perceived calmness in their movements.

Vaginal infections Leucorrhoea which indicates an infection such as thrush can be treated with a local wash of boiled water and 2% tea tree oil which is antibacterial, antiviral and antifungal. There are now proprietary preparations of tea tree creams and pessaries in regulated doses which midwives may prefer to recommend.

Blackwell, writing in the *Lancet* in 1991, describes the case of a woman who presented with anaerobic vaginosis but who declined the conventional treatment of metronidazole. She treated herself with tea tree pessaries which proved to be effective in resolving the problem, which did not recur.

Pruritus without confirmed infection can be eased by using a vulval wash of lavender or camomile, or adding this to the bath or bidet. Once again, those midwives unsure in their usage of essential oils could suggest a strong solution of camomile tea for the vulval wash, and mothers could of course prepare this for themselves.

Conclusion Aromatherapy provides a wonderful array of pleasant-smelling aids to the midwife's normal practice if used cautiously and responsibly. Of all the complementary therapies enjoying a resurgence of popularity, aromatherapy is perhaps the one in which midwives are most interested. The use of touch enables a return to the nurturing which has, to a certain extent, been lost in the last decade in an attempt to justify the increased use of technology.

Aromatherapy should in no way be considered an alternative to conventional treatment, but as a complement, as an additional tool for symptom relief, to resolve so many of the conditions which midwives already treat.

Midwives have much to offer women in their care and must be mindful not to abuse their privileged position. As with any other innovation it is the overenthusiastic midwife, trying to force through aromatherapy, perhaps with inadequate knowledge, poor quality oils or liberal doses who will meet resistance from colleagues. Judicious introduction of 'safe' essential oils, in consultation with medical staff, will enable midwives to demonstrate their effectiveness and gain their acceptance alongside other therapeutic substances. Perhaps in the not too distant future we shall see aromatherapy as an integral component of midwifery practice. It certainly merits consideration. In the meantime this chapter may have served to interest and enthuse readers sufficiently to learn more so that they can be the innovators we need. Good luck!

Training to be an aromatherapist

There is a great number of courses in aromatherapy, of variable quality. Midwives wishing to pursue an aromatherapy qualification should investigate carefully to find the training programme which suits them best.

Although there is no nationally prescribed standard for aromatherapy training, many centres are approved by one of the self-regulating bodies which belong to the Aromatherapy Organisations Council. Those which offer a recognised 'kitemark' such as the International Federation of Aromatherapists (IFA) or the International Society of Professional Aromatherapists (ISPA) are recommended, although midwives should still ascertain if a particular course is appropriate to their needs.

There is also a move towards improving the academic level of many of the courses to diploma and degree standard, such as those offered at the Universities of Greenwich, Middlesex and Westminster in London.

It should also be stressed that, while a 10-week evening class in aromatherapy will provide sufficient background for the safe treatment of family and friends, it is not adequate preparation for professional use. The dangers to clients, and to the midwife's professional registration, of 'dabbling' in aromatherapy cannot be emphasised enough.

References

Abraham M, Devi N S, Sheela R 1979 Inhibiting effect of jasmine flowers on lactation. *Indian Journal of Medical Research* 69: 88–92

Acolet D, Modi N, Giannakoulopoulos X et al. 1993 Changes in plasma cortisol and catecholamine concentrations in response to massage in preterm infants. *Archives of Diseases in Childhood (Fetal and Neonatal Edition)* 68(1): 29–31

Adamson-Macedo E N, de Roiste A, Wilson A et al. 1997 Systematic gentle/light stroking and maternal random touching of ventilated preterm: a preliminary study. *International Journal of Prenatal and Perinatal Psychology and Medicine* 9(1): 17–31

Adamson-Macedo E N, Dattani I, Wilson A et al. 1993 A small sample follow-up study of children who received tactile stimulation after preterm birth: intelligence and achievements. *Journal of Reproductive and Infant Psychology* 11(3): 165–168

Appleton S M 1997 Handle with care: an investigation of the handling received by preterm infants in intensive care. *Journal of Neonatal Nursing* 3(3): 23–27

Arcier M 1992 *Aromatherapy*. Hamlyn, London

Avery M D, van Arsdale L 1987 Perineal massage: effect on the incidence of episiotomy and laceration in a nulliparous population. *Journal of Nurse-Midwifery* 32(3): 181–184

Bakerink J A, Gospe S M, Dimand R J, Eldridge M W 1996 Multiple organ failure after ingestion of pennyroyal oil from herbal tea in two infants. *Pediatrics* 98(5): 944–947

Balacs T 1992a Safety in pregnancy. *International Journal of Aromatherapy* 4(1): 12–15

Balacs T 1992b Peppermint pharmacology. *International Journal of Aromatherapy*, Spring: 22–25

Beccara M A D 1995 Melaleuca oil poisoning in a 17-month old. *Veterinary and Human Toxicology* 37(6): 557–558

Belaiche P 1995 Treatment of vaginal infections of Candida Albicans with the essential oil of Melaleuca alternifolia (Cheel). *Phytotherapy* 15: 13–15

Blackwell A L 1991 Letters—anaerobic vaginosis. *Lancet* 337 (February): 2

Bond C 1996 Massage for babies with special needs. *Health Professional Digest* 12: 13–14

Brandao F M 1986 Occupational allergy to lavender oil. *Contact Dermatitis* 15(4): 249–250

Burns E, Blamey C 1994 Using aromatherapy in childbirth. *Nursing Times* 90(9): 54–60

Carson C F, Riley T V 1994 The antimicrobial effect of tea tree oil. *Medical Journal of Australia* 160: 236

Dale A, Cornwell S 1994 The role of lavender oil in relieving perineal discomfort following childbirth: a blind randomised clinical trial. *Journal of Advanced Nursing* 19(1): 89–96

De Groot A C 1996 Airborne allergic contact dermatitis from tea tree oil. *Contact Dermatitis* 35(5): 304–305

De Groot A C, Weyland J W 1993 Contact allergy to tea tree oil. *Contact Dermatitis* 28(2): 309

Delgado I F, De Almeida Nogueira C M, Souza C A M et al. 1993 Peri- and postnatal developmental toxicity of beta-myrcene in the rat. *Food and Chemical Toxicology* 31(9): 623–628

Dellinger-Bavolek J 1996 Infant massage: communicating love through touch. *International Journal of Childbirth Education* 11(4): 34–37

de Roiste A, Bushnell I W R 1995 The immediate gastric effects of a tactile stimulation programme on premature infants. *Journal of Reproductive and Infant Psychology* 13(1): 57–62

Ferrell-Torry A T, Glick O J 1993 The use of therapeutic massage as a nursing intervention to modify anxiety and the perception of cancer pain. *Cancer Nursing* 16(2): 93–101

Field T M, Morrow C, Vaideon C et al. 1993 Massage reduces anxiety in child and adolescent psychiatric patients. *International Journal of Alternative and Complemental Medicine* 11(7): 22–27

Fraser J, Kerr J R 1993 Psychophysiological effects of back massage on elderly institutionalised patients. *Journal of Advanced Nursing* 18: 238–245

Graef P, Price-Douglas W 1997 An educational program for cuddlers. *MCN— American Journal of Maternal/Child Nursing* 22(1): 48–49

Hagan S 1992 Aromatherapy and its benefits to people who are HIV positive. *Aromatherapy World,* Summer: 20–21, 8

Halbardier B 1995 A change in perspective. *Neonatal Network* 14(3): 79

Harrison L 1997 Research utilisation: handling preterm infants in the NICU. *Neonatal Network* 16(3): 65–69

Harrison L L, Leeper J D, Yoon M 1990 Effect of early parent touch on preterm infants' heart rates and arterial oxygen saturation levels. *Journal of Advanced Nursing* 15(8): 877–885

Holmes P 1992 Lavender oil. *International Journal of Aromatherapy* 4(2): 20–22

Jacobs M R, Hornfeldt C S 1994 Melaleuca oil poisoning. *Clinical Toxicology* 32(4): 461–464

Jaeger W et al. 1992 Evidence of the sedative effect of neroli oil, citronellal and phenylethyl acetate on mice. *Journal of Essential Oil Research* 4: 387–394

Jirovetz L, Buchbauer G, Jager W et al. 1992 Analysis of fragrance compounds in blood samples of mice by gas chromatography, mass spectometry, GC/FTIR and GC/AES after inhalation of sandalwood oil. *Biomedical Chromatography* 6(3): 133–134

Johanson R B, Spencer S A, Rolfe P et al. 1992 Effects of post-delivery care on neonatal body temperature. *Acta Paediatrica* 81(11): 859–863

Kuhn C M, Schanberg S M, Field T et al. 1992 Tactile-kinesthetic stimulation effects on sympathetic and adrenocorticol function in preterm infants. *Journal of Pediatrics* 119(3): 434–440

Labrecque M, Marcoux S, Pinault J J et al. 1994 Prevention of perineal trauma by perineal massage during pregnancy: a pilot study. *Birth* 21(1): 20–25

Lawless J 1992 *Encyclopaedia of Essential Oils.* Element Books, Shaftesbury, UK

McArdle M 1992 Letter—Rosewood in pre-eclampsia. *International Journal of Aromatherapy* 4(1):33

McGeorge B C, Steele M C 1991 Allergic contact dermatitis of the nipple from Roman chamomile ointment. *Contact Dermatitis* 24(2): 139–140

Mennella J A, Johnson A, Beauchamp G K 1995 Garlic ingestion by pregnant women alters the odor of amniotic fluid. *Chemical Senses* 20(2): 207–209

Minchin M 1994 Geranium. When there were no more cabbage leaves. *Australian Lactation Consultants' Association (ALCA) News* 5(1): 8–10

Mynaugh P A 1991 A randomized study of two methods of teaching perineal massage: effects on practice rates, episiotomy rates and perineal lacerations. *Birth* 18(3): 153–9

Nakagawa M, Nagai H, Inui T 1992 Evaluation of drowsiness by EEGs—odors controlling drowsiness. *Fragrance Journal* 20(10): 68–72

Nogueira A C, Carvalho R R, Souza C A M et al. 1995 Study on the embryofeto-toxicity of citral in the rat. *Toxicology* 96(2): 105–113

Olowe S A, Ransome-Kuti P 1980 The risk of jaundice in glucose-6-phosphate dehydrogenase-deficient babies exposed to menthol. *Acta Paediatrica Scandinavica* 69(3): 341–345

Pages N et al. 1990 Essential oils and their teratogenic potential: essential oil of *Eucalyptus globulus*—a preliminary study. *Plantes Medicinales et Phytotherapie* 24(1): 21–26

Pages N, Fournier G, Baduel C et al. 1996 Sabinyl acetate, the main component of Juniperus sabina L'Herit essential oil, is responsible for anti-implantation effect. *Phytotherapy Research* 10(7): 438–440

Porter S J 1996 The use of massage for neonates requiring special care. *Complementary Therapies in Nursing and Midwifery* 2(4): 93–96

Rademaker M 1994 Allergic contact dermatitis from lavender fragrance in Difflam gel. *Contact Dermatitis* 31(1): 58–59

Raman A, Weir U, Bloomfield S F 1995 Antimicrobial effects of tea tree oil and its major components on *Staphylococcus aureus, Staph. epidermidis* and *Propionibacterium acnes*. *Letters in Applied Microbiology* 21: 242–245

Reed L, Norfolk L 1993 Aromatherapy in midwifery. *Aromatherapy World*, Summer, 12–15

Sapsford C 1993 Committee communication —research. *Aromatherapy World,* Summer: 6

Scafidi F A, Field T, Schanberg S M 1993 Factors that predict which preterm infants benefit most from massage therapy. *Developmental and Behavioral Pediatrics* 14(3): 176–180

Sellar W 1992 *The Directory of Essential Oils.* C. W. Daniel, Saffron Walden, UK

Selvaag E, Erikson B, Thune P 1994 Contact allergy due to tea tree oil and cross-sensitisation to colophony. *Contact Dermatitis* 31: 124–125

Selvaag E, Holm J-O, Thune P 1995 Allergic contact dermatitis in an aromatherapist with multiple sensitisations to essential oils. *Contact Dermatitis* 33: 354–355

Shrivastav P, Goerge K, Balasubramaniam N et al. 1988 Suppression of puerperal lactation using jasmine flowers (Jasminum sambac). *Australian and New Zealand Journal of Obstetrics and Gynaecology* 28(1): 68–71

Southwell I A, Freeman S, Rubel D 1997 Skin irritancy of tea tree oil. *Journal of Essential Oil Research* 9: 47–52

Steele J 1992 Environmental fragrancing. *International Journal of Aromatherapy* 4(2): 8–11

Stevenson C 1992 Orange blossom evaluation. *International Journal of Aromatherapy* 4(3): 22–24

Stewart N 1987 New ways to beat sickness. *Mother.* May

Tiran D 1996 *Aromatherapy in Midwifery Practice.* Baillière Tindall, London

Tisserand R (ed.) 1993 *Gattefossé's Aromatherapy.* C W. Daniel, Saffron Walden, UK

Tisserand R, Balacs T 1995 *Essential Oil Safety: A Guide for Health Professionals.* Churchill Livingstone, Edinburgh

United Kingdom Central Council 1991 *Midwives' Rules.* UKCC, London

United Kingdom Central Council 1992a *Guidelines for Administration of Medicines.* UKCC, London

United Kingdom Central Council 1992b *Scope of Professional Practice.* UKCC, London

Valnet J 1980 *The Practice of Aromatherapy.* English translation by Tisserand R (1982). C. W. Daniel, Saffron Walden, UK

van Ketel W G 1982 Allergy to Matricaria chamomilla. *Contact Dermatitis* 8(2): 143

Walker P 1995 *Baby Massage.* Judy Piatkus Publishers, London

Weiss J 1973 Camphorated oil intoxication during pregnancy. *Paediatrics* 52: 713–714

Worwood V 1990 *The Fragrant Pharmacy.* Bantam Books, London

Young J 1997 To touch or not to touch. *Modern Midwife* 7(6): 10–14

Zarno V 1994 Candidiasis. *International Journal of Aromatherapy* 6(2): 20–23

Further reading

Lavabre M 1990 *Aromatherapy Workbook.* Healing Arts Press, Rochester, USA

Maxwell Hudson C 1988 *The Complete Book of Massage.* Dorling Kindersley, London

Westwood C 1991 *Aromatherapy: A Guide to Home Use.* Amberwood

Denise Tiran

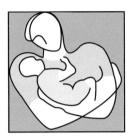

Chapter 8 **Reflexology in Midwifery Practice**

Reflexology or reflex zone therapy involves a sophisticated form of foot massage or manipulation in which the feet represent a map of the whole body. Working on the feet, or the hands which correspond accordingly, parts of the body distal to the feet can be treated. Although reflexology is not a diagnostic tool it is possible to detect changes in physiological function, e.g. stages of the menstrual cycle, as well as areas of disorder or disease which may be present in the body, or to have an indication of previous and even potential problems which may arise in a given area.

The history of reflexology

Reflexology, reflex zone therapy and the metamorphic technique all evolved from the ancient Chinese system of medicine used thousands of years ago. In acupuncture, needles are inserted into a point on the body distal to the source of a particular health problem, in the belief that they are linked by energy lines called meridians. So too, in reflexology, is there the theory of energy pathways linking the feet and hands to the rest of the body. While many Western reflexology authorities feel that these are not the same as the meridians of acupuncture, some believe they are identical.

Other therapists support the theory that reflex points in the feet act as nerve receptors for all the organs of the body, in an attempt to explain in more Westernised terms how reflexology works. This 'neurotheory' is supported by Frankel (1997) who measured baroreceptor reflex sensitivity in three groups of subjects who received either reflexology or foot massage or no intervention, indicating sensory nervous system stimulation of the feet in the first two groups.

In practice the right foot relates to the right side of the body and the left foot relates to the left side; the dorsum represents the front of the body including the musculature, and the soles of the feet represent the back of the body and the internal organs. Kevin and Barbara Kunz (1984, p. 10) state that the exception to this rule is the cerebral and central nervous systems which are controlled by the opposite side of the brain and thus the reflex areas on the feet for these parts of the body should be on the opposite foot. This concept may support the nerve receptor theory but no mention of it is made by other writers (Marquardt, 1983; Wagner, 1987; Goodwin, 1988; Hall, 1991).

Egyptian tomb paintings have depicted scenes of what appears to be foot massage and it is also thought that primitive tribes elsewhere in the world used similar techniques. Very little is documented about reflexology after this time until its resurgence at the end of the nineteenth century. The four main protagonists of the twentieth century were William Fitzgerald, Eunice Ingham, Hanne Marquardt and Doreen Bayly.

Fitzgerald, an American doctor at the turn of the century, was an ear, nose and throat specialist who observed that patients' perceptions of pain could be affected by pressing elsewhere on their bodies. He had discovered Red Indian tribes practising zone therapy and explored the principle further, developing and refining it into a system of treatment which he used within his medical practice, to great scepticism from his colleagues.

His research led him to divide the body into ten longitudinal zones running from head to toes and fingers (Fig. 8.1). It is interesting to note that at this time the feet were not singled out for any special significance but that effective treatment could be given through pressure on the hands, feet, tongue and lips. It is the theory of the ten longitudinal zones which enables the therapist to treat any disorder within a specific zone by working on either the hand or the foot in the same zone. This is of particular relevance when it is not possible to work on a client's feet, due to infection or perhaps an amputation, and the therapist would then work on the hands in the same zones as he or she would have treated on the feet.

Another doctor, J. S. Riley, also used reflex zone therapy extensively but his main claim to fame is as the teacher of Eunice Ingham. In the 1930s Mrs Ingham, an American masseuse, was the first person to use reflexology as it is used today. She devised the special 'grip' technique and refined the therapy to one in which almost all treatment can be carried out on the feet or the hands. Her compression massage was thought to be a way of working on crystalline deposits under the skin which result from excess calcium and uric acid when the metabolism is disrupted. The reflexology technique

Fig. 8.1. The ten longitudinal zones of the body.

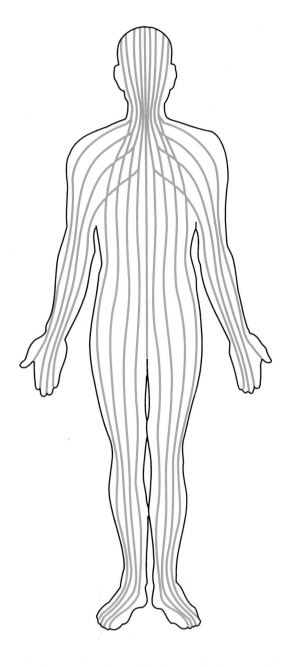

aimed to disperse these crystals and facilitate their excretion through the blood and lymphatic processes.

A pupil of Eunice Ingham's was Hanne Marquardt, a German, who added the concept of transverse body zones to the existing theory of longitudinal zones. These transverse zones correspond to the shoulder girdle, the waist and the pelvic floor, and related transverse zones can be described in the feet (Fig. 8.2).

Fig. 8.2. The transverse zones of the body and feet.

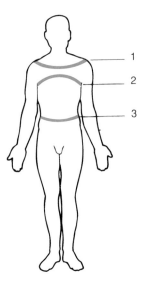

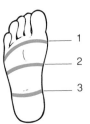

Fig. 8.2. The transverse zones of the body and feet.

The person credited with bringing reflexology to Britain is Doreen Bayly, who persevered against her critics to demonstrate the many benefits of the treatment and established the first British reflexology training institution.

Another reflexologist, working in the 1960s, Robert St. John, discovered that the inner edge of the foot, which represents the spinal zone, also corresponds to the prenatal period. He thus surmised that by working on this part of the feet, energy blockages which occurred during fetal life could be released—this became known as prenatal therapy or the Metamorphic Technique (Fig. 8.3).

Therapists do not aim to treat illness but rather to stimulate the innate capacity of the body to rebalance itself towards optimum health. St. John's most famous pupil, Gaston St. Pierre, investigated the technique further and is considered one of the leading authorities on the subject today (Cohen, 1987; Lambert, 1988).

It is not the aim of this chapter to consider in detail the metamorphic technique but suggestions for further reading are given at the end of the chapter.

How does reflexology/reflex zone therapy work?

Reflexology or reflex zone therapy of the feet can be used to highlight areas of the body in which past, current or potential energy disturbance may be present. This may be identified visually, manually or as a result of the recipient's response to the treatment.

On examination of the feet the therapist may be able to observe discoloration, dryness or rashes on the skin surface or oedema and swelling of certain areas which may or may not be diagnostically significant. Minute tactile examination over the entire surface of both feet may elicit the presence of crystalline deposits, resistance and tension or pitting oedema. If

Fig. 8.3. The spinal zones of the feet which relate to the prenatal period in the Metamorphic Technique.

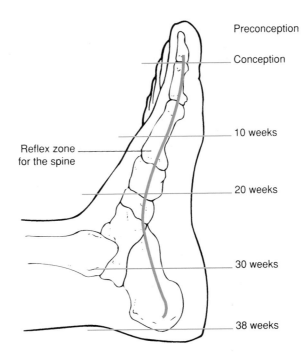

Preconception

Conception

10 weeks

Reflex zone
for the spine

20 weeks

30 weeks

38 weeks

there is disorder or disease in the body the client may experience a bruised feeling on palpation of the feet, or a pinpricking sensation 'as if the therapist is sticking her nail into the foot' while working on those areas which relate to the affected organs. Either of these responses may indicate energy disturbance but is not a diagnosis of disease in itself. Occasionally when visual evidence is present but the client feels no discomfort at all in that part of the foot, this may be more indicative of disease than a bruised or pinpricking sensation. However as a general rule, the sharp sensation highlights possible acute or current disorder while the bruised feeling identifies previous or chronic problems.

Reflexology can also be performed regularly for stress relief and relaxation and for maintenance of optimum health. It is with this in mind that it becomes such a useful adjunct to normal midwifery or nursing practice, as it can truly be used as a complement to any other orthodox treatment.

Reflexology is performed using the special 'grip' sequence devised by Eunice Ingham in which the therapist's thumbs or fingers move across the feet covering every minute point. This is sometimes called 'thumb walking' (Kunz and Kunz, 1984, p. 23), 'massage' (Hall, 1991, p. 103) or perhaps the most descriptive, 'caterpillar crawling' (Wagner, 1987, p. 44). The purpose of the technique is to activate the body's self-healing capacity by stimulating the reflex points, or to calm and relax zones which indicate an acute disturbance in the body. The former is achieved by an intermittent pressure of the thumb or, in the case of sedation, by a sustained continuous pressure on the relevant reflex point for up to 2 minutes. An example of the latter can be seen in someone suffering an occipital headache. The large toe on each foot represents the head in miniature, with the occipital zone being on the back of the big toe at the junction between the toe and the foot (Fig. 8.4). This point is likely to be painful to touch in someone with an occipital headache, but continuous pressure is sustained until the discomfort in the toes is alleviated—this should be reflected by an easing of the headache.

Logically frontal headache would be relieved by applying the same technique to the relevant part on the dorsum of each toe. There is however one major difference between reflexology and reflex zone therapy, in that whereas the former treats symptomatically, the latter attempts to treat causatively. Therefore a reflex zone therapist treating the same occipital headache would explore both feet and treat any part of the foot which was either painful to touch or which visually demonstrated disorder. This might include, for example, the zones to the kidneys if the cause of the headache was renal hypertension.

Location of specific zones on the feet is easier if the two feet are placed together and a picture of the body is superimposed upon them. However because of the diminutiveness of the feet in relation to the size of the whole body care must be taken that the correct organ zone has been identified. Working one eighth of an inch off the intended zone could mean that an entirely different body organ is being treated. This is especially significant in midwifery when working on the heels, which represent the zones to the reproductive organs (Fig. 8.5).

Fig. 8.4. Reflex zones to the head (see also Fig. 8.8).

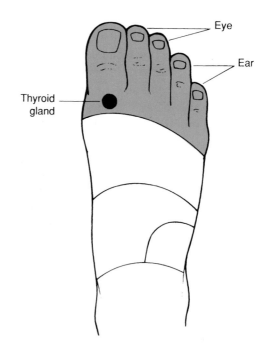

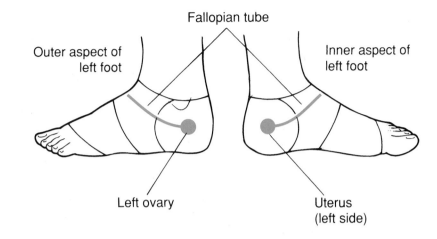

Fig. 8.5. The reflex zones to the female reproductive system (left side).

Fallopian tube

Outer aspect of left foot

Inner aspect of left foot

Left ovary

Uterus (left side)

A knowledge of the position of reflex zones is useful when applying simple massage to the feet. It can be seen that the heels represent the pelvic area, and it is this part on which vigorous brisk massage is contraindicated in early pregnancy, to avoid any potential risk of spontaneous abortion (see Chapter 7, Massage and Aromatherapy).

Some reflexologists include the use of 'tools' in their practice, such as elastic bands or clothes pegs, to apply continuous pressure to certain areas of hands or feet, or combs to create friction on specific zones (Hall, 1991, p. 17). However, it is generally considered that the relationship between client and therapist, and the sensitivity of the reflexologist in detecting nuances in the recipient, are of paramount importance and result in a more effective treatment. For this reason nothing other than the bare unencumbered hands of the therapist should be used to perform the treatment—not even oils or creams are required, although some therapists use a small amount of talcum powder to avoid friction of skin to skin contact. Other 'gadgets' claiming to stimulate reflexology points are also to be avoided as these may overstimulate and cause pain. In addition the individuality of every foot cannot be identified by a standard piece of equipment such as a reflexology sandal, which may put pressure incorrectly on the feet and serve to aggravate existing conditions or even initiate others which are latent.

The theory that pressures on the feet from shoes or specific conditions such as corns, verrucae or athlete's foot may indirectly stimulate disorder elsewhere in the body is often reported anecdotally by therapists, and is worthy of further investigation.

Vera, a middle-aged woman who received regular reflexology for relaxation, developed a verruca on the upper surface of her left second toe, which incidentally represents the zone for the left eye. On questioning her it emerged that she had also begun to suffer 'spots' in front of her left eye which had commenced at about the same time as the verruca first appeared.

It is wise to avoid direct reflexology to infected areas so Vera was given essential oil of tea tree to use (one drop neat applied to the centre of the verruca daily and confined by a corn plaster; see Chapter 7). She used the tea tree oil for 5 days, when she began to see an improvement in the size of the verruca—and the severity of the visual disturbance lessened. A further 10 days of tea tree application had virtually eliminated the verruca, and the 'spots' before her eyes did not recur after the eighth day.

This does raise the question of whether the situation would have resolved itself spontaneously, for no empirical evidence exists to prove otherwise. However, many reflexologists recount similar instances, and it would seem to confirm the theory of the interrelationship between the feet and the rest of the body. Franz Wagner (1987, pp. 52–53) identifies several potential problems as a result of common foot complaints, including previous, existing or latent disease, injuries, hyperactive or hypoactive organ functioning, or merely excessive exhaustion or tiredness. The theory is supported by Kunz and Kunz (1984, p. 19). Marquardt (1983, p. 74–75) goes further, giving a variety of examples with suggestions as to their specific potential outcomes. These include: hallux valgus causing problems of the cervical spine and thyroid gland; fallen arches/flat feet leading to spinal column disorders; and pelvic and hip conditions arising from injury to or congestion of the malleoli and heels.

In midwifery the supposition that an intravenous cannula inserted into the back of the hand, which is over the zone relating to the breast, may impair the onset of lactation is also worth investigating. Certainly the converse is true in that women with inadequate lactation can be helped by stimulation of these zones on the hands and the feet (Fig. 8.6).

Contraindications to treatment

It is obviously impractical to attempt to work on someone's feet if there are major problems of the lower limbs, such as severely varicosed veins or ulcers, thrombosis or fungal infections, although unilateral disorders can be treated on the opposite limb. It is also feasible to work on the reflex zones to the hands (see Fig. 8.1), although deeper manipulation may be necessary as the hands are less sensitive to therapy than the feet.

If a person has an acute infectious disease or is pyrexial it is also advisable to refrain from giving a full treatment, yet simple sedation techniques can be very soothing to someone emotionally and physically stressed by serious illness. Similarly if the client has carcinoma, multiple sclerosis or a condition requiring surgery, reflexology will not eliminate the cause of the illness. It

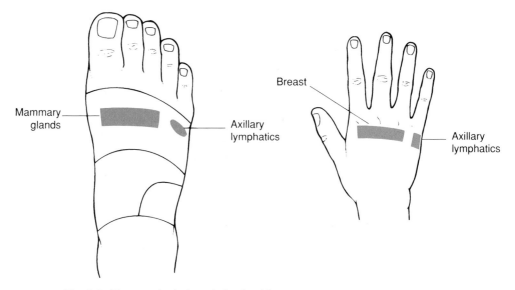

Fig. 8.6. *The zones for the breast in hand and foot.*

will however relax and calm the person, activate excretory organs, stimulate the respiratory system and may dramatically reduce pain.

In pregnancy, reflexology or reflex zone therapy is only contraindicated if there is a risk of fetal loss, although Kunz and Kunz (1984, p. 82) dispute this, stating that 'miscarriage is a reaction of the body, NOT a response to reflexology'. Great care should be taken however during the first trimester and with the first treatment at any time during pregnancy, but reflexology can be a very pleasurable means of relaxing both the mother and fetus, and enabling the woman's body to find its own equilibrium.

Reactions to reflexology treatment

A variety of positive and negative reactions can occur during, after or between treatments. These arise as a result of the activation of the body's innate self-healing capacity and demonstrate that toxins are being eliminated in an attempt to attain homeostasis. Often there is a healing crisis in which the person appears to get worse before getting better, as the body 'kick starts' itself into action.

All reactions occurring at any time during the course of treatment should be recorded, however insignificant or unrelated they may seem.

While administering the reflexology treatment it is important to observe the client for responses to the massage—whether they appear calm and re-laxed, agitated, in pain or frightened. Occasionally the person may start to perspire or complain of feeling hot and/or cold—this is often as pressure is applied to reflex zones relating to diseased or disordered organs in the body. However it may be even more significant if the therapist is aware of possible disorder by observation or manipulation of the feet while the client feels

*Fig. 8.7. The reflex zones
for the solar plexus (left
side).*

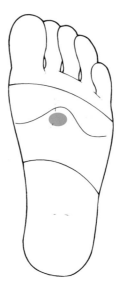

nothing and does not respond at all. If reactions do occur during treatment, simple stroking of the feet and 'harmonising' grips can be used until the symptoms subside. For example, the reflex zone for the solar plexus (Fig. 8.7) can be treated by sustained pressure and will help to calm the client down. This area can also be treated as part of a session for relaxation.

Between treatments, if a client is receiving a course of reflexology, other reactions may occur but are not always recognised as such. These may include improvement in the texture and tone of the skin due to improved circulation; alternatively skin eruptions in the form of spots and rashes may present as the body attempts to rid itself of toxins (the so-called 'healing crisis'). Most clients report sleeping better, although some complain of remembering vivid dreams. Activation of the excretory processes often results in increased diuresis or bowel action, sometimes accompanied by an unusual, somewhat unpleasant odour of either urine or faeces; other secretory processes are stimulated leading to extra mucus production in the respiratory tract or vagina. A few people become feverish, not symptomatic of illness, but rather as a natural defence mechanism, and the fever should not be suppressed by antibiotics. Indeed it has been seen in some clients that latent, perhaps previously suppressed or inadequately treated illness, may surface; completion of a course of reflexology should resolve the problem. Many clients experience mood changes, usually positive, as a response to treatment, and report a sense of relaxation and calm. This is what makes reflexology such a valuable aid to the treatment of stress-related conditions.

Some authorities, such as Wagner (1987, p. 56), suggest that the therapist may also experience reactions due to the energy flow between therapist and the client. This may take the form of tiredness and yawning, nausea or headache, and throbbing of the hands and fingers. Wagner recommends that thorough washing of the hands followed by brisk shaking and rubbing of the lower arms should resolve the situation.

The use of reflexology/reflex zone therapy during pregnancy, labour and puerperium

Reflexology can be extremely beneficial for expectant, labouring or newly delivered women, and for their babies, both to treat a variety of specific conditions and to aid relaxation and induce sleep. Some women enjoy regular sessions throughout their pregnancies which help to alleviate the adverse effects of physiological changes as they arise, by triggering the body's self-healing and self-regulating capacities.

It is also thought to be useful in cases of infertility or subfertility when treatment of the reflex zones for the pituitary gland and ovaries may stimulate ovulation. This would normally be carried out in conjunction with other treatment such as dietary advice, relaxation exercises and the recommendation to sit in alternate hot and cold baths, with the water level above the waist, in an attempt to improve pelvic lymphatic and nerve supplies.

Identification of the pituitary gland reflex zone (Fig. 8.8) is vital to the use of reflexology in midwifery, as so much of physiology is dependent on pituitary activity.

Throughout pregnancy it is wise to work very gently over the reflex zone to the uterus, although the zone should not be sedated by sustained pressure on the area—this would have the effect of 'sedating' the pregnancy and possibly creating difficulties for maternal and fetal health.

Contraindications Contraindications to reflex zone therapy in pregnancy include major placental disturbance such as placenta praevia or abruption,

Fig. 8.8. The reflex zone for the pituitary gland.

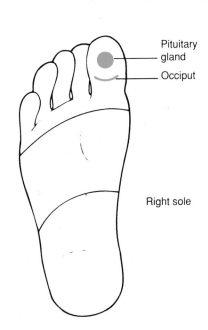

Pituitary gland

Occiput

Right sole

ectopic pregnancy, threatened abortion, pyrexia or infection and any unstable pregnancy about which the therapist is unsure.

An additional condition which some therapists would avoid treating with reflexology is pre-eclampsia, although gentle harmonising stroking movements may lower the blood pressure sufficiently to prevent eclampsia. Yangsheng (1995) describes the successful reduction of blood pressure in a multigravida. Treatment of the kidney zones may also be of use but this should be done with caution to avoid exacerbating renal dysfunction.

Nausea and vomiting Nausea and vomiting of the first trimester may respond to reflexology in conjunction with other treatments as outlined elsewhere in this book. Harmonising massage strokes and sedation of the solar plexus zone may generally relax the mother and treatment of the reflex zones for the endocrine system can relieve severe hyperemesis of hormonal aetiology. Sickness associated with migraine may also be relieved as the reflexology is effective in treating the headache.

Constipation Constipation responds wonderfully well to reflexology and can be performed antenatally and postnatally as well as on neonates and infants. The arches of the feet correspond to the gastrointestinal tract and clockwise massage of these areas with the thumbs can be very effective (Fig. 8.9). A qualified therapist would also treat the zone for the liver, but the novice may achieve good results simply by circular massage—it would be acceptable for midwives with limited experience of reflexology to attempt massage of the arches rather than the specific reflexology technique. The author has treated a woman, 22 weeks pregnant, who had not had

Fig. 8.9. The reflex zones for the intestines—massage in a clockwise direction to stimulate peristalsis (both feet).

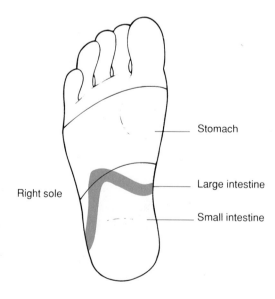

Stomach

Large intestine

Right sole

Small intestine

her bowels open for three weeks. After two sessions of reflexology she was able to defecate three times a week.

Haemorrhoids Varicosities, particularly haemorrhoids, can be treated successfully with reflexology, before and after delivery. Sedation of the rectal reflex zone and stimulation of the lymphatic system and intestinal zones will ease discomfort, aid defecation and may reduce swelling of prolapsed haemorrhoids.

Backache Backache due to the effects of relaxin may be relieved by working on the spinal zones along the inner edges of the feet, as well as sedation of the zones for the sacroiliac joint and abdominal musculature. If the problem is exacerbated by laxity of the symphysis pubis, gentle work on the pituitary gland zone should rebalance the hormonal output.

Oedema Physiological ankle oedema can be resolved to a certain extent by working on the reflex zones to the lymphatic system, kidneys, liver and gastrointestinal tract regularly.

Heartburn Heartburn may be alleviated by stimulating the zones for the oesophagus, stomach and intestines and sedating the zones relating to the solar plexus and diaphragm and cardiac sphincter.

Cystitis Most authorities (Kunz and Kunz, 1984, p. 132; Wagner, 1987, p. 139; Hall, 1991, p. 145) suggest that the symptoms of cystitis, pyelitis and nephritis can be treated with reflex zone therapy, but great care must be taken by even the most experienced reflexologist when dealing with this condition in a pregnant woman. The therapist must also be certain to work only in the direction of the urinary tract from the kidneys to the ureters and then the bladder to avoid spreading any infection in the opposite direction. Wagner (1987, p. 139) urges discretion in any client in whom renal calculi are suspected, for inadvertently enthusiastic treatment may dislodge a loose stone, moving it to a position where it causes a blockage and a subsequent deterioration in renal function.

Frequency of micturition, however, due to pressure from the growing uterus or engaged presenting part, may be improved by gentle reflexology to the urinary tract zones.

Anxiety Anxious or depressed mothers may enjoy receiving regular reflexology from a qualified practitioner throughout pregnancy. This would alleviate insomnia, reduce stress, and may provide an opportunity to discuss in detail their fears and worries. As with other tactile one-to-one therapies, practitioners are advised to be competent in identifying and resolving or referring psychological problems.

Insomnia For those women in whom an active fetus at night prevents sleep, reflexology can help by not only relaxing the mother but also the fetus. Midwives on night duty in an antenatal ward could utilise simple foot massage as a means of facilitating sleep for inpatients. If the mothers are hypertensive, without impending eclampsia, this would help to reduce blood pressure as well.

Induction Technically, labour can be induced by stimulating the zones to the pituitary gland and uterus, but the midwife-reflexologist must not exceed the limits of her practice by attempting this without the express permission of the obstetrician. However, the same treatment could be used in cases where labour needs to be accelerated or when the membranes rupture but spontaneous contractions do not follow.

Pain Pain in labour can be reduced by gentle work all over the feet but paying particular attention to the reflex zones for the uterus, pituitary gland, lymphatic system and other pelvic organs. For the midwife not qualified in reflex zone therapy, simple foot massage will serve to warm the feet, as labouring women quite literally suffer from cold feet as energy is directed elsewhere. Vigorous rubbing of each heel between the midwife's two palms can ease discomfort and enhance uterine action, while encouraging the mother to massage briskly around her wrists for 2 minutes every hour may also be helpful. The wrists and across the top of the ankles correspond to the Fallopian tubes and reproductive lymphatics and this action helps to relieve pelvic congestion. A casual study by Motha and McGrath (1993) of the effects of reflexology on 64 women showed that it was effective in treating a range of symptoms of pregnancy, including backache, heartburn and hypertension. Labour length also appeared to be significantly reduced. Feder et al. (1993) also demonstrated the value of reflex zone therapy for labouring women.

Contractions Uterine action can be regulated with reflexology, either stimulating or sedating according to whether the contractions are inadequate or excessive. In the event of incoordinate activity, harmonising grips and treatment of the zones to the pituitary and other endocrine glands should help.

Micturition For women unable to pass urine, reflexology can initiate micturition and save the mother from the potential complications of catheterisation. This is also an especially effective means of treating retention following delivery or Caesarean section.

Janet, a 25-year-old primigravida, went into labour spontaneously at 38½ weeks' gestation and was admitted to the labour suite after 3 hours of regular painful uterine contractions at home. On examination the cervix was found to be 4 centimetres dilated, partially effaced and soft.

She progressed to full dilatation within 2½ hours. However, the relative speed of the first stage had meant that she had only passed urine once, just before leaving home for the maternity unit, and she had continued to drink water throughout her labour. Janet felt a strong urge to push spontaneously but after 1¼ hours of active pushing the presenting part was still at the level of the ischial spines, and on examination per vaginam the bladder was found to be full although Janet was unable to pass urine herself.

The midwife in attendance, a qualified reflexologist, asked if she could treat Janet's feet, to which she readily agreed. Stimulation of the zones to the urinary tract resulted in an almost instantaneous urge to pass urine, and the voiding of 450 ml. Emptying of the bladder facilitated descent of the presenting part, and Janet was delivered of a 3.8 kg boy just 20 minutes later.

Hyperventilation Reflexology can be effective in regulating the breathing of a mother who hyperventilates in labour, particularly in a prolonged second stage, by working on the zones to the solar plexus and respiratory tract.

Cephalopelvic disproportion If mild cephalopelvic disproportion is thought to be the cause of delay in the second stage, treatment of the zones to the pelvic joints and ligaments has been found in practice to create a little extra 'give' in the pelvic canal, sufficient to facilitate a vaginal delivery rather than Caesarean section.

Retained placenta Retained placenta also responds to treatment with reflex zone therapy, with stimulation of the uterine and pituitary gland zones on the feet. Community midwives qualified in reflex zone therapy in the author's area of work have utilised their skills on several occasions to avoid transfer to hospital of a mother who has delivered at home but in whom the placenta is slow to separate. Although these are anecdotal accounts without controls, the subject is worthy of research and could serve as a simple means of dealing with a situation which normally requires medical attention, but with which the midwife is trained to cope in an emergency.

Cynthia, a gravida four, insisted on a home birth despite complications in previous pregnancies—mild hypertension, postmaturity and haemorrhage during the third stage of her last labour. Two midwives were allocated to provide continuity of care, and the pregnancy progressed normally apart from fluctuating blood pressure readings up to 100 mmHg diastolic towards term.

Labour commenced spontaneously at 42 weeks' gestation and full dilatation was confirmed after 6 hours. An uncomplicated birth of a healthy girl was achieved following 35 minutes of spontaneous pushing. However no further contractions occurred and a period of 40 minutes elapsed with the placenta still in situ. The midwife urged Cynthia to put the baby to the breast, but she did not want to suck so nipple stimulation was started in an attempt to make the uterus contract. This had no effect, and by now 65 minutes had passed.

The supporting midwife was nearing the end of her training as a reflexologist and asked if she could treat Cynthia's feet. Contractions recommenced after 5 minutes followed by separation and delivery of the placenta 3 minutes later.

In this case reflexology had been used as a last resort before calling medical aid because the midwife was not fully qualified, but she knew enough to justify what she was doing as an accountable midwife. In the future she would attempt to treat a mother's feet earlier to reduce the interval between birth of the baby and separation of the placenta.

Subinvolution If a mother is found to have retained products of conception or subinvolution, reflex zone treatment of the feet can facilitate the physiological process and avoid the need for evacuation of retained products.

Perineal discomfort may be alleviated by working on the zones to the pelvic floor; other discomforts of the postnatal period such as uterine 'after-pains', backache, especially after epidural anaesthesia, headache and shoulder pain from poor positioning during breastfeeding may also be relieved.

Haemorrhoids can be treated to reduce pain and swelling when they have prolapsed by working on the reflex zones to the rectum and the lymphatic system.

For breastfeeding mothers reflex zone therapy is extremely useful in encouraging lactation, relieving engorged breasts, in particular venous engorgement, and stimulating milk flow to prevent stasis in the axillae. Jie and Tianjun (1995) report the successful stimulation of lactation with reflexology in 10 women. As mentioned earlier in this chapter, mothers who have had an intravenous cannula inserted into the back of the hand in labour may be slow to start lactating. Midwives, even those not trained in reflexology, can massage the dorsum of each foot and the back of each hand, which should work on the reflex zones to the breasts; a qualified practitioner would also treat the pituitary zone (see Fig. 8.8).

Depression The relaxation and de-stressing effects obtained from reflexology are useful in helping women suffering from postnatal 'blues' and may be effective in those with puerperal depression. Any mother would benefit from having a few sessions of reflexology after delivery, for at least it is calming and relaxing, and it may prevent or treat physiological disorders or pathological conditions which arise in the early postnatal period (Fig. 8.10). Although no research specific to postpartum mood changes was found, reflexology has been shown, in a randomised, controlled trial, to be effective in treating a range of symptoms associated with premenstrual syndrome (Oleson and Flocco, 1993).

Research into reflex zone therapy/ reflexology

While reflexology purports to be a complete discipline in its own right it must be acknowledged that there is not a substantial body of knowledge with which to support it, although this situation is gradually changing. Much of the discussion in this chapter is of unsubstantiated claims purely from anecdotal evidence. This fact would seem to undermine to some extent the value of reflexology/zone therapy, and without research to underpin theories the situation is unlikely to change. Reflexology is often used as a complement to other therapies, either for diagnosis (although this is not the aim of the therapy) or as an option available to practitioners who are qualified in other therapies.

In preparation for this chapter extensive international searches of relevant literature were made, but they yielded little in the way of specific research into reflex zone therapy/reflexology. Much of what has been written is descriptive, without significant reference to other authorities. Numerous reports of successful reflexology treatments come from China, but these are in no way controlled trials. Unfortunately, therefore, their potential value is lost in the continued debate about the validity of trials which are not randomised, controlled and double-blinded.

It was interesting to note that the few research trials conducted into reflexology were in countries where complementary medicine is more accepted, and the research findings were published in non-English journals (Eriksen, 1992; Ferrer de Diso, 1993; Eichelberger, 1993). Much of the English language literature is written by nurses attempting to describe the benefits to nursing/midwifery practice from their personal practice (Barron, 1990; Evans, 1990; Levin, 1992; Lockett, 1992; Tattam, 1992). What was fascinating to discover was that the two international searches classified reflexology or reflexotherapy with some aspects of acupuncture. This poses the question of whether reflexology truly is considered to work on the same energy pathways as acupuncture, or whether those who compiled the databases assumed a relationship.

The lack of research is worrying, although the author is aware of several projects in progress around the UK. There are many aspects of the use of reflex zone therapy in midwifery which would be well worth evaluating, such as for constipation, retention of urine, inadequate lactation or engorged breasts, induction or acceleration of labour and many more. The difficulty, as always with manual therapies and as mentioned above, is the impossibility of carrying out randomised double-blind controlled trials, as it is obvious that the client would know whether or not the treatment was carried out. However, randomisation of who receives conventional treatment or reflexology is possible, and this probably has to be the way forward.

Reflexology/reflex zone therapy is expanding and being incorporated into the practice of midwives and nurses, although it is of concern that they believe they can practise reflexology on clients and patients without attending a reputable and credible course of instruction. Readers are referred to the section on accountability in Chapter 1 and are advised to investigate potential courses thoroughly before joining them.

However, the value of reflexology/reflex zone therapy is constantly being demonstrated in practice, and it is certainly a therapy which complements conventional midwifery care well. There is considerable strength of feeling amongst practitioners that the therapy needs further integration into orthodox care, especially within the National Health Service. This must be the optimum means of achieving greater credibility for the therapy. Healthcare practitioners who add it to their current skills will be better

Fig. 8.10. Reflexology in the postnatal period. (Courtesy of Nursing Times.)

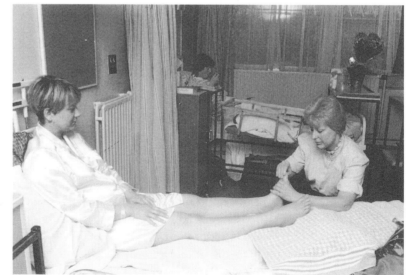

placed to provide a more comprehensive range of treatments, supported by their in-depth knowledge of anatomy and physiology, health and disease. Finally the opportunities presented to these practitioners to conduct research into reflexology should work towards developing the theoretical background on which the therapy is based. Only in this way will reflexology be fully accepted as an integral part of British health care.

Training in reflex zone therapy/ reflexology

There are as yet no national standards for reflexology training although many of the reputable schools are moving towards the National Occupational Standards. Midwives considering the practice of reflexology should thoroughly scrutinise a variety of courses.

References

Barron H 1990 Towards better health with reflexology. *Nursing Standard* 4(40): 32–33

Cohen N 1987 Massage is the message. *Nursing Times* 83(19): 19–20

Eichelberger G 1993 *Studie uber Fussreflexzonenmassage—Alternative zu Pillen.* (Study on foot reflex zone massage—alternative to tablets). *Krankenpfl-Soins Infirm* 86(5): 61–63 (in German)

Eriksen L 1992 *Zoneterapi mod kronisk forstoppelse* (Zone therapy in chronic constipation). *Sygeplejersken* 92(26): 7 (in Danish)

Evans M 1990 Reflex zone therapy for mothers. *Nursing Times* 86(4): 29–31

Feder E, Liisberg G B, Lenstrup C et al. 1993 Zone therapy in relation to birth. *Proceedings of International Confederation of Midwives 23rd International Congress* 2: 651–656

Ferrer de Diso M 1993 *Energia y reflexologia como tratamiento holistico* (Energy and reflexology as holistic treatment). *Rev Enferm* 16(174): 65–67 (in Spanish)

Frankel B S M 1997 The effect of

reflexology on baroreceptor reflex sensitivity, blood pressure and sinus arrhythmia. *Complementary Therapies in Medicine* 5: 80–84

Goodwin H 1988 Reflex zone therapy. In: Rankin Box D (ed.) *Complementary Health Therapies—a Guide for Nurses and the Caring Professions*: 59–84. Croom Helm, London

Hall N M 1991 *Reflexology: a Way to Better Health*. Gateway Books, Bath, UK

Jie Z, Tianjun Z 1995 Foot reflexology in the treatment of hypogalactia. Chinese Medical Research Institute

Kunz K, Kunz B 1984 *The Complete Guide to Foot Reflexology*. Thorsons, London

Lambert M 1988 *Finding Your Feet (Metamorphic Technique)*. M. & J. Lambert (Publ.)

Levin S 1992 Why homeopathy, wherefore reflexology? *Nursing (South Africa)* 7(8): 38–39

Lockett J 1992 Reflexology—a nursing tool? *Australian Nurse Journal* 22(1): 14–15

Marquardt H 1983 *Reflex Zone Therapy of the Feet*. Thorsons, London

Motha G, McGrath J 1993 The effects of reflexology on labour outcome. *Journal of Association of Reflexologists*: 2–4

Oleson T, Flocco W 1993 Randomized controlled study of premenstrual symptoms treated with ear, hand and foot reflexology. *Obstetrics and Gynecology* 82(6): 906–911

Reflexions (1993) Reflexology around the world. *Journal of the International Association of Reflexologists* 2(1): 14–17

Tattam A 1992 The gentle touch. *Nursing Times* 88(32): 16–17

Wagner F 1987 *Reflex Zone Massage*. Thorsons, London

Yangsheng X 1995 *Hypertension of pregnancy treated with foot reflexology—a case report*. Foot Reflexology Service Center, Ankang City, Shaanxi, China

Further reading

Dougans I, Ellis S 1991 *Reflexology—Foot Massage for Total Health*. Element Books, Shaftesbury, UK.

Ingham E D 1938, revised 1984 *Stories the Feet can Tell*. Ingham Publishing Inc., Florida, USA

Elise Johnson

Chapter 9 **Shiatsu**

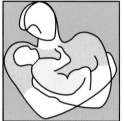

Shiatsu is a Japanese word meaning 'finger pressure'. It has evolved from an earlier form of Japanese massage called Anma (or Tuina in China). In order to comprehend the principles behind shiatsu we have to understand those of Chinese Medicine, which was introduced to Japan as early as the sixth century by a Buddhist monk. The Japanese then developed their own method of manual healing, particularly concentrating on techniques of abdominal diagnosis and treatment. Shiatsu is actually a twentieth-century art, since newer western medical knowledge of anatomy and physiology and physiotherapy techniques have been incorporated into it. It was recognised in Japan in 1964 as opposed to the former Anma massage, and has spread rapidly to the west since then. Now there are over 300 qualified therapists throughout the United Kingdom and this number is increasing all the time.

Details of the therapy

Unlike its predecessor Anma, which consisted of many techniques such as pushing and pulling strokes, tapping, rubbing, stroking and squeezing, done directly on the skin, shiatsu uses simple pressure and holding techniques in combination with gentle stretching, and is performed through loose fitting clothing. A qualified shiatsu practitioner will take a full case history and then make a diagnosis before treatment. There are several forms of diagnoses (as there are styles of treatment). Many concentrate on 'hara' or palpation of the abdomen in order to assess the relative energy in each of the internal organs. In other forms of shiatsu, pulses are taken. Whatever the style of diagnosis and treatment, they are all based on traditional Chinese Medicine. The practitioner will then apply pressure, with either thumbs, fingers, elbows or knees along meridians (energy lines) and points in the body, according to the diagnosis made. This application of pressure tonifies, sedates, or 'moves' the 'Ki' (energy) in the body. Further refinements of treatment are carried out according to what the practitioner feels energetically in the body. Recipients feel a variety of sensations while receiving shiatsu, described commonly as a 'good hurt', dull aching, or pain disappearing under the therapist's fingers, as the energy is being rebalanced in the body.

How traditional Chinese medicine works

Energy, known as 'Qi' in Chinese, 'Ki' in Japanese, is considered to be the motive force of all life. Without Ki there is no life. In ancient times it was noted that even though Ki flowed everywhere in the body, sometimes it seemed to flow near the surface. When there was illness, when the flow of Ki was disturbed, sometimes it manifested in the superficial areas of the body as pain, swelling, irritation and redness. It was then found that by rubbing or pressing these areas, one could eradicate the illness itself, even an internal one. These observations were systematised and the basis of meridians and points was founded. Therapies emerged such as acupuncture, moxibustion, cupping and massage. Whereas acupuncture utilizes needles to adjust the Ki energy, moxa uses heat and cupping uses cups, shiatsu, on the other hand, uses touch to adjust the internal energies of the body. Since imbalance of Ki precedes obvious symptoms of a disease, shiatsu (like all Oriental medicine) has a preventative role in the treatment of disease. However, the most common syndromes which shiatsu does help to treat are conditions such as musculoskeletal problems (for example lumbago, fibrositis and sciatica), headaches and migraine, respiratory ailments, including coughs, catarrh and asthma, stress and tension, insomnia and digestive disorders. The gynaecological conditions that can be treated include infertility and menstrual problems. The common disorders of pregnancy which are amenable to treatment by shiatsu will be discussed later in this chapter.

The Western explanation

In order to examine the physiological effects of finger pressure or shiatsu on the body, we have to examine the nature of connective tissue. Research done by two independent researchers in Japan, Yoshio Nagahama and Hiroshi Motoyama, has concluded that the meridians lie in the connective tissue, and more specifically in the superficial fascia.

An interesting insight into the nature of connective tissue is provided by James Oschman from Natural Science of Healing.

The connective tissue and fascia form a mechanical continuum, extending throughout the animal body, even into the innermost parts of each cell. All the great systems of the body—the circulation, the nervous system, the musculoskeletal system, the digestive tract, the various organs—are sheathed in connective tissue. This matrix determines the overall shape of the organism as well as the detailed architecture of its parts. All movements, of the body as a whole, or of its smallest parts, are created by tensions carried through the connective tissue fabric. Each tension, each compression, each movement causes the crystalline lattices of the connective tissues to generate bioelectric signals that are precisely characteristic of those tensions, compressions, and movements. The fabric is a semiconducting communication network that can convey the bioelectric signals between every part of the body and every other part. This communication network within the fascia is none other than the meridian system of traditional Oriental medicine, with its countless extensions into every part of the body. As these signals flow through the tissues, their biomagnetic counterparts extend the stories they tell into the space around the body. The mechanical, bioelectric, and biomagnetic signals travelling through the connective tissue network, and through the space around the body, tell the various cells how to form and reform the tissue architecture in response to the tensions, compressions, and movements we make.

While this theory shows that connective tissue is capable of communication and energy conduction in the form of electron and proton transfer, it follows that the application of pressure anywhere in the body will generate small electric currents. This is explained more easily by the following scenario. Pressure applied to tissues can help to transform the tissue. Work done on organic gels, part of the cytoplasm of cells, shows that pressure will cause the gel to become a solution. Therefore, particle accumulations trapped in the gel state may be released at the same time as the gel becomes more hydrated. Hydration will make the tissue more energetically conductive. Shiatsu massage will not only induce small electric currents that will be conducted away from the point of pressure, but it will also help rearrange the tissues, making them more conductive (Matsumoto and Birch, 1988). The electric currents will have many physiological effects, just as they do in acupuncture, such as an increase in microcirculation and vasomotion that will increase oxygenation of the tissues, and will help flush toxins and waste products, improving their overall function (see also Chapter 5). The end result of all this is that physiologically, shiatsu massage has the ability to regulate nerve function, strengthen the body's resistance to disease, flush out the tissue, improve circulation of blood, and make joints more flexible.

Contra-indications to shiatsu treatments

In general, most conditions are amenable to shiatsu treatment. Some conditions that are contraindicated include active skin diseases, burns, fractures (above or below the site is permitted), fever, herniated vertebral discs, infectious diseases, open sores or scars, osteoporosis, tumours or cancers, although it is effective for pain relief, thrombosis and varicosities (above or below the site is permitted).

During pregnancy there are few contraindications for shiatsu, but rather specific areas of the body on which to avoid pressure. Points to be avoided are Gall Bladder 21 (Fig. 9.1), Large Intestine 4 (Fig. 9.2), Spleen 6 (Fig. 9.3) and Liver 3 (Fig. 9.4). Only gentle work is advised on the lower back and sacrum, while the lower inner leg around Sp6 location should be

Fig. 9.1. Gall Bladder 21.

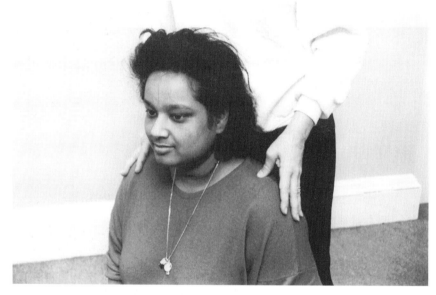

Fig. 9.2. Large Intestine 4.

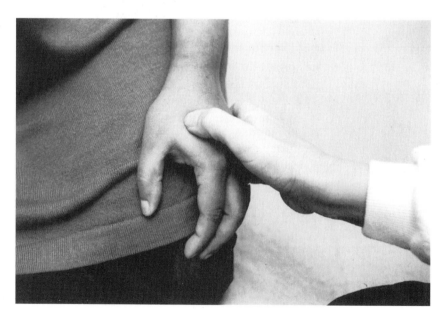

Fig. 9.3. Spleen 6.

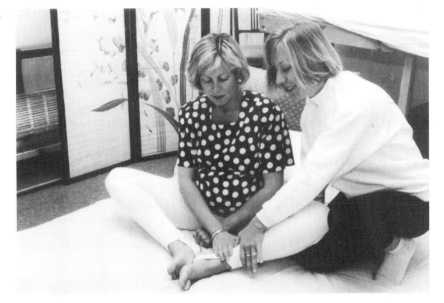

Fig. 9.4. Liver 3.

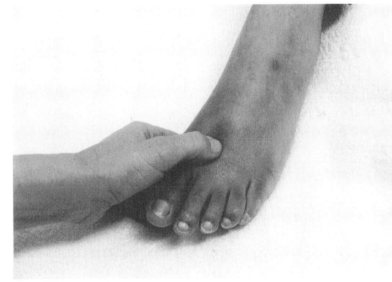

avoided, especially during the first trimester. Shiatsu is not advised in the first trimester if there has been a history of miscarriage or if there are signs of imminent miscarriage. Force must never be used when giving shiatsu treatment and the therapist should use body weight to lean into a point or meridian when applying pressure, rather than muscle power.

Uses in pregnancy   Midwives would find a knowledge of shiatsu techniques a very useful adjunct to their normal practice. However while certain simple techniques can be learnt and used in conjunction with massage and other manual therapies, the midwife as always must recognise her limitations. Shiatsu can be enormously beneficial for pregnancy, labour and the puerperium, but unless the midwife is fully trained she should refrain from using some of the more involved techniques. Referral to a qualified, reputable practitioner would be preferable.

The remainder of this chapter deals with the application of shiatsu to pregnancy and childbirth in order to demonstrate the effectiveness of the therapy for the women in the care of midwives. If there is any doubt as to whether or not the midwife should be attempting the shiatsu movements, she should refer the woman to a practitioner.

Shiatsu—conditions of pregnancy which can be helped

- Breathlessness
- Haemorrhoids
- Nausea and vomiting
- Carpal tunnel syndrome
- Heartburn
- Oedema
- Chronic cough
- Increased frequency of micturition and vaginal discharge
- Cramps
- Insomnia
- Pain—lumbar and sacral
- Headaches
- Tiredness

Why is shiatsu of benefit in pregnancy?

Since shiatsu is a physical 'hands on' therapy, it can be extremely useful during pregnancy, which is a very emotional time for women, due to hormonal changes. Physical touch can be very reassuring and calming. In terms of Oriental medicine, pregnancy together with the postnatal period is considered to be one of the 'gateways of change'. These occur at times of great hormonal fluctuations and are held to be stages where great care should be taken with one's health, because during them it is possible either to strengthen or weaken one's constitution to a great degree. One sees this when, for example, a mother develops a condition after one pregnancy which disappears after a subsequent one. By having shiatsu during a 'gateway of change', a woman's Ki can be bolstered, thereby preventing any pathology from developing.

Shiatsu allows the woman's Ki to flow freely during pregnancy, and

---

Gateways of change are birth, perinatal period (for the baby), puberty, onset of regular sexual activity—'marriage' in the texts, pregnancy, labour and the postnatal period, and the menopause

(From course notes, JCM Seminars, London 1981)

facilitates relaxation. This is important for the mother and fetus, as she is advised to 'modify her mental outlook and lifestyle in order to ensure healthy development of her baby' (Zhejiang College of Traditional Chinese Medicine, 1987). In practical terms today, this means to be calm and free from emotional upsets. The Japanese call this fetal education or 'Tai Kyo'. In the Orient it is traditionally thought that one-third of a person's ultimate social, physical, and mental functioning is determined by their experiences in the uterus (Ohashi, 1983). It is also thought that fetal education is embodied in the effort to remain quiet. The fetus will grow in peace if there is a well-regulated circulation of Ki. Therefore it is most important for a mother to maintain a stable and smooth circulation of Ki so that the infant may gain a bright and cheerful disposition. This is surely one of shiatsu's real strengths, to enable the mother's Ki to flow, with the resultant relaxation and relief of fatigue.

Shiatsu is also very useful in pregnancy because of its ability to tonify the body's Ki, for it is the Ki energy of the Kidney primarily and the Stomach and Spleen that most often becomes depleted during pregnancy. (It should be noted that in terms of Oriental medicine the organs and their functions are not identical to the Western definition of organ function, but have a much wider meaning. For example, this is why we use the capital letters 'K' in Kidney and 'S' in Stomach and Spleen to denote Chinese function and meaning. It is not within the scope of this chapter to go into the full Oriental physiology of the organs, since that would entail a complete course of study in itself, but see the further reading list.) Most of the pathologies or conditions of pregnancy can be helped by addressing these deficiencies in the shiatsu treatment.

The Kidney energy of the mother provides the primary source of energy for the fetus growing within her, so it becomes utilised from the moment of conception. The mother's Kidney energy reserves will be drained further if she overworks and does not rest enough. Hence a variety of symptoms or disorders will occur such as lower backache, oedema, fatigue, breathlessness, chronic coughs, anxiety and insomnia, vaginitis and cystitis. It is interesting to note that in Oriental medicine, as indeed in other complementary therapies, recognition is given to the relevance of all symptoms, even those which in Western terms seem coincidental, for example coughs.

The Spleen, with help from the Stomach, is the organ which is responsible for the production of Blood. Nourishment of the baby both during and after pregnancy depends on an adequate supply of the woman's Blood. In pregnancy Blood nourishes the fetus via the placenta, and afterwards the Blood helps make breastmilk. Therefore, the mother's Blood is constantly nourishing the baby and tonification of the mother's Spleen energy is necessary. Symptoms of imbalances in these organs are as follows: constipation, spasms in the legs, haemorrhoids, heartburn, nausea and vomiting and oedema.

Generally it is considered safe to receive shiatsu from the beginning of pregnancy, with a caution not to use any of the contraindicated points. The areas of the lower inner leg, and strong pressure on the lower back and sacrum, should be avoided.

Pregnant women will benefit from weekly shiatsu sessions with a qualified therapist with the relevant experience.

The following antenatal conditions during the 40-week gestation period are all suitable for shiatsu treatment, either during the antenatal examination given by the midwife if she is appropriately trained or during a complete shiatsu session given by a shiatsu therapist. (Aetiologies of each condition are explained below in terms of Oriental medicine.)

Breathlessness Not only does this occur by reason of the size of the pregnant abdomen which takes up so much room, but in terms of Oriental medicine the Lungs are strongly related to proper functioning of Kidney Ki. Therefore during a session with a qualified practitioner, working the Kidney meridian throughout the body will support the function of the Lungs, which will also be assisted by opening up the chest with work on the Lung 1 point (Fig. 9.5). This is extremely effective to relieve breathlessness, especially during the last trimester. Midwives can also try pressure on Pericardium 6 (Fig. 9.6), which is a point that affects the chest.

Chronic coughs Many times while working with pregnant women one sees clients with chronic coughs. Treatment should be sought from a shiatsu therapist to tonify the woman's energy, since often this weakness in the lungs in Oriental medicine is caused by weakened Kidney energy.

Fig. 9.5. Lung 1.

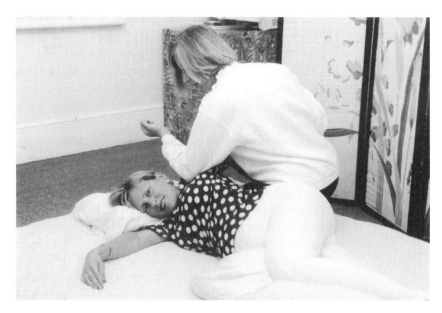

Fig. 9.6. Pericardium 6.

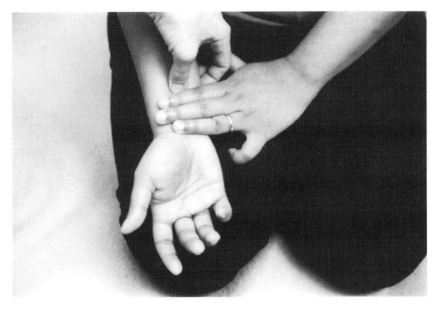

Carpal tunnel syndrome Oedema during pregnancy is seen in Oriental medicine as a disorder occurring as a result of a deficiency of Spleen and Kidney energies causing retention of body fluid. Work on the Masanaga's meridians of Spleen and Kidney channels in the affected arm will help. Another effective technique is work on the Masanaga Kidney channel of the leg. Midwives mastering the fundamentals of shiatsu can perform this latter method and locally work Pericardium 6. Press firmly for 7–10 seconds, three times.

Constipation One of the reasons in Oriental medicine for constipation is the mother's depletion of Stomach and Spleen energy. The midwife could work gently but firmly down the Stomach meridian concentrating on pressing Stomach 36 (St 36) (Fig. 9.7), for 7–10 seconds, three times. Self shiatsu on Stomach meridian (Fig. 9.8) is also helpful.

Cramps Leg cramps, or spasms of the gastrocnemius muscles, occur in the leg muscles through deficiency of Blood nourishing the tissues and deficiency of Kidney energy. Regular shiatsu can be a preventative or first aid treatment. Pressure to Stomach, Gallbladder and Bladder channels in the leg will help cure cramps. Midwives could demonstrate the Bladder 57 (Fig. 9.9) point while dorsiflexing the foot slowly, which the woman could press during a spasm.

Haemorrhoids One reason for haemorrhoids to occur in pregnancy is due to the taxing of the Spleen energy. This is because in Oriental medicine

Fig. 9.7. Stomach 36. One of the pressures which can relieve constipation.

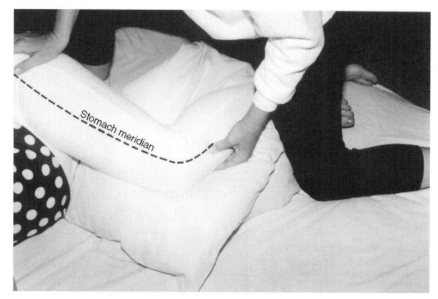

Fig. 9.8. Self shiatsu on stomach meridian to relieve constipation.

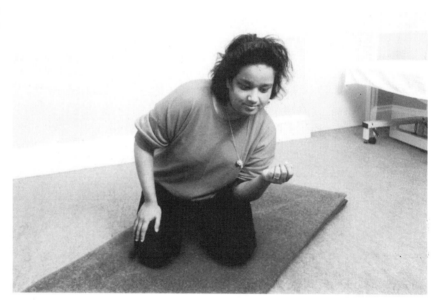

one of the functions of the Spleen is to hold Blood in the blood vessels, and to support the organs.

First aid techniques are as follows:

- Gentle but firm pressure on Governing Vessel 20 (Fig. 9.10), pressing firmly for 7–10 seconds, three times.
- Similar pressure on Bladder 57, Bladder 58 and Bladder 17. In the postnatal period Spleen energy can be improved by pressure on Bladder 57 and Governing Vessel 20 (GV 20).

Fig. 9.9. Bladder 57—may help to ease cramps.

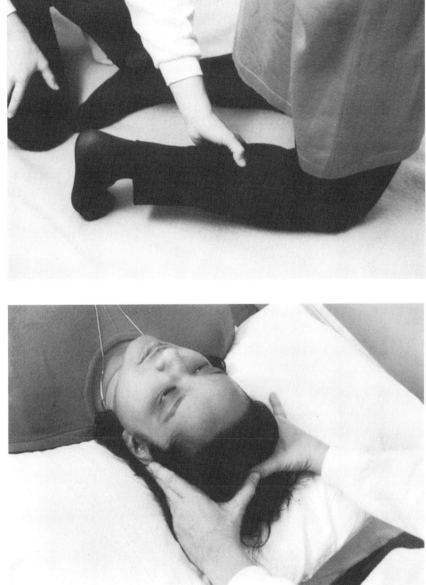

Fig. 9.10. Governing Vessel 20—first aid for haemorrhoids.

Shiatsu is effective on points such as GV 20, and Bladder 57, which effectively tonify Spleen energy.

Heartburn This can be very problematic in late pregnancy and a frequent source of discomfort which is very responsive to shiatsu treatment. Besides Western medical advice on avoidance of fried and fatty foods and eating small frequent meals (this is practical advice to mothers with weak Stomach Ki also), shiatsu treatment is very effective. Heartburn occurs according to

Oriental medicine because of the weakening of Stomach Ki, which thereby is caused to rebel and travel upwards, causing heartburn.

Symptomatic treatment is as follows. Work Stomach meridian firmly. Midwives with some shiatsu training can do this effectively. The shiatsu-trained midwife could also teach the mother to work Conception Vessel 22 and work down the Bladder channel (Fig. 9.11). Press Stomach 36, and Pericardium 6.

Suzie was a 34-year-old with two other children aged 3 and 1, who came for shiatsu treatment at 33 weeks' gestation. She had been suffering from severe heartburn with acid regurgitation most often in the day, and especially on eating. The diagnosis in the session was weak Stomach and Spleen energy. The meridian was felt to be very depleted in the leg and was very sensitive to touch, especially Stomach 36. Slow, gentle but tonifying firm pressure was administered to the Stomach, Kidney and the Spleen meridian (avoiding strong pressure on the inner lower leg) with great sensitivity displayed by Suzie. Symptoms improved immediately after treatment and relief lasted for about 4–5 days. Self shiatsu at home on the Stomach meridian and Conception Vessel 22 also improved symptoms. Several more sessions before the end of the pregnancy kept the symptoms down to a minimum.

Increased frequency of micturition and increased vaginal discharge

Both of these conditions can often be found in the first few weeks of

Fig. 9.11. Working down the Bladder channel concentrating on the associated points of the stomach and spleen.

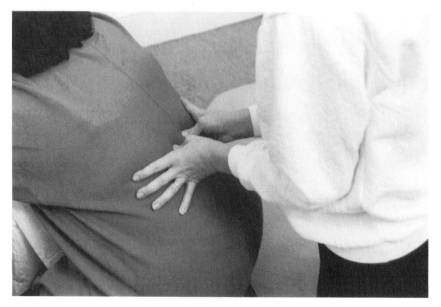

pregnancy and also the last trimester. These occur because in terms of Oriental medicine there is a switch of the mother's Kidney energy as it is redirected towards the fetus. Typical symptoms include frequent, copious micturition, heavy legs, bloating in the first few weeks of pregnancy, and increased vaginal discharge. Sometimes a first aid measure which can be performed by the midwife involves working on the Kidney channel in the leg, both Masanaga and the traditional location.

Insomnia This is commonly experienced at the end of pregnancy because of increased movements of the fetus and frequency of micturition. 'Over-thinking' and anxiety about the expected baby often cause insomnia and if this is the case, regular shiatsu sessions with a therapist can help by enabling the mother to relax. Sessions are recommended to be performed in the evening and it is best to include a lot of work on head, neck and shoulders.

Nausea and vomiting In terms of Oriental medicine there are several reasons for this condition. It occurs due to depletion of Stomach Ki during the time that the pregnant woman is nourishing the baby. The natural direction of the Stomach energy in the body is in a downwards flow, but when the Stomach energy is weak there is a tendency for it to 'rebel' upwards, hence nausea occurs. Alternatively it may be due to the fact that the Liver energy stagnates (usually because of weakening of the mother's Kidney energy in supporting the growing fetus) and leads to rebellious Stomach Ki. This stagnation of Liver Ki happens as a result of the sudden cessation of menstruation when one becomes pregnant. There is a swift change in metabolism which causes the Liver Ki to stagnate, which in turn 'invades the Stomach and Spleen', hence once again nausea occurs.

In practice, whatever the aetiology, the midwife can assist in tonifying the mother's Stomach meridian down the leg with gentle but strong focus on Stomach 36 and by pressing firmly for 7–10 seconds, three times.

Research by Dundee et al. (1988) showed efficacy of the use of the Pericardium 6 point in the reduction of troublesome sickness. This work has been replicated by others (Barsoum et al., 1990; Dundee and Yang, 1990; Price et al., 1991; De Aloysio and Penacchioni, 1992; Evans et al., 1993; Belluomini et al., 1994). The work of Stein et al. (1997) demonstrated the effectiveness of P6 acupressure compared to intravenous meta-clopramide in preventing nausea and vomiting during spinal anaesthesia for Caesarean section.

It is now possible for mothers to purchase wristbands from health stores and chemists which are designed to work on the P6 acupressure point, in order to relieve sickness. Midwives may prefer to advise mothers to use these or perform shiatsu themselves on Pericardium 6. A shiatsu therapist will work down the Bladder channel with the woman either sitting or lying on her side (Fig. 9.12). Treating the Bladder channel will not only tonify

Fig. 9.12. Treating the Bladder channel will tonify the stomach and spleen energies.

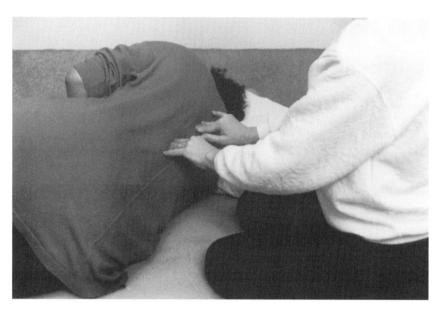

the Stomach and Spleen energies via their associated points, but will also tonify the Kidneys because of the strong relationship between the Bladder and Kidneys in Oriental medicine.

Mothers can be advised to eat biscuits frequently because this stimulates peristalsis which descends the Stomach Ki that is rebelling.

Amanda was 10 weeks pregnant when she came for shiatsu treatment and was feeling quite nauseous, although not actually vomiting. Her symptoms were better for eating, worse with fatigue. She was always running around after her 2-year-old and 4-year-old children. She was anaemic and quite tired and had been prescribed iron tablets. Occasionally if she was very tired she would feel nauseous in the evening, at about 5 p.m. After the first treatment, which consisted of Stomach meridian work, pressure on Stomach 36, Bladder meridian work and Pericardium 6 pressure, she felt immediate relief which lasted for about 4 days. She was advised to drink ginger root tea, which has the effect of warming the Stomach and Spleen, thereby strengthening it.

She was also advised to rest more, eat frequent small meals, and to avoid rich, greasy food which further aggravates stagnation of Liver energy. After the next week of similar treatment, relief went on for 6 days. She was advised to make rice congee, which is a rice soup made from six parts water to one part rice and is cooked slowly for several hours. Camomile tea was advised for settling the stomach instead of tea or coffee. This advice was heeded and Amanda managed to cope with the reduced nausea until her body had adjusted to the hormonal changes of early pregnancy.

Oedema Oedema is a disorder, in terms of Oriental medicine, occurring in pregnant women with depletion of Spleen and Kidney energy, causing retention of body fluid which further depletes the Spleen and Kidney energy. The Spleen and Kidney energies become drained or exhausted towards the end of pregnancy, and thus the function of transportation and transformation of body fluids becomes impaired and fluid accumulates in the tissues, primarily in the extremities and lower half of the body. This condition is ideally suited for treatment by the shiatsu practitioner on all Kidney meridian locations in the body, especially Masanaga locations in the leg. Midwives could try working the Bladder meridian (Fig. 9.13) with the woman sitting or lying on her side. Alternatively first aid treatment involving pressing points Kidney 7, Stomach 36, Bladder 23 and Kidney 3 can be effective.

Most of the severe cases that this author has treated have been found in women aged 35 and over. This is not surprising since Kidney energy naturally declines with age. Also, many cases of oedema were found in women who did not rest enough. Kidney energy becomes depleted through over-work and not resting.

Loretta, a journalist aged 38, was in her third trimester and suffering from severe oedema of pretibial areas and ankles, forcing her to buy larger sized shoes. Her blood pressure was

Fig. 9.13. Bladder
meridian.

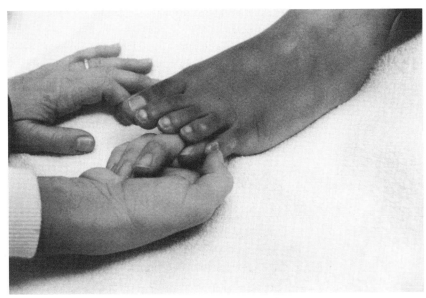

within normal limits, she had no headaches but had slight proteinuria. She was under considerable pressure of deadlines for her newsletter, drank one or two cups of coffee daily, and attended various after work conferences.

One shiatsu session focused on the traditional Kidney meridian location in the leg, and Masanaga location, and also in the arms and chest, after which there was significant reduction of oedema. Advice for more rest was somewhat adhered to, as was the advice to stop drinking coffee. Weekly sessions controlled the oedema from progressing further and indeed markedly improved it.

Lumbo-sacral pain and sciatica This is found frequently because of the increase in weight on the mother's spine and due to Kidney Ki deficiency, which governs the lower back. Consequently, deficiency of Kidney energy causes lower back pain. Mothers will often instinctively rub the pain to make it better and it is for this very reason that shiatsu is so recommended for this pain. Work by an experienced shiatsu therapist is recommended. This will involve working on the Bladder channel of the back, in side or 'sitting position', with focus on Bladder 23, and also firm but gentle pressure on the Masanaga Kidney meridian in the sacral area, upper thigh and lower leg. This is of particular value in labour, and work on the Bladder channel could be performed by the midwife or taught to the birth companion.

Headache Headaches should be treated by a shiatsu practitioner who can assess the cause and treat the mother accordingly, although chronic tension headaches in 21 non-pregnant subjects were successfully treated with acupressure combined with head massage by Puustjarvi et al. (1990). However the midwife should be vigilant in observing the mother for pre-eclampsia and would normally seek advice, in the first place, from the obstetrician.

Tiredness This is very responsive to complete shiatsu treatment by a qualified practitioner. Weekly sessions are extremely beneficial, especially during the last six weeks of pregnancy. Work will be focused on the Kidney, Stomach, and Spleen channels.

Uses in labour

Uses of shiatsu in labour

- Induction for prolonged pregnancy
- Augmentation of contractions
- As an analgesic
- Expulsion of the placenta

The midwife should be familiar with the ways in which a qualified shiatsu practitioner can help the mother, as some women may wish to be accompanied by their practitioner in labour. Teamwork is vitally important and communication early in pregnancy will help to develop the partnership.

Midwives are able to use a limited number of simple shiatsu techniques if they can justify their use, but may wish to refer to an expert for specific conditions and appropriate treatment.

Induction for prolonged pregnancy and acceleration of labour   Shiatsu techniques are a favourable method of inducing labour for postmaturity. Firstly, if anxiety is a factor, complete shiatsu sessions in the week during which the mother is overdue will help to foster relaxation and tonify her energy. The shiatsu practitioner will then use all the points previously contraindicated: strong downwards pressure on Gall Bladder 21, then pressure on Spleen 6, Bladder 67 and Large Intestine 4. These points can be pressed safely from the estimated due date onwards, and this treatment is most effective if performed daily. Midwives should remember that induction of labour falls outside their normal practice and therefore only those who have shiatsu training should perform these techniques after consultation with medical staff.

Augmentation of contractions   If the first stage of labour has started and the contractions have begun to slow down, then pressure on Spleen 6, Large Intestine 4, together with Bladder 31, Liver 3 and Gall Bladder 21 can help to stimulate uterine activity. Strong thumb pressure on all the points is required, as well as strong downward palm pressure on sacral points (Fig. 9.14).

Fig. 9.14. Sacral point pressure may augment contractions.

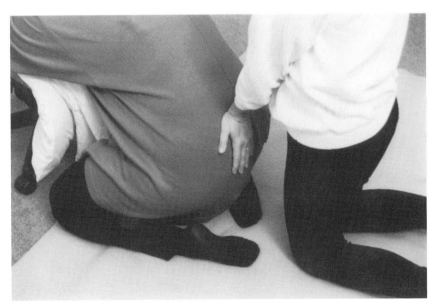

Exhaustion during labour If the woman becomes exhausted during labour, work on the Stomach meridian and Bladder meridian on the back and legs between contractions can be helpful. The reason for this is two-fold; it will not only revitalise tired legs but will also increase the vital energy of the woman to enable sufficiently strong contractions to occur for dilatation of the cervix.

Analgesia in the first stage of labour If labour is prolonged, shiatsu pain-relieving techniques should be supplemented between contractions. Pressure to Gall Bladder 30, Gall Bladder 31, Stomach 36, and Bladder 60 points will help to restore circulation and relax leg muscles (Fig. 9.15). For effective pain relief during a contraction, strong pressure on Bladder 60 is very useful and effective. Additional points of Spleen 6, Large Intestine 4, Liver 3 and Conception Vessel 4 are also beneficial.

Analgesia in occipito-posterior position Shiatsu is an excellent analgesic for the occipito-posterior position, which is regularly associated with very tedious and painful labour. The midwife could perform this technique and should use strong downward palm pressure or thumb pressure into the sacral foramen at the beginning of the contraction, maintaining it to the height of the contraction till it subsides. This can be done with the woman in either a standing position, sitting leaning over a beanbag, or lying on her side (Fig. 9.16).

Ester, a 33-year-old shiatsu therapist, was in her second pregnancy. Following spontaneous rupture of membranes at

Fig. 9.15. Bladder 60—pressure can be effective for pain relief in labour.

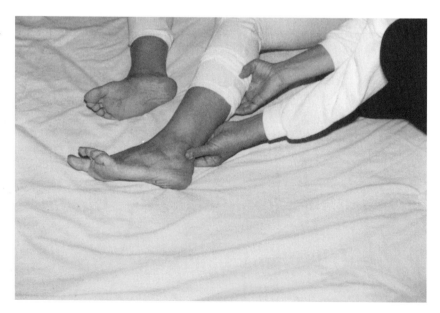

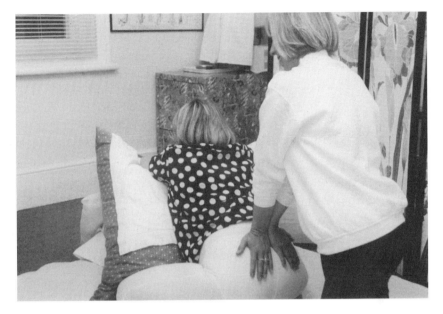

Fig. 9.16. Easing the sacral pain of an occipito-posterior position.

term, she arrived at hospital in established labour. She remained ambulant until contractions were occurring every 2 minutes. On vaginal examination the cervix was found to be 2 cm dilated. The midwife suggested that Ester enter the birthing pool for pain relief and relaxation. Ester asked her husband to use strong palm pressure on her sacrum as she hung on to the side of the pool. Once she left the pool, her husband continued applying thumb pressure around the sacral grooves while she was on all fours, and leaning over the beanbag chair.

Ester found this technique, combined initially with water then on 'all fours', to be very effective in easing the pain and she delivered a 3.5 kg baby in the 'all fours' position with no trauma to the perineum.

Analgesia in the second stage of labour During the second stage one midwife can support the mother's occiput with pressure around the occipital ridge with one hand and another person can use very strong pressure on the Bladder 67 point, squeezing between thumb and index finger or using the nail to press the point. If it is impossible for one person to do this, two people can do it between them. Bladder 67 runs down both legs from the sacrum along the same lines as the autonomic nerves. Intense pressure applied here tends to block sensation in the sacral and pelvic area, thus relieving pain.

Retention of the placenta Midwives could, with limited training, and in an emergency, press on Gall Bladder 21, Bladder 60, Large Intestine 4, and

Spleen 6 points to facilitate separation of the placenta. However, without adequate training this could be a case of a little knowledge being dangerous. If a shiatsu practitioner is present in the labour room she or he could apply treatment which would be effective in separating and expelling the placenta. It should be recognised too that the mother who is accompanied by a shiatsu practitioner is likely to want to avoid active management of the third stage. It is therefore possible that except in cases of a morbidly adherent placenta, patience and time will work naturally and shiatsu may not be required.

Shiatsu in the puerperium

Uses of shiatsu in the puerperium

- Postnatal depression
- Insufficient breast milk
- General relaxation
- Constipation

Postnatal depression The woman who is susceptible to the 'blues' or extreme tiredness would be advised to consult a qualified therapist as soon as she feels able. The practitioner may treat the woman even while she is breastfeeding, lying on her side. The importance of adequate rest during the puerperium cannot be emphasised enough. The postnatal period, described earlier as one of the 'gateways of change', is a crucial time in a woman's life, when she must take care of herself and replenish all the energy given out during the birth process. The Chinese place so much importance on this period that they also call it 'doing 40 days', where the mother is advised only to care for the baby and to rest; all members of the family and community members take on responsibility for the household chores, so that the mother will fully recover her energy. This is not always possible to achieve today, but the midwife should encourage the woman to rest more. The euphoric energy immediately felt after birth soon wears off and the true state of energy of the mother emerges. Rest, plus several shiatsu sessions, can help to boost the mother's Ki so that postnatal depression is less likely to develop. If rest is not possible during the night because of an unhappy, crying infant, shiatsu for the neonate may be helpful.

Insufficient breast milk One of the reasons for this condition is depletion of the mother's Blood after birth and exhaustion of energy. Shiatsu sessions from a qualified therapist will aid relaxation in order to build the mother's Ki. Concentration on work on the Stomach and Spleen meridians will help build up quality reserves of milk, as will work on the Kidney meridian which helps build vital energy.

Shiatsu massage for the neonate

Shiatsu baby massage is actually a combination of Swedish massage and shiatsu techniques, mainly done directly on the baby's skin using oil. In many cases the relaxation of the baby achieved through the massage will help the mother to rest and relax as well. Learning how to massage the infant can be extremely useful to both mother and baby. If the neonate is happy and relaxed it will sleep, thereby enabling the mother to rest.

In terms of Chinese medicine a woman's Ki and blood go into making breast milk. Exhausted mothers do not make adequate breast milk. The baby may suck and suck and still not be adequately satisfied; the consequent intake of air in such excessive breast feeding will create colic, leading to pain and crying. The mother naturally tends to try to feed the baby more in order to satisfy him or her, leading to more severe colic. A vicious cycle is produced and the mother will find herself drained through having to get up constantly during the night to try to placate the baby. Conversely if the baby is happy and relaxed with the help of massage, the mother can rest and produce adequate quantities of breast milk to satisfy the baby.

In Dr Montague's book *Touching* (Montague, 1971), he writes:

…the more we learn about the effects of cutaneous (skin) stimulation, the more pervasively significant for healthy development do we find it to be. Stimulation of the skin, cuddling, rocking, massage—increases cardiac output, promotes respiration and develops the efficiency of the gastrointestinal functions of the infant.

Conditions helped by shiatsu baby massage

Shiatsu baby massage: conditions helped

- Colic
- Sleeplessness
- Vomiting, possetting
- Constipation
- Diarrhoea

Colic In the early days there are many occasions when the baby will cry and not settle. For the breastfeeding mother requiring analgesia this may be explained in terms of Chinese medicine as 'cold producing' (Scott, 1991). This 'cold' is then transferred to the mother's milk and passes through to the baby via breastfeeding. Cold contracts, and it is this that produces the pain in the infant's digestive system. Other foods that are cold in nature are bananas, dairy products, grapes and their derivatives, e.g. champagne! When such foods are eaten by the breastfeeding mother, the cold quality of them is also transferred to the baby via the breast milk, thereby causing digestive pain to the infant.

When abdominal massage is performed on the baby in combination with the techniques below it will help to 'move and warm' the Ki of the abdomen and strengthen the digestion, thereby relieving colic (Fig. 9.17).

The shiatsu practitioner, appropriately trained midwife or the mother

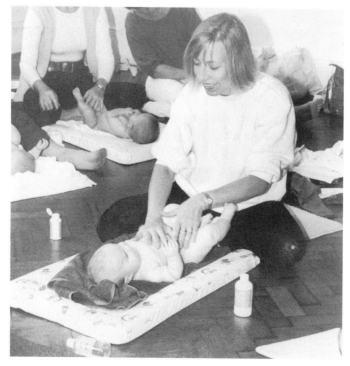

Fig. 9.17. Abdominal massage for the relief of neonatal colic.

should use relaxed fingertips and hands to massage the abdomen in a clockwise direction, hand over hand, following the natural flow of peristalsis of the digestive tract. With the pad of the index finger, gently press Conception Vessel 12 three times, then massage with the fingertips the left side of the baby's abdomen over the descending colon. This process is repeated three times followed by clockwise abdominal massage. Massage up the infant's Spleen meridian in the inner leg and down the Stomach meridian on the lateral thigh. Press point Stomach 36 gently three times.

Sleeplessness   A complete daily body shiatsu massage can help relax the baby and increase circulation, fostering sleep. This is most effective to induce sleep an hour after the last feed before bedtime.

Vomiting and possetting   Where there is no organic malfunction of the digestive tract such as pyloric stenosis or hiatus hernia, then shiatsu massage can help the baby who vomits. In addition to daily massage, the techniques described for the treatment of colic, with the addition of the point Stomach 34, can be helpful. The mother should be advised to keep the infant in as upright a position as possible directly after a feed.

Information about mother and baby shiatsu massage classes (Fig. 9.18) is available through the Shiatsu Society.

Conditions amenable to shiatsu baby massage during the first and second years of life

- Constipation
- Diarrhoea
- Teething
- Earache
- Restlessness

- Bedwetting
- Poor appetite
- Insomnia
- Excess catarrh
- Coughs

Fig. 9.18. Mother and baby shiatsu massage class.

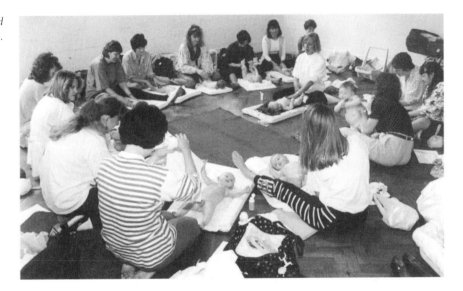

Conclusion   Although a full shiatsu training is 3 years long it would be useful for one or two midwives within a maternity unit to undertake that training. They would be able to offer at least a limited service to mothers. Other midwives could attend specific short courses for midwives to enable them to learn the techniques sufficiently to use them safely as a complement to their normal midwifery practice.

Midwives may also wish to forge links with local reputable shiatsu practitioners with experience and a special interest in dealing with mothers and their babies. Practitioners could be encouraged to communicate with the maternity unit and could be invited to conduct ante- or postnatal classes with the midwives. Shiatsu has a great deal to offer for pregnancy, labour and the postnatal and neonatal period. It is a non-invasive and pleasurably relaxing treatment. Midwives can work to increase their understanding of its value for mothers and babies so that clients can obtain the best care possible.

Training

As yet there is no licensing of shiatsu practitioners, therefore legally anyone can practise shiatsu. The Shiatsu Society has been set up to ensure standards of practice. This is an umbrella organisation for all the styles of shiatsu and includes the National Professional Practitioners' Register (set up in 1986) and Assessment Panel. Being a member of the Shiatsu Society (MRSS) guarantees a certain level of competence in practice. The Society's guidelines for training stipulate a minimum study period of 500 hours over a period of at least 3 years. This includes study in Western medicine including anatomy, physiology, and pathology. In order to qualify for inclusion on the Professional Register and to gain MRSS designation, candidates must pass theoretical and practical examinations.

Shiatsu training includes exercises to develop and maintain one's own Ki such as Qi-Gong, lower abdominal breathing and meditation; learning the basis of oriental diagnosis and principles of oriental medical theory; Zen shiatsu theory; shiatsu techniques, use of hara, location of classical and Masanaga meridians, and tsubo function and location; and Western medical study of anatomy, physiology and pathology.

Midwives interested in gaining a professional qualification should contact The Shiatsu Society for further information.

Introductory courses offered by most schools can assist in the fundamental use of one's bodyweight in giving shiatsu.

References

Barsoum G, Perry E P, Fraser I A 1990 Postoperative nausea is relieved by acupressure. *Journal of the Royal Society of Medicine* 83: 86–89

Belluomini J, Litt R C, Lee K A et al. 1994 Acupressure for nausea and vomiting of pregnancy: a randomized blinded study. *Obstetrics and Gynaecology* 84(2): 245–248

De Aloysio D, Penacchioni P 1992 Morning sickness control in early pregnancy by Neiguan point acupressure. *Obstetrics and Gynaecology* 80(5): 852–854

Dundee J W et al. 1988 P6 acupressure reduces morning sickness. *Journal of the Royal Society of Medicine* 81: 456–57

Dundee J W, Yang J 1990 Prolongation of the anti-emetic action of P6 acupuncture by acupressure in patients having cancer chemotherapy. *Journal of the Royal Society of Medicine* 83: 360–362

Evans A T, Samuels S N, Marshall C et al. 1993 Suppression of pregnancy-induced nausea and vomiting with sensory afferent stimulation. *Journal of Reproductive Medicine* 38(8): 303–306

Matsumoto K, Birch S 1988 *Hara Diagnosis: Reflections on the Sea*. Paradigm Publications, MA, USA

Montague A 1971 *Touching*. Harper and Row, New York

Ohashi W 1983 *Natural Childbirth the Eastern Way*. Ballantine Books, New York

Oschman J 1987 *The Connective Tissue and Myofascial Systems*. Aspen Research Institute, Berkeley, CA, USA

Puustjarvi K, Airaksinen O, Pontinen P J 1990 The effects of massage in patients with chronic tension headache. *Acupuncture and Electrotherapy Research* 15: 159–162

Scott J 1991 *Acupuncture in the Treatment of Children*. Eastland Press Inc., USA

Stein D J, Birnbach D J, Danzer B I et al. 1997 Acupressure versus intravenous metoclopramide to prevent nausea and vomiting during spinal anesthesia for caesarean section. *Anesthesia and Analgesia* 84(2): 342–345

Zhejiang College of Traditional Chinese Medicine (ed. B. Flaws) 1987 *Handbook of Traditional Chinese Gynaecology*. Blue Poppy Press, Boulder, CO, USA

Further reading

Flaws R 1983 *The Path of Pregnancy*. Paradigm

Lundberg 1992 *The Book of Shiatsu*. Gaia Books Ltd

Maciocia G 1989 *Foundations of Chinese Medicine*. Churchill Livingstone, Edinburgh

Masunaga, S, Ohashi, W 1977 *Zen Shiatsu*. Japan Publications, New York

Ross J P 1984 *Zang Fu, The Organ Systems of Traditional Chinese Medicine*. Churchill Livingstone, Edinburgh

Fiona Mantle

Chapter 10

The Role of Hypnosis in Pregnancy and Childbirth

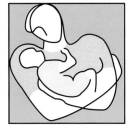

The quest for pain relief in childbirth is as old as time, and through the ages a range of methods has been used in spite of the condemnation of the Christian church. In 1591, for example, Eufame MacLayne was burnt at the stake for requesting pain relief in labour (Brann, 1995). All civilisations have used mind-altering substances either for religious purposes, for enjoyment or for the relief of pain. The main disadvantage to most of these methods as a form of analgesia in childbirth is the concomitant effect on the baby. On the other hand, hypnosis has been used since ancient times as a mind-altering modality and in addition it has the advantage, as far as is known, of being completely safe for both the mother and baby. Hypnosis is usually described as a state of deep physical relaxation with an alert mind producing alpha waves, and it is in this state that critical faculties are suspended and the subconscious mind can be more readily accessed. A similar stage of altered consciousness can also be found in meditation, relaxation and daydreaming. Since most people spend a certain amount of their waking life daydreaming, hypnosis can be said to be a state which occurs naturally. However, in spite of its name hypnotherapy is not a therapy in its own right but a method of delivering a conventional therapy more effectively; an adjunct employed to enhance the effect of an established treatment. The role of hypnosis is probably best explained as putting this daydreaming state to therapeutic use. Key to the daydreaming state is the tuning out of external stimuli; focus of concentration is narrowed and the subject's range of attention is selective, but when cued to an external stimulus the person 'comes to'. This phenomenon is familiar to many people who have had the experience of completing a frequently-travelled route with little recollection of the intervening journey. This has been referred to as 'highway trance'. It has long been debated whether there is, in fact, a separate, distinguishable state of hypnosis (since no physiological differences have been identified between this and other mind–altering states) or whether it is simply the extension of an everyday experience induced by the hypnotherapist. Heap (1996) elegantly summarises the arguments by suggesting that hypnosis is a complex psychological phenomenon based on the interaction of two people—the hypnotist and the subject, in which the former uses verbal suggestions to bring about changes in the subject at the behavioural, cognitive, emotional and physiological levels. The common conception of the hypnotist using a long preamble including progressive relaxation as a way of inducing a trance is now considered unnecessary, except to meet the subject's expectations and enhance motivation (Kirsch, 1991). However, these traditional procedures are excellent ways of reducing tension and arousal which subjects can learn for themselves and are therefore useful as a self-help tool and a coping mechanism.

Heap (1996) points out that the experience of hypnosis is highly subjective and can be accounted for by a wide range of psychological concepts such as compliance (Wagstaff, 1981: 91) or role play (Coe and Sarbin, 1991), and Edmonston (1981) has viewed it as a deep form of relaxation. As Heap (1996) suggests, part of the ongoing problem of understanding hypnosis is the lack of a universally accepted definition, although the effects of hypnosis are real enough to provide a working modality. If we take the concept of the daydreaming state as a non–technical working definition it begs the question as to who can be hypnotised. There are standard scales of hypnotic susceptibility available, but they tend to be used for research purposes where standardisation is important and are rarely useful in the clinical situation. Generally speaking, good hypnotic subjects tend to be creative and imaginative, for example, although in practice most people can attain a useful level of hypnotic trance. Hypnosis is not a means of domination, the surrendering of the will to the therapist, but is best described as a partnership in practice. It can be seen from this description of the phenomenon that it is an entirely natural and empowering process which, when applied to pregnancy and childbirth, allows the woman to work with her body rather than against it during labour.

Antenatal care Although most people associate hypnosis with relief of pain in labour it also has a wider role to play in physical and psychological preparation for childbirth. It can be a very valuable tool in the treatment of antenatal stress or anxiety by using post-hypnotic suggestions, guided imagery or self-hypnosis. Benson (1975) noted that many stressors and potential stressors, which occur naturally in everyday life, can be reduced to manageable levels by the use of only 20 minutes of relaxation a day. Hartland (1982) suggests a range of methods of inducing the hypnotic state including eye fixation, progressive relaxation and trance deepening techniques. Techniques for dealing with stress and anxiety include inducing a state of relaxation in response to the adverse stimuli, which is a more manageable approach than progressive relaxation for which the client is usually required to be sitting or lying down. Another technique which can be used very successfully is the clenched hand technique (Stein, 1963) which involves the identification of a situation which arouses feelings of anxiety followed by identification of a calming, relaxed situation. Under hypnosis the client is conditioned to associate positive feelings with the clenched hand of her choice, a technique which can later be used consciously in situations which produce anxiety.

As well as dealing with emotional difficulties in pregnancy, hypnosis can help with some of the physiological symptoms which women experience. For example, hypnosis has been shown to be useful in regulating autonomic responses such as vasodilation in the treatment of warts, reducing of itching in eczema and modifying allergic responses. Similarly by dealing with the emotional aspect of physiopathology, hypnosis can help to alleviate constipation, nausea and insomnia. Walker et al. (1988) used the 'cued controlled' relaxation with ego strengthening suggestions and gain of control over the nausea associated with chemotherapy patients.

A review of the literature on hyperemesis gravidarum offered by Torem (1994) indicates that emotional factors are implicated in the condition. Fuchs et al. (1980) used hypnosis with positive suggestions in the treatment of 138 pregnant women with hyperemesis gravidarum, with group hypnosis producing better results than individual sessions. Goldman (1990) describes an approach to the problem which involves the removal of any fears about hypnosis along with an explanation of the role of the vomiting centre in the brain and how it works, coupled with a general discussion about the value of good nutrition in pregnancy. Goldman also uses guided imagery, with the mother imagining herself eating, enjoying and retaining familiar foods in a relaxed environment where she feels safe and secure. Harmon et al. (1990) used cued response so that if a woman felt nauseous she would sit down and rest until the nausea diminished. Torem (1994) goes on to describe five case studies which utilised a range of hypnotic techniques. For the treatment of constipation Hartland (1982) used suggestions of warmth in the stomach and bowels together with strengthening of intestinal muscles, a technique which can be successful especially if combined with a planned time for evacuation. Learning relaxation techniques can also facilitate onset and quality of sleep.

Hypnosis has traditionally been associated with helping people to give up smoking. Unfortunately it has not always lived up to its reputation, and in spite of the obvious cause for motivation Valbo and Eide (1996) found that using hypnosis to help mothers to stop smoking during their pregnancy was unsuccessful. The method used included two sessions, backed up with a cassette, enhancing the women's wish to give up smoking. However, this superficial approach does nothing to uncover the subconscious reasons for smoking, which are deep-seated and multi-factorial.

During the antenatal period mothers undergo a range of medical investigations and examinations and, to deal with the fear of these procedures, hypnosis follows the usual principles of alleviation of anxiety, discomfort and pain by suggestion and imagery. Kohen (1980) describes the use of relaxation and well-being as well as distraction and disassociation in the treatment of four cases of women undergoing gynaecological examinations.

On a very hopeful note, Omar et al. (1986) describe the use of hypnosis in the treatment of preterm labour. Thirty-nine mothers with a history of preterm labour were given sessions of hypnotic relaxation in addition to pharmacological intervention, together with a cassette tape to use at home, whilst the control group of 70 women was given pharmacological intervention alone. The rate of pregnancy prolongation was significantly higher in the hypnosis group than in the control group who were given medication alone. The advantage of this intervention was demonstrated by the improved infant birth weight in the experimental group. However, there is no evidence that hypnosis has any effect in the treatment of post-date pregnancies (Omar and Sirkovitz, 1987).

On the other hand, hypnosis proved to be of value in the treatment of breech presentation as Mehl (1994) has demonstrated. One hundred women with a breech presentation at 37 and 40 weeks gestation were matched with a comparison group for obstetric and sociological histories. The experimental group underwent hypnosis which included suggestions for relaxation and the reduction of feelings of fear and anxiety. Hypnosis was provided up until the mother delivered or cephalic version occurred. Successful outcome was measured by either the baby spontaneously converting or external cephalic version being achieved. The results were significant in that the vertex presentation occurred in 81% of the intervention group compared with 48% of the control group, and the investigators concluded that suitably motivated subjects could be treated successfully. They further suggest that psycho-physiological factors might influence the occurrence of breech presentation and that this might explain the frequency of cephalic version following hypnosis.

Mental and physical trauma when associated with childbirth can have long-term repercussions whether it is a result of miscarriage, stillbirth or insensitive handling of unexpected interventions. These previous experiences can spoil the enjoyment of the mother for the next pregnancy. Fortunately there is a range of therapeutic interventions which can help to alleviate this trauma and dissociate the previous pregnancy from the present one so that the mother can approach labour in a more positive way. These techniques usually involve the use of regression to the previous incident, the restructuring or closure of the event, and dismissal. One very good method of doing this is to view the event again as a mental videotape or stage play. The advantage of the video approach is that the client can rewind and re-run the 'tape' as often as she wishes until the scenario is suitably adjusted. The 'video' is then turned off or, in the case of the theatre stage, the curtains are drawn over the incident. In this way a miscarriage or previous traumatic delivery can be separated out from the present pregnancy and whilst the mother will not forget the incident it can be suggested that it will no longer cause her any emotional upset since it is 'in the past'. Occasionally problems can arise when the client's emotions impede the restructuring or the client feels that they are unable to revisit the incident because it was too traumatic. In these circumstances another technique can be used, called the bubble technique. This involves imagining a safe, protective, but clear shell around oneself to isolate and protect.

Care in labour   Although Grantly Dick-Read, who identified the fear–tension–pain syndrome, denied that his method of education, relaxation and suggestion for childbirth had anything to do with hypnosis it is clear that much of his technique involved a hypnotic approach. His methods involved teaching mothers the physiological mechanics of labour coupled with deep relaxation techniques as well as the suggestion that the mother would be calm and relaxed and, therefore, feel no pain. Heron and Abramson (1952) identified several advantages of hypnosis over other methods of analgesia in childbirth. They point out that it has the facility to increase the mother's ability to relax both mentally and physically and that the mother can be taught how to gain control over her bodily functions, thus reducing the tension and fear which contribute to pain.

Since hypnosis does not involve the use of any adverse substances it has no known effect on maternal or fetal respiratory function, whereas the side-effects of most conventional forms of analgesia are prejudicial to the baby. In addition hypnosis may shorten the first stage of labour, thus preventing the mother from becoming too tired (although it may lengthen the second stage slightly); it has no depressing effect on uterine contractions and does not appear to interfere in any way with normal labour. Any additional analgesia which may be requested by the mother can usually be given in reduced dosages. Mothers feel more relaxed and alert following hypnosis as opposed to conventional drugs, and lactation can be stimulated and facilitated by direct suggestion under hypnosis with cued responses being given to the mother to use at home. Objections to the use of hypnosis as a form of analgesia usually revolve around issues of religion, or fear of loss of autonomy, which is easily countered by a good explanation of the nature of hypnosis, the susceptibility of the client and the varying degrees of analgesia which can be obtained.

Early hypnosis techniques mentioned by Hartland (1982) concentrated on obtaining complete analgesia, utilising the suggestion that the mother would fall into a deep sleep as soon as the baby was born and forget about what had happened! A more modern approach emphasises the mother's control over her body and emotions and stresses the role of hypnosis in the antenatal period.

Hilgard and Hilgard (1983) discuss eight hypnotic techniques which can be usefully employed in labour. Hypnosis during pregnancy can provide a valuable medium for the mother to rehearse the labour, to become familiar with it and to increase her confidence in her ability to cope. Hilgard and Hilgard also suggest that by going through the process of labour perceptions are changed, and that mothers look forward to the experience with confidence and are able to anticipate a pleasurable outcome. Relaxation has been discussed earlier, but its continuing value must be acknowledged. Symptom substitution reduces the perception of pain by substituting the experience of pain with something else. Akin to this is the technique of symptom displacement. Hilgard and Hilgard suggest that a good substitution during labour might be the transferring of the rhythmic contractions of the uterus to the clenching and unclenching of the hand in time to the contractions. Direct suggestion might be in the form of the mother imagining that she is experiencing no pain from the waist down. Transfer of location of analgesia, a technique which is derived from dentistry, involves the mother inducing numbness in her fingers and transferring this sensation to her abdomen. In using disassociation the mother imagines she is elsewhere and views what is happening from there. All these techniques also include a post-hypnotic suggestion of confidence, happiness and well-being.

Effects on labour

As Mairs (1995) points out, the quality and quantity of a person's experience of pain is the result of a variety of factors which include the underlying cause of the pain, the person's cultural background and the ethos of that culture to pain. In addition to the previous experience of pain, other factors include physical and emotional well-being or ill health. Modern theories of pain and greater insight into the nature of pain (which considers the psychological factors to be extremely important) suggest that hypnotic interventions, when used properly, can modify the client's perception of pain in more than one of its components (Gibson and Heap, 1991). The use of hypnosis in the treatment of anxiety has been discussed earlier in the chapter and it is this which contributes most to the alleviation of pain. Heap and Dryden (1993) point out that it is not just the induction of very deep relaxation which influences pain perception (although clearly it reduces tension) but the fact that hypnosis can help clients to manage their anxiety in a variety of very positive ways which is instrumental to pain relief, particularly in maternity care. There is a considerable body of evidence to suggest that hypnosis can have a very positive effect on the whole experience of labour. Davidson (1962) and Connelly (1989) noted that hypnotic preparation of mothers resulted in less requirement for analgesia. Barber (1986) suggests that altering the perception of pain is the most important weapon in dealing with it and suggests that it is a shift of consciousness which allows this to happen. Even though mothers look upon childbirth as an essentially positive experience they do experience a certain level of anxiety and, since the link between anxiety and pain is well established, any mechanism which reduces the mother's levels of anxiety will help to reduce the pain. This has been demonstrated in a number of studies. Jenkins and Pritchard (1993) found that overall, mothers who were hypnotised used less analgesia, with some women requiring none at all. The length of the first stage of labour in hypnotised primigravidae compared favourably with the non-hypnotised multiparae. In the study, hypnosis was also associated with a 25% shorter mean second stage in primigravidae but indicated no difference between the two parous groups. In spite of the hypnosis, the mean duration of the second stage in the primigravidae was still longer than that in multiparae in both groups. The authors concluded that the results indicated that the advantages of hypnosis during labour and delivery are considerably more than those of relaxation alone and that hypnosis has additional benefits in the reduced amount of analgesia required and a shorter period of labour. It must be emphasised that the results refer to normal labour and that the main effect of the hypnosis is the higher levels of relaxation which can be achieved. Harmon et al. (1990) used a randomised control trial with hypnosis subjects and controls who had already enrolled into childbirth education classes. Both groups were offered additional childbirth preparation, one group having hypnosis and the control group a standard relaxation tape. Results indicated that labour was shorter in stage one for the hypnosis group, who also used less medication and had more spontaneous deliveries and higher Apgar scores than the control. The authors believe that these positive outcomes were the result of the hypnosis; specifically, the women had reduced perceptions of pain rather than being able to tolerate pain better, a point made by Grantly Dick-Read some 50 years ago. Mairs (1995) studied 28 primigravid women whose experiences were compared with 27 primigravidae who did not use hypnosis. All the women were volunteers who were already attending antenatal classes and were between 26 and 37 weeks pregnant. In this particular study, there was no significant difference between the hypnosis and the non-hypnosis group in drug usage and the duration of labour. However, the study did show that hypnosis helped to alleviate the anxieties around unplanned caesarean section. The subjects filled in a pre-birth questionnaire and were asked to rate, on a ten point scale, their anticipated levels of anxiety and pain for three time periods: early labour, delivery and postnatal. A postnatal questionnaire completed 2–14 days postnatally documented their actual perceptions of pain and anxiety on a ten point scale. Results showed that there was no difference between the groups on levels of anticipated pain, but the subjects who used hypnosis experienced less pain during labour. Although experience of pain during incision for episiotomy was not significantly different, less post-episiotomy pain was felt by the hypnosis group. The hypnosis group reported feeling more control over their anxiety, which may have influenced their perception of pain and increased their ability to cope.

Safety

Bearing in mind that hypnosis is a naturally occurring phenomenon which we have all experienced many times during our lives it can be assumed that there is no intrinsic danger when used by an appropriately qualified professional who acknowledges the parameters of professional practice. Careful history-taking is vital; for example, before suggesting that the client visualise a country scene it is advisable to check that they do not suffer from hayfever, and any phobias or situations which might cause distress need to be ascertained. The worst side-effect is usually that the client falls asleep during the treatment. The one group of people for whom hypnosis is contraindicated are those who have any history of psychosis.

Non-therapeutic hypnosis and its misuse From time to time, usually as a result of the totally inappropriate use of hypnosis for so called 'entertainment', a court case occurs which casts doubt upon the safety of hypnosis as a useful therapy. In these instances the subject is invited on to the stage without any psychological or physical assessment relating to past history or present state, and is then induced to behave in a way which incites ridicule and humiliation in front of friends and often a wider audience. This in itself is enough to damage seriously the integrity of the person's self-image and result in feelings of insecurity, depression and distrust of friends and family. It is not the hypnosis itself which has caused the trauma but the way in which it has been used.

Conclusion

Hypnosis is a gentle, safe and effective therapy which can, after appropriate training, be used by midwives and health visitors within the scope of professional practice. It has a range of applications to maternity care, both physical and psychological, which can be of considerable benefit to mothers and bring professional satisfaction to the practitioner.

Training

The British Society of Experimental and Clinical Hypnosis runs diploma and M.Sc. courses at London and Sheffield Universities and will accept membership from healthcare professionals who subscribe to a code of professional practice, such as nurses, midwives and health visitors.

References

Barber J 1986 Hypnotic analgesia. In: Holtzman A, Turk D (eds) *A Handbook of Psychological Treatments*. Academic Press, New York

Benson H 1975 *The Relaxation Response*. Aron, New York

Brann L 1995 The role of hypnosis in obstetrics. *The Diplomate* 2, 2: 95

Coe W, Sarbin T 1991 Role theory. Hypnosis from a dramaturgical and narrational perspective. In: Lynn S, Rhue J (eds) *Theories of Hypnosis, General Models and Perspectives*. Guildford Press, New York

Connelly D 1989 A comparison of drug usage between mothers who have trained in self hypnosis and those who have no hypnosis training. Presentation to the Irish Branch of the British Society of Experimental and Clinical Hypnosis, Belfast.

Davidson J 1962 An assessment of the value of hypnosis in pregnancy and labour. *British Medical Journal* 11: 951

Edmonston W 1981 Hypnosis and Relaxation: Modern Verification of an Old Equation. Wiley, New York

Fuchs K, Paldi H, Abramovici H et al. 1980 Treatment of hyperemesis gravidarum by hypnosis. *International Journal of Clinical and Experimental Hypnosis* 28: 313

Goldman L 1990 Control of hyperemesis. In: Hammond D (ed.) *Handbook of Hypnotic Suggestions and Metaphors*. Norton, New York

Harmon T, Hynan M, Tyre T 1990 Improved obstetric outcomes using hypnotic analgesia and skill mastery combined with childbirth education. *Journal of Consulting and Clinical Psychology* 58, 5: 525

Hartland J 1982 *Medical and Dental Hypnosis and Its Clinical Applications*. Baillière Tindall, London

Heap M, Dryden W 1993 *Hypnotherapy: a Handbook*. Open University, Milton Keynes, UK

Heap M 1996 Special hypnosis supplement. *The Psychologist* 9, 11: 498

Heron W, Abramson M 1952 Hypnosis in obstetrics. In: Le Con A (ed.) *Experimental Hypnosis*. Macmillan, New York

Hilgard E, Hilgard J 1983 *Hypnosis in the Relief of Pain*. Kaufmann Inc., Los Altos, CA, USA

Jenkins M, Pritchard M 1993 Hypnosis: practical applications and theoretical considerations in normal labour. *British Journal of Obstetrics and Gynaecology* 100: 221

Kirsch I 1991 The social learning theory of hypnosis. In: Lynn S, Rhue J (eds) *Theories of Hypnosis, Current Models and Perspectives*. Guildford Press, New York

Kohen D 1980 Relaxation/mental imagery (self hypnosis) and pelvic examinations in adolescents. *Developmental and Behavioural Paediatrics* 1: 180

Mairs D 1995 Hypnosis and pain in childbirth. *Contemporary Hypnosis* 12, 2: 11

Mehl L 1994 Hypnosis and conversion of the breech to vertex presentation. *Archives of Family Medicine* 3, 10: 881

Omar H, Friedlander D, Palti Z 1986 Hypnotic relaxation in the treatment of premature labour. *Psychosomatic Medicine* 48, 5: 351

Omar H, Sirkovitz A 1987 Failure of hypnotic relaxation in the treatment of post-term pregnancies. *Psychosomatic Medicine* 49(6): 606

Stein C 1963 The clenched fist technique as a hypnotic procedure in clinical psychotherapy. *American Journal of Clinical Hypnosis* 6: 113

Torem M 1994 Hypnotherapeutic techniques in the treatment of hyperemesis gravidarum. *American Journal of Clinical Hypnosis* 37, 1: 1

Valbo A, Eide T 1996 Smoking cessation in pregnancy; the effects of hypnosis in a randomised study. *Addictive Behaviours* 21, 1: 29

Walker L, Dawson A, Pollet S et al. 1988 Hypnotherapy for chemotherapy side effects. *British Journal of Experimental and Clinical Hypnosis* 5: 79

Wagstaff G 1981 *Hypnosis Compliance and Belief.* Harvester Press, Brighton, UK

Wagstaff G 1991 Compliance, belief and semantics in hypnosis. A non state socio-cognitive perspective. In: Lynn S, Rhue J (eds) *Theories of Hypnosis, Current Models and Perspectives.* Guildford Press, New York

Dianne Garland

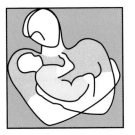

Chapter 11
The Uses of Hydrotherapy in Today's Midwifery Practice

Continuing advances in medical technology have totally altered both the nature and pattern of care offered to pregnant women today. The tide of social change in care provision will, in the next few years, move the power base from professionals to clients, particularly as a result of the most recent report on 'Changing childbirth' (Department of Health, 1993).

For many years pioneers of alternative maternity care have been striving to develop a gentler approach to labour and delivery. Frederick LeBoyer's *Birth Without Violence* (1975) attempted to affect the way in which obstetrics was practised in Western countries. The technological age was advancing and LeBoyer's work was a starting point on the long road to change. Although the book was written nearly 25 years ago his words still have as much relevance today as they did then:

'We were wondering about how best to prepare the child ... now we can see it's not the child that needs to be prepared. It is ourselves. It is our eyes that need to open, our blindness that has to stop. If we used just a little intelligence how simple things could be.'

Another French pioneer brought to the forefront the continuing medicalisation of childbirth and the need to relearn our cultural and social skills that are linked to childbirth. In *Entering the World* (1984) Michel Odent supported the theory that a known caregiver and an environment conducive to regaining and retaining a sense of dignity and identity would do much to enhance a woman's labour and delivery.

Midwives wishing to implement the use of water for labour and delivery are likely already to respect these values and attitudes for the care of women. For those who seek a deeper spiritual philosophy for the use of water the writings of Michel Odent (1990) and S. Ray (1986) can lead them into a fascinating exploration of birth.

Water does seem to possess powers of recuperation, for example visitors to Niagara or Victoria Falls cannot fail to be inspired by the strength and beauty of the cascading water. For many people their holidays are spent by water, by the sea or mountain lakes, or even skiing, on frozen water. At the end of a long tiring day many people will seek seclusion and relaxation by taking a bath. Is it so surprising therefore that many women find water for labour so inviting?

Aquanatal swimming

It is not a prerequisite that women considering the use of water during labour should attend prenatal or 'aquanatal' classes. However, these sessions at which exercises to music are practised in the pool may help women to determine whether or not they like the flotation sensation, as this environment may require a period of adjustment (Garland and Ford, 1989).

Exercising in water (Figs 11.1, 11.2) can be a pleasurable experience and a social event for pregnant and newly delivered women. It is a way of empowering them to regain control over their bodies and, as Oudshoorn (1990) writes, is designed to maintain general condition and muscle function and improve circulation. The mothers are encouraged to practise relaxation techniques, and controlled breathing and floating in water facilitates this.

Fig. 11.1. Aquanatal exercises.

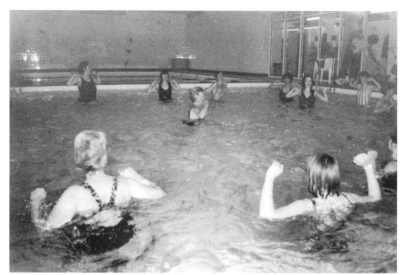

Fig. 11.2. Aquanatal relaxation.

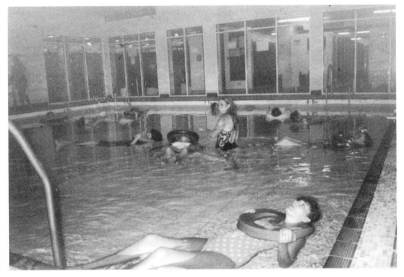

The combination of practising exercises and the water tension means it is especially effective in relieving aches and pains such as backache or the throbbing of varicosities.

In addition for some women, negative perceptions of self-image related to their enlarging shape may be overcome while in the water. Mothers-to-be gain a freedom of movement they may not have felt for some time, particularly towards term. In a non-threatening environment the 'hidden' body is free to move and relax without the full force of gravity.

Aquanatal classes may replace or augment conventional parent education classes, but in either case, being with other women with similar interests in the use of water for labour and delivery can facilitate a sharing of fears and aspirations about the situation. Where there are mothers present who have delivered previously in water this can also be helpful. There are several physiological advantages of exercising in water during pregnancy. It is thought that uterine blood flow may be increased as a result of increased central blood flow due to extravascular fluid being pushed into the vascular spaces by the hydrostatic force of the water. This in turn encourages diuresis and can assist in reducing oedema (Katz, 1996). McMurray et al. (1993), Katz (1996) and Watson et al. (1991) found that the thermoregulatory effect of the water resulted in fewer fetal heart rate changes than in women who exercised on land.

Postnatally it may be possible to continue the classes, or perhaps to run them concurrently for ante-and postnatal mothers. This may be a way of encouraging the women to continue postnatal exercises and so facilitate the shedding of extra weight and adipose tissue acquired during pregnancy (Baddeley, 1993).

Before commencing aquanatal classes midwives should consider the following issues:

- Pool suitability—graduated pools with a shallow and a deep end are preferable to enable non-swimmers to join in and to provide variation in water pressure for different exercises.
- The temperature of the water should be between 29°C and 30°C as this reduces tension and relaxes muscles. If the water is too hot the women may feel dizzy and faint or if it is too cool they may be susceptible to muscle cramps.
- Arranging for exclusive use of the pool during classes facilitates a more relaxed environment and ensures privacy. Clarification should be sought as to the cost of hiring the pool and whether this will include the entrance fee for the mothers or if they will need to pay for themselves.
- There should be at least two midwives present for the classes, one to demonstrate the various exercises at the side of the pool and one to be in the pool assisting the women. The midwives should hold either Amateur Swimming Association or specific 'Aquafit' certificates as well as a life saving certificate if there is no other life saver at the pool.
- Midwives must refer to the relevant professional documents such as the UKCC's *Code of Practice* (1994) and *Scope of Practice* (1992).
- It may be necessary to review personal indemnity insurance cover as midwives may be conducting these classes outside their normal work parameters, perhaps because of their own interest, and would be considered to be working independently.
- Carrying out a local survey of mothers' wishes will determine the demand for aquanatal classes; various means of advertising the classes should be utilised.
- Careful screening of mothers wishing to commence the classes should ensure that anyone with a medical or obstetric problem obtains the approval of the obstetrician to do so.
- It may be necessary to arrange creche facilities.
- A portable, battery-operated cassette player should be available for music.
- There should also be a variety of flotation aids available such as rubber rings and inflatable neck supports.
- Comfortable swimwear is essential for mothers and midwives.

The use of water for labour and delivery

The demand to set up a waterbirth service has often come from the consumers, and midwives should of course act as the mothers' advocate, but it is easy to become so enthusiastic that the importance of adequate planning can be overlooked. The *Midwives' Rules and Code of Practice* states that 'some developments in midwifery care can become an integral part of the role of the midwife' (UKCC, 1998). The Code emphasises that each midwife should acquire competence in new skills through adequate preparation.

Midwives spend a great deal of time, following qualification, in developing advanced skills and knowledge, and this section of the code addresses this in relation to water labour and birth.

In some maternity units delivering babies under water is seen as an extension of normal midwifery practice with practitioners regaining 'lost' skills such as physiological third stage management. Midwives are expected to seek out appropriate opportunities for gaining experience. Managers and supervisors in other centres have decided that this aspect of care should be viewed as part of the scope of practice (UKCC, 1992), and specify a requirement for midwives to attend lectures and conduct a certain number of waterbirths under supervision. Each unit must develop the most appropriate way of training its staff, in conjunction with the midwives themselves, supervisors of midwives and medical colleagues. Many excellent study days and opportunities for networking are now available and midwives should scan the professional journals for relevant advertisements.

Midwives are also advised to communicate with those from other units where waterbirths are an established part of the maternity service, in order to share achievements and examine potential or actual problems. Skill sharing is of paramount importance, locally, regionally and nationally, and because of the sporadic availability of waterbirths so far, issues common to several units can be identified.

Similarly there needs to be good teamwork between the midwives and medical staff right from the start of the project. Some units have been able to devise protocols for waterbirths jointly with midwives, obstetricians, paediatricians and microbiologists in the planning groups. Increasingly units offering waterbirths are developing policies to cover as many issues as possible.

Reviewing currently available literature, both on maternal and neonatal physiology and on recent research trials, can enable revision of basic theory relevant to the practice of waterbirth and an exploration of statistical evidence on a variety of issues (Brown, 1982; Gradert et al., 1987; Dane, 1987; Milner, 1988).

Simulation exercises are a useful means of discussing the management of practicalities such as assisting the mother in and out of the tub, or dealing with obstetric and paediatric problems in the bathroom, such as haemorrhage or shoulder dystocia. Positioning of necessary equipment in the bathroom, and health and safety issues such as care of the midwife's back, can also be considered. If possible, observation of a colleague conducting a delivery with the mother in water is a valuable exercise. Reflecting on the episode may raise additional issues.

Suitable facilities for conducting water labours and deliveries Some units who have attempted to set up facilities for waterbirths have experienced major difficulties with finding suitable tubs and adequate space in which to put them. Several types of tubs are now available, both portable and those which can be installed into the plumbing system in the unit. The tubs may differ in shape and size but have similarities regarding depth, temperature maintenance and cleansing. Some units have specified the ease and speed of water drainage as being important in the event of maternal problems, but in reality it is more practical to ask the mother to leave the water rather than attempt to drain the tub.

When selecting a tub suitable for the labour ward, the following factors need to be considered:

* The weight of the pool when full of water, remembering that one gallon weighs ten pounds, and waterbirth tubs hold 100 gallons. It may be necessary to involve the engineers and building and works departments in hospitals. The weight of the tub has posed a particular problem for women who have hired pools for use at a home birth, only to find that the floor was not substantial enough to support the tub.
* The depth and width of the tub to allow the midwife easy access to the mother whilst providing space for the mother to move around in the water.
* Systems for filling and draining the pool and for filtering out debris such as meconium, blood and membranes. It may be necessary to check with the hospital engineers, especially for tubs which drain into the main hospital drainage system. A plastic, easily sterilised sieve or small fishing net could be used to remove some debris.
* Thermostatic control in order to maintain the water temperature (portable tubs usually have a thermo-cover included to maintain the heat until full). A thermometer such as those used in aquaria will help the midwife to check the temperature of the water once the mother is in the tub.
* A policy for cleaning the tub after use to avoid the risk of cross-infection. Disposable liners may be available for certain types of tub.
* Local availability of the tubs with an opportunity to observe the ease and speed of preparing them prior to hire or purchase.
* Cost—and the source of funding. In some units midwives have entered enthusiastically into innovative methods of fundraising.

If the midwife is caring for a mother anticipating a water birth in the home it is normally the responsibility of the family to sort out the practical details and arrange for hire and arrival of the tub. This would include checking structural support of floors, covering, with child safety covers, of electrical sockets in the relevant room to avoid the effects of humidity, and insurance of the building and the contents in case of disasters.

An additional source of water may also be required in the home as most domestic water tanks hold between 40 and 70 gallons, compared with the 100-gallon waterbirth tub.

Other useful equipment Although continuous routine fetal monitoring should be unnecessary for women in the bath, a monitor suitable for use in water will be needed for auscultating the fetal heart. A battery-operated mucus extractor may also be required.

Floatation aids to ensure the mother's comfort should be available, and a battery-operated cassette player to enable the mother to listen to music will add to her comfort.

Fans to keep the mother and midwife cool can also be useful. Some waterbirthing equipment is shown in Fig. 11.3.

Preparation of mothers who wish to use water for labour and birth As stated previously, aquanatal exercise is not a vital prerequisite for water labour and birth, but it is important to plan the care and discuss with the parents the relevant mutually-agreed 'ground rules' for the event. For example the mother will need to understand that if the midwife requests her to leave the tub it is for a matter of safety. Parents should be offered sufficient information to enable them to make an informed choice about waterbirth, as with any other aspect of their care. Midwives should recognise that acknowledging their own limitations is not an admission of inadequacy but rather enables parents to understand the parameters of the situation and engenders a feeling of trust and confidence. This is particularly so in the early days as units work to establish a waterbirth service. Some maternity units offer special waterbirth classes for interested parents to enable them to find out information and to discuss practicalities with midwives and with other parents. Other units see their waterbirth service as a normal part of the care available to all low-risk women and incorporate the relevant information into conventional parent education classes.

Fig. 11.3. Waterbirthing equipment.

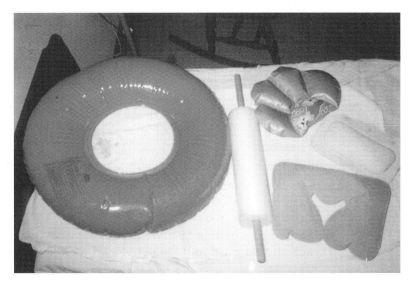

Criteria for agreeing mothers suitable for water labour and delivery

In conjunction with the obstetric team it is important to identify selection criteria and to adhere to these when introducing the concept of waterbirth to parents.

Details of the medical and obstetric history should be examined to elicit any existing or potential problems. Towards term the progress of the current pregnancy should be reviewed and decisions made, according to locally agreed criteria, about mothers with complications such as hypertension, haemorrhage or anaemia.

Whilst women within a very wide spectrum of normality are recorded as labouring and delivering in water, there have also been anecdotal accounts of water deliveries of breech presentations, twins, and women who have had a previous Caesarean section. Individual units must identify those criteria for 'normality' which are most appropriate, and may reflect other policies within that unit, for example the care of a woman with a uterine scar.

Policies and guidelines

Before introducing a service of water labour and births it is important to draw up protocols. Adverse publicity in 1993 regarding the temperature of the water has resulted in units working together to design universal guidelines.

Maternity units such as Maidstone in Kent have been offering waterbirths for several years and have adapted their protocol in response to suggestions from midwives, mothers and medical staff and after reflection on early experiences. The following points for possible guidelines are based on those currently available at the Maidstone unit.

It is considered that the clinical judgement of the midwife is paramount; if a midwife feels it is necessary to ask a mother to leave a water tub for medical reasons the mother must understand the situation. This is explained at parent education classes and when parents are seen individually about their wishes for a water labour.

The unit's guidelines reflect the criteria of 'normality' as specified by the midwives, obstetricians and paediatricians. It is preferred that there should be no known or envisaged problems in labour and that the gestation of pregnancy should be at least 37 weeks. Mothers requiring induction of labour with either amniotomy or prostin pessaries may use the tubs if there are no other known problems. Labour needs to be established before immersion to facilitate the enhancement of uterine activity, which does not seem to occur if the woman is in early labour (Lenstrup et al., 1987).

Although women whose diastolic blood pressure is more than 90 mmHg at the onset of labour are generally discouraged from using the tubs, those who have had mild hypertension in pregnancy may use them, as evidence suggests that relaxing in water can reduce blood pressure. Mothers who have had a previous caesarean section are not offered hydrotherapy as the effects of intrauterine pressure changes as a result of immersion in water have not been evaluated. Once the membranes have ruptured the mother may stay in the tub for up to 24 hours, as is the practice with other women without obstetric complications, although experience has shown that women do not normally need more than 5 hours in the water to complete their labours.

As the water is primarily used as a means of relieving pain in labour (Kroska and Carroll, 1982; Brown, 1982; Dane, 1987; Milner, 1988) the only other form of analgesia offered to mothers in the tubs is inhalational analgesia.

All maternal and fetal observations need to be carried out as agreed, with a monitor suitable for use in water being available (Fig. 11.4); a baseline cardiotocograph may be useful in case of problems later in the labour (Gibb, 1992). Some other waterbirthing equipment is shown in Fig. 11.5.

In order to keep the mother as comfortable as possible the flotation aids can be used to support her head and neck, and she should be encouraged to drink plenty to avoid dehydration in the warm room. Midwives too should be allowed to drink frequently as the room will naturally be even warmer than the normal labour rooms. These aspects must be discussed before waterbirths are commenced, particularly in units where there is a policy of fluid restriction in labour.

To prevent the risk of infection and to keep the water clear enough to observe any blood or meconium passed from the vagina, a sieve should be used to remove debris. As with other deliveries it is recommended that gloves are worn for any necessary examinations per vaginam. The temperature of the water is maintained between 33°C and 40°C in the first stage and at a constant 37–37.5°C in the second stage, during which period it

Fig. 11.4. Monitor.

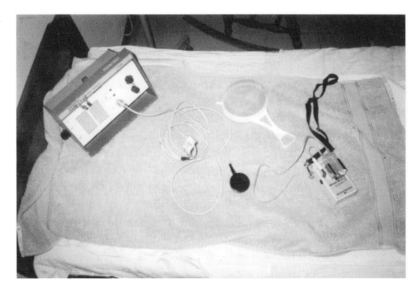

Fig. 11.5. Other waterbirthing equipment.

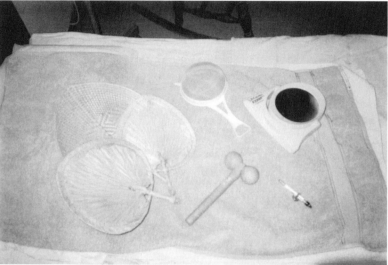

is recorded quarter-hourly. It is likely that initiation of respiration in the baby may occur if the temperature is cooler than this in the second stage.

Due to the effects of water on skin elasticity it is probable that minimal control of the fetal presenting part will be required in the second stage and that perineal trauma will be slight. However when suturing is required it may be necessary to delay the procedure as the tissues of the perineum may initially be saturated with water.

As the baby is delivered he or she should be kept totally under the water to prevent respiration in response to the colder air, but he should be brought to the surface promptly as hypoxia may occur if the placenta begins to separate while the baby is submerged. There is no evidence to suggest a risk of water embolism, so if the mother wishes the cord can be clamped and cut after it has stopped pulsating. However, under no circumstances should the cord be under water when it is clamped and cut.

Most women should be able to expel the placenta spontaneously if the first and second stages have been normal; therefore it should not be necessary to administer an oxytocic drug. Third stage management may vary according to the condition and wishes of the mother, but it is often preferred that either the mother leaves the tub or the water is drained out. If the mother remains in the water for the third stage, blood clots will need to be collected using a sieve and estimated as either less than or more than 500 ml, as it is not feasible to record the blood loss any more accurately than this.

In an emergency the mother should be asked to leave the water for appropriate treatment.

The Maidstone unit does not have a second midwife present at deliveries in water as it is not normal policy to do so for any normal delivery, unless the midwife requires assistance or is working with a colleague for educational purposes.

Midwives should take account of their own positions when leaning over the tubs. Balaskas and Gordon (1990) suggest that midwives should undertake back strengthening exercises in an attempt to prevent injury, and certainly the health and safety issues should be considered in advance.

The need for research and audit Reports that two babies had died as a result of their mothers delivering in water hit the headlines in late 1993 (*Daily Telegraph* 15/10/93) and *Sunday Times*, 17/10/93) and attention was drawn to the lack of reliable research and audit. Some units are actually auditing their own statistics, and some have been published (Burns and Greenish, 1993; Garland and Jones, 1994). It is noticeable that certain accepted medical practices have been adopted without initial research or later evaluation, yet this is a popular criticism levelled at any complementary therapy or alternative strategy in midwifery or nursing.

The need for reliable audit was highlighted by McGraw (1989):

> Throughout the struggles over [these] innovations in childbirth, proponents have all too often made broad sweeping and unsupported claims about the lasting benefits of these changes. Similarly opponents have frequently predicted dire calamities, also with limited supporting evidence, if such innovations are adopted ... It is naive to assume that mere anecdotal evidence or assertions that [their] innovation is more natural will lead to its adoption by a medical profession that prides itself on its objectivity and scientific methods.

This statement, written years ago, appears as relevant today as it did then. Whilst it is true that little pure research exists, much has been written by consumers and professionals. Only through research and audit in units where the service is already offered can water labour and birth be shown to be a safe option for low risk women. Such aspects as outcomes of labour, neonatal Apgar scores, and the rate of complications such as postpartum haemorrhage and maternal or neonatal infections, need to be identified and evaluated. Subjective data on client expectations and satisfaction would be especially valuable in the light of the *Changing Childbirth* report (Department of Health, 1993). In this report the Expert Committee highlighted the need for research into many aspects of midwifery, stating:

> There is a long history in maternity services of well intentioned changes which are not backed up with proper research based evidence to support their introduction ... This is also true for other techniques and practices such as water birth, homeopathy and aromatherapy ... where women express a wish for a particular form of care which has no proven benefits, this fact must be discussed with them openly and fairly.

Waterbirth has much to offer as a means of relaxation and analgesia in labour, and there may be other, as yet undiscovered, benefits to mothers and babies. It is certainly an additional choice for mothers, allowing them greater freedom and control in the labour and delivery.

References

Baddeley S 1993 Aquanatal advantages. *Modern Midwife* July/August

Balaskas J, Gordon Y 1990 *Water Birth.* Unwin, London

Brown C 1982 Therapeutic effects of bathing during labour. *Journal of Nurse-Midwifery* 27(1): 13–16

Burns E, Greenish K 1993 Pooling information. *Nursing Times* 89: 8

Daily Telegraph (15/10/93) Health chief alerted after babies die during water births.

Dane S 1987 Help for mums in labour. *Evening Telegraph* (Peterborough) 9/2/87

Department of Health 1993 *Changing Childbirth.* HMSO, London

Garland D, Ford L 1989 An aqua birth concept. *Midwives Chronicle* July

Garland D, Jones K 1994 Waterbirth, 'first stage' immersion or non immersion? *British Journal of Midwifery* 2(3)

Gibb D 1992 *Fetal Monitoring in Practice.* Butterworth Heinemann, London

Gradert Y, Hertel C, Lenstrup C, Bach F W, Christensen N J, Roseno H 1987 Warm tub bath during labor: effects on plasma catecholamine on endorphin-like immunoreactivity concentrations in the infants at birth. *Acta Obstetrica et Gynaecologica Scandinavica*, 66(8): 681–683

Katz V L 1996 Water exercise in pregnancy. *Seminars in Perinatology* 20(4): 285–291

Kroska R, Carroll M 1982 Use of water in labor. *Birth* 9(1): 47

LeBoyer F 1975 *Birth Without Violence.* Mandarin, London

Lenstrup C. et al. 1987 Warm tub bath during delivery. *Acta Obstetrica et Gynaecologica Scandinavica* 66(8): 709–712

McGraw R 1989 Recent innovation in childbirth. *Journal of Nurse-Midwifery* 34: 4

McMurray R G, Katz V L, Meyer-Goodwin W E et al. 1993 Thermoregulation of pregnant women during aerobic exercise on land and in water. *American Journal of Perinatology* 10(2): 178–182

Milner I 1988 Water baths for pain relief in labour. *Nursing Times* 84(1): 38–40

Odent M 1984 *Entering the World.* Marion Boyars, London

Odent M 1990 *Water and Sexuality* Arkana, USA

Oudshoorn C 1990 Swimming classes for pregnant women. ICM paper

Ray S 1985 *Ideal Birth.* Celestial Arts

Sunday Times (17/10/93) Fears grow over water births as more babies die.

United Kingdom Central Council 1992 *The Scope of Professional Practice*. UKCC, London

United Kingdom Central Council 1998 *Midwives' Rules and Code of Practice*. UKCC, London

Watson W J, Katz V L, Hackney A C et al. 1991 Fetal responses to maximal swimming and cyclin exercise during pregnancy. *Obstetrics and Gynaecology* 77(3): 382–386

Further reading

Artol R 1991 *Exercises in Pregnancy*, 2nd edn. Williams & Wilkins, Baltimore

Garland D 1996 *Waterbirth: an Attitude to Care*. Hale Books for Midwives, London

Hawksworth C 1994 *Aquanatal Exercises*. Hale Books for Midwives, London

McCandlish R et al. 1993 Immersion in water during labour and birth. *Birth* 20: 2

Sue Mack, Dianne Steele

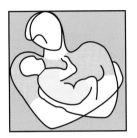

Chapter 12 Complementary Therapies for the Relief of Physical and Emotional Stress

What is stress? There cannot be life without stress. It is the physiological/psychological spur that makes us get up and go and carries us through the day. Positive stress, coped with by the individual, can produce a feeling of satisfaction, happiness or even euphoria. Negative stress, not coped with, can produce illness, fatigue or breakdown. Thus it is both the kind of stress, its origin and intensity, and the coping mechanism of the individual that determines the effect of stress.

The word stress comes from the Old French *estresse*, which means narrowness or oppression; this is exactly how many people would describe the feeling of being stressed.

Stress may be best defined from its effects. We may consider this on a simple cause and effect model, that is stress ⇒ strain. Noise may lead to headache, conflict may result in anger. This system while offering a simple explanation takes no account of the individual's response to stress.

We share with all animals a primitive physiological response to stress, the fight/flight mechanism. This is triggered whatever the stressor, and is not within our control. Hans Seyle (Seyle, 1956), an endocrinologist, studied the physiological effects of stress and developed a theory he called the General Adaptation Syndrome (GAS) to describe the common human response. The three stages of GAS are first alarm, secondly resistance and finally exhaustion. Thus many stimuli result in the same pattern of response.

This is in part affected by the interpretation of the stimuli by the individual. The alarm phase provokes a quick response including lowered blood pressure and tachychardia. The resistance phase is the body's fight back. There is increasing production of adrenocorticotrophic hormones, with raised blood pressure and heart rate. If this is prolonged and the adaptation required too great, the body becomes increasingly vulnerable and exhaustion follows. Here it is the adaptation to stress, the coping mechanism, that affects the outcome.

A cognitive model of stress (Lazarus 1966) includes the importance of thought, experience and the meaning of stress to the individual. Thus stress and adaptation may vary over time and in different situations for the same individual. The career woman who manages a demanding work schedule may find great difficulty in coping with her demanding infant.

To be able to deal adequately with negative stress we need to be able to recognise it, activate our coping skills appropriately and act on them, with help and support where available.

Why is stress important?

Stress, or our maladaptive response to stress, has been implicated in many illnesses as well as the damaging attempts we make to relieve it by the use of cigarettes, drugs and alcohol.

The body's response to any stress is to release adrenalin and noradrenalin from the adrenal gland into the bloodstream, thus speeding up reflexes, increasing heart rate and blood pressure. This gives an immediate boost to our performance, but if not used as energy, has serious implications for cardio-vascular disease. Thyroid hormones released also charge our metabolism but if they continue to be produced, can lead to exhaustion and collapse. The cholesterol released from the liver when the body is under stress gives short term energy but can increase blood cholesterol levels with risk of arteriosclerosis.

It has been shown that psychological stress does impair the efficiency of the immune system (Jabaaij, 1993). Dutch researchers found that people experiencing stress produce significantly lower titres of antibodies to hepatitis B vaccine than do non-stressed subjects.

Excess stress response has been implicated in heart disease, stroke, problems of the digestive tract and migraine. Studies in heart disease, where most research has been done, have shown the physiological benefits of stress reduction teaching on those most at risk (Patel, 1987).

Studies of patients in hospital also show that those who felt most in control and relaxed not only had fewer emotional problems but also had a shorter recovery time.

In relation to pregnancy, a Danish study showed the effects of distress on preterm delivery (Hedegaard, 1993). In a population of 8719 women there was found to be a significant relationship between distress, established using a general health questionnaire, at 30 weeks' gestation and preterm delivery. No relationship was found with preterm delivery and distress at 16 weeks' gestation. This study obviously has implications for the management of stress in pregnant women, particularly in the later weeks.

This research has not been confirmed by other studies, however, one of which found anxiety more common in women who did not go into labour until 42 weeks (Sharma et al., 1993).

Managing stress   The first approach to stress management is the recognition of stress. Some people deny its existence for them ('I just carry on, nothing ever bothers me') or believe that they need it to function ('I can only work for exams when the adrenalin is pumping'). Yet for everyone, as we have seen, there is a level at which we stop functioning well under stress. We start to get headaches or sore muscles, we forget to do things we knew we should get done, we become irritable and feel others are putting unreasonable demands on us. All these are signs of too much stress, of not managing our time or our resources to the benefit of ourselves.

What we most notice when we are stressed is change. Change in our feelings, behaviour and mood. Change is also one of the triggers of stress. Any alteration in our circumstances requires us to make some adaptation in response. In order to reduce stress we must begin by knowing how to recognise the symptoms and identify some of the causes. These symptoms may be physical, mental, emotional or produce behavioural changes. How the individual responds will depend on personality, experience and learned coping mechanisms. For some women physical symptoms may be ignored, and to somatise their symptoms will not produce any reduction in stress. They do not easily allow themselves to be sick. For others sickness may be the only refuge from overwhelming psychological pressure. Whilst none of the individual symptoms listed in Table 12.1 are exclusive to stress, taken together they may show that someone is not coping well.

It is clear that many of these changes may occur normally in pregnancy; there is a natural increase in the size and activity of the adrenal glands, nausea is frequently experienced and concentration may be affected by the change in focus from external to internal concerns. However, it is the cluster of symptoms and the individual's own feeling of stress that are important.

The cause of the stress may come from outside ourselves or from within. External stresses such as poverty or poor housing or isolation, as well as particular life events, may seem obvious causes of stress. The threat to which we are responding is more clear even if change seems difficult or impossible. The Holmes and Rahe Schedule of Life Events (Holmes and Rahe, 1967) charts the possible seriousness of an event: for example the death of a spouse is rated as 100 and divorce as 73. Whilst pregnancy scores 40 it may have a very different effect on the woman for whom it is a planned and wanted

Table 12.1.
Stress
symptoms:
examples

Physical stress symptoms	Emotional stress symptoms	Mental stress symptoms	Behavioural changes
Tense muscles	Anxiety	Difficulty making decisions	Increased smoking or drinking
Dry mouth	Irritability	Difficulty concentrating	Appetite changes
Nausea	Feeling depressed	Memory lapse	Sleep pattern changes
Palpitations	Feeling insecure	Feeling under pressure	
Dizziness	Crying		
Sweaty hands	Feelings of guilt		
Diarrhoea			

event and the woman for whom it may be unplanned, unwanted or both. In his research into depression in women, Brown (1978) found that it is probably the meaning of the event for the person that is important in establishing the level of tension and subsequent depression. Internal stress results from our perception of a situation. If something is perceived as threatening we activate our fight/flight response. It is often fear that frightens us. We may cope well with real situations but live in fear of what is imagined or dreaded. We most often feel frightened or stressed when we feel helpless. If we feel unable to respond to the perceived threat, we feel vulnerable and undefended. We may look outside ourselves for protection or guidance and our expectation of others to look after us may be unrealistically high. Personality too affects our ability to adapt to and reduce stress. Cardiologists Friedman and Rosenman (1974) in the course of their research into cardiovascular disease, found those whom they described as having Type A personalities to be at greater risk of heart disease. These people were very competitive, striving, easily angered and quick in movement. When they learned to relax more they became no more at risk than matched controls.

Since we cannot entirely avoid stress or change our personalities easily, we need to be able to recognise when the stress is becoming damaging, learn to activate our coping skills and how to reduce the effects.

Stress in pregnancy

Pregnancy may be the time of greatest change in a woman's life. A first pregnancy is a journey into the unknown, when every map seems to show a different route. The journey is also taken carrying all our history and experience and the feelings and expectations of others. It represents change not just in income and expenditure, home and social life, but change in self-image from woman to mother, man to father. It brings with it a loss of our old self and life with uncertain gains, a testing of our skills, maturity and the strength of our relationships. Such enormous changes may make us feel vulnerable, and we need time and support to adapt to them. If there are other pressures in our lives this adaptation may be complicated, delayed or extremely difficult.

A woman in her second and subsequent pregnancies also faces changes; how to assimilate another child into the pattern of life, how to help her other children to adjust, as well as financial and social implications.

Pregnancy also causes physical stress. Because these are such common experiences, nausea, vomiting, fatigue and sleeplessness may be marginalised by both the woman and health professionals. She may feel that it is wrong to complain about these things, that they are the lot of the pregnant woman, but for her they may be distressing and disabling. They may be taken as a positive sign of pregnancy and almost welcomed, but they may be resented and feared, affecting her feelings about the infant who may be felt to be causing the discomfort.

Signs of stress, depression and anxiety are commonly found in normal populations of women attending antenatal clinics. One study in South London showed 35% of women attending for the first time had high negative scores for depression on the General Health Questionnaire (Sharpe, 1988).

Other studies have found high levels of worry, mood lability and insomnia (Raphael-Leff, 1991). Some of these are socio-economic in origin and not easily amenable to change, but many relate to the pregnancy itself. There are the doubts expressed about motherhood, the unanswerable question of 'What will it be like?' as well as the very understandable fears of women who have experienced previous problem pregnancies or for whom this pregnancy is unwanted or untimely. There are also particular anxieties that arise at different times throughout the pregnancy.

Conception   Now that for many women conception and pregnancy are an option, there may be stress around making that choice and why we make it. The reasons for choosing to have a child at all, or at that time, may well affect her feelings about being pregnant and there may be many pressures on a woman to become pregnant and to choose to continue the pregnancy. These may be her own anxieties about 'the biological clock', or pressure from others to fulfil some need of their own. She may find it difficult to tell anyone about whether she chose to be pregnant and assumptions may be made that she is pleased, when her feelings are ambiguous or confused. It can then be difficult to admit to feelings of ambiguity or uncertainty. This may be true of the first or subsequent pregnancies. The woman who is pregnant through aided conception may also have issues about whether or whom to tell. What motherhood means to that woman may be very relevant to how she feels about the changes in her body and her self-image.

Joanne was a 35-year-old single woman in a senior management post in industry. She became pregnant by her married lover when not using contraception. The response of her partner was to assume that she would seek abortion immediately. When she said that she wanted time to consider options, he withdrew and never made further contact. She was distressed to find that some friends also assumed that she would not continue the pregnancy. Her elderly widowed mother, whilst apparently offering support, rehearsed all the difficulties of single parenthood and reflected on her own difficulties postnatally. Joanne was left feeling that her choice to continue the pregnancy was selfish and unthinking. She began to feel depressed and unwell, concentration at work was difficult and she became uninterested in food although nausea was a minor problem. She felt she had to be positive about the pregnancy when talking to midwives and doctors as so many people had been so negative, and a junior doctor had expressed some surprise at her wanting to start a family 'in her circumstances'. She also feared that this negativity might in some way harm the baby. It was only when she could admit her own ambivalence about coping with single motherhood, and her anger at the response of her partner and some of her friends, that she could look at the reality of her situation and begin to feel more in control of making the changes that were needed. When the baby was delivered early, although well, she again felt that she might have been in some way responsible because she had been uncertain about whether or not she wanted her. Her doubts about her ability to mother affected her feelings of cabability in handling her daughter.

First trimester   This is the phase of 'becoming pregnant'. A woman's mood may depend on how she feels about being pregnant. She may spend some days totally involved with the pregnancy and her hopes and fears, and others almost unaware of her state. Her response to the physical discomforts of early pregnancy may also be affected by her reaction to being pregnant. If she has experienced previous difficulties in pregnancy or the loss of a baby through miscarriage or stillbirth, these early weeks may be fraught with danger and she may be unwilling even to talk about the pregnancy until she is certain it will continue. Those women afraid of pregnancy or of its implications for their future may even deny the pregnancy to themselves and apparently live their lives as normal.

Early pregnancy may also see the resurfacing of painful past conflicts or experiences. The vulnerability and the enforced changed self-image of pregnancy may arouse many infantile responses that seemed well hidden. The woman's own relationship with her mother, her own childhood anger and frustration, may surface in a way that feels overwhelming.

Ellen approached her GP asking for a termination of pregnancy at twelve weeks. She was feeling extremely unwell with constant sickness and abdominal pain. She had not been able to work as a secretary for more than occasional days since two weeks into the pregnancy. The illness and disability were the only reasons she gave her doctor for seeking termination, and refused to consider remedies the GP suggested. The GP was uncertain about this and referred Ellen to the counsellor. In the first session, the counsellor encouraged Ellen to discuss the whole situation of the pregnancy including her partner's reaction and the effect it might have on her whole life and the plans she had made. Ellen denied any anxieties about the future, insisting that it was only the sickness that had made her decide to seek termination. She did however agree to another counselling session later that week. The counsellor was aware of the need to explore the situation quickly, given the time constraints. The fact that Ellen had readily agreed to another session suggested that she did want to talk about her situation. In the second session the counsellor addressed this apparent ambivalence, her determination to seek abortion and her willingness to continue counselling. Ellen said that she had recognised the need for counselling after it had been lacking in the past. When the counsellor pressed this Ellen began to talk about a previous termination when she was 17 years old. She had told no one about this and tried to put it out of her mind. She felt she had been successful in doing this until she became pregnant again. She now believed that the sickness and pain that she was experiencing was retribution for ending the previous pregnancy and that she had no right to become a mother, as she had killed her other child. When she was able to look at the situation she had been in when she made the decision to terminate the first time, she agreed that she could not have coped with a pregnancy in a violent, abusive relationship with no family support. In trying to deny the first pregnancy, she had also denied the awful situation in which she, as a refugee and homeless, had been living.

Second trimester   At this stage the woman becomes more aware of the baby as an individual, the demands from within become more obvious and her focus becomes more internal. This may be difficult for those around her, particularly a partner, when she seems to be absorbed by the baby and they may feel excluded. Now the pregnancy also becomes public property and the woman is on the receiving end of comment, advice and warnings. There is often a very strong feeling of nurturing the baby at this stage, particularly as activity increases and so does appetite. If she has doubts about whether she is doing the right thing or if her physical health is poor, she may have great anxiety about protecting and nurturing her baby properly.

Third trimester   A woman's coping resources may be very stretched by this stage of pregnancy. She may need help, for the first time since infancy, with simple tasks; she may tire easily and may feel very dependent. If she has had to stop work she may also feel isolated and withdrawn. It is a transition period from being the woman you know to the mother you are uncertain about becoming.

Depending on how she has felt about being pregnant or during the pregnancy, the woman may anticipate the end of it with relief or regret. She may enjoy the last weeks of not being a parent or be eagerly anticipating beginning. Some women who have doubts about their ability to be a good mother may become preoccupied with this during the last few weeks. Others may have great anxiety about the labour itself. If they have experienced difficulties and anxieties before or if they do not feel confident in the professionals they have met antenatally they may dread the whole experience. They may also be concerned about whether they will 'behave well' during labour or if they will 'let themselves down' by seeming out of control or by upsetting or angering those who attend them.

Postnatal period   If all has gone well the immediate postnatal reaction may be one of relief and joy, exhaustion and elation. Later the woman will need to learn or relearn the skills of mothering. If this is accompanied by doubts about her ability to mother or by physical problems this early pressure may be quickly lost in the need just to get by. Women are not always sure how they should feel postnatally and may suffer a lot of discomfort unnecessarily.

Between a half and two-thirds of women suffer from the 'blues' in the days after delivery. This may be related to the immense hormonal changes that the woman experiences but also to the upheaval of new motherhood. Other new mothers experience a more serious depression that will require professional help. It is estimated that one in ten women suffer from clinical depression after giving birth but fewer than a third are actually recognised or treated.

The father's or partner's reaction to the birth and arrival of the baby may be very important in affecting the mother's state of mind. If they are positive and felt to be supportive the woman may find this transition to motherhood much eased, but if the partner has their own issues about coping with parenthood and what they see to be this new role, they may be demanding that the mother help them to adjust. Some men take over the care of the child as a way of establishing their role and women may sometimes see this as threatening to their own position and feel marginalised in their caring for the baby.

The resumption of sexual relations may also be stressful for some new mothers. They may feel sore and uncomfortable physically, be afraid of damaging the perineum or simply not feel very sexual. Some women find great difficulty in combining the role of mother and lover and may need help to think through their own responses. For those women for whom this becomes a continuing problem it may be necessary to seek out professional counselling.

Reducing the stress

Since stress has both mental and physical causes and psychological and somatic effects, we should consider a range of therapies that deal with both.

Exercise as a means of reducing stress It is well documented that physical activity can enhance health and well-being and reduce mortality (Bouchard, 1994). Exercise is known to stimulate the release of endorphins and encephalins which serve as the body's own anti-stressor, boosting a sense of well-being and acting as a natural antidepressant. Exercise has many physiological effects including prevention of coronary heart disease and hypertension, obesity and diabetes mellitus, osteoporosis and musculoskeletal disorders and certain types of cancer. A survey by the Health Education Authority (1993) found that people engaged in physical activity primarily to reduce stress, to enable them to feel in good shape, to improve their general health and self-esteem. Conversely those whose lifestyles were sedentary had negative views, regarding physical activity as unpleasant and difficult, that it was pointless to undertake small amounts of exercise and too late to start; this was particularly so of people who had previously had a negative experience of physical activity (HEA, 1993). Guidelines on the frequency and duration of exercise (non-pregnant), sufficient to protect against coronary heart disease, were produced by the American College of Sports Medicine (ACSM, 1990) and adopted around the world. Initial guidelines suggested at least three sessions per week of vigorous activity lasting 20–40 minutes, although more recent thinking recommends thirty minutes of moderately intensive activity at least four to five times weekly (Killoran, 1995).

No guidelines specific to exercise during pregnancy exist, and advice is based on limited research findings, coupled with a knowledge of the physio-logical changes which occur. It would be wise to incorporate into the booking history details of the expectant mother's exercise pattern, including the number of years she has been exercising and whether this has been con-sistent or intermittent, the type, frequency, duration and level of physical activity and her general lifestyle such as walking to work. This should provide a background on which to base any further discussion regarding exercise intentions during pregnancy and the puerperium.

During pregnancy women are aware of altered body image and concerned about body weight, muscle tone and shape. Many women embark on pregnancy having been accustomed to regular physical exercise; others may feel the need to take up a physical activity to help them cope with the discomforts of pregnancy and to prepare them for the birth, at a time when they are more receptive to health promotion advice. However, despite the acknowledged physiological and psychological benefits of exercise, inappropriate or inaccurate advice about activity can be harmful to either mother or fetus and it is therefore important to ensure that the advice given is as up-to-date and as research-based as possible.

There are three classifications of the activities which women undertake in pregnancy:

- 'Physical activity' is defined by Caspersen (1985) as any musculoskeletal bodily movement which results in energy expenditure, including activities of daily living such as work and leisure as well as both aerobic and anaerobic sports.
- 'Exercise' is perceived as non-competitive, structured leisure activities involving repetitive body movements such as aerobics, walking, cycling, swimming, dancing and jogging, generally undertaken as a means of improving health, reducing stress and maintaining fitness.
- 'Sport' involves structured physical activity, governed by rules and tending to be competitive in nature, such as team games.

A woman's physical fitness will be determined by lifestyle factors, heredity and the amount and type of physical activity which she takes. Aerobic fitness relates to cardiorespiratory ability to supply oxygen and energy during physical activity and eliminate waste products created during the exercise. Anaerobic exercise is very intense and, as a result of exceeding oxygen availability, causes the muscle cells to revert to anaerobic metabolism. This type of exercise can only be maintained for short periods of time due to the production of lactic acid from the anaerobic metabolism within the cells, which requires oxygen to remove it. Anaerobic exercise includes sprinting, jumping and weighlifting. Whilst research into anaerobic exercise in pregnant women is unethical, investigations into gestational aerobic fitness can determine the potential dangers of anaerobic exercise (Wallace, 1987).

The intensity, duration and frequency of exercise sessions in pregnancy should be at a level where it does not cause pain, shortness of breath or fatigue and women should be encouraged to be responsive to their bodies to avoid injury or trauma. Inactive women can safely and gradually begin aerobic exercise during pregnancy such as walking, cycling and swimming but activities where bending, jumping, running and twisting are likely

Table 12.2. Physical activities in pregnancy

Activities safe throughout pregnancy	Activities that may become unsafe during pregnancy	Activities considered unsafe throughout pregnancy
Walking	Golf	Scuba diving (any use of compressed air)
Swimming	Racket sports	Contact sports, e.g. boxing/judo, football/rugby, weightlifting
Cycling	Gymnastics	Competitive events
Jogging	Weight training	
Yoga	Horseriding	Sauna (jacuzzi, whirlpool)
Aerobics, land or water	Netball	Dangerous sports, e.g. parachuting, paragliding, bungie jumping, rock climbing, potholing
Racket sports	Downhill ski-ing	
Cross-country ski-ing	Waterski-ing	
Tai-chi	Running	
	Any sports involving balance	

This table is not definitive.

to cause injury should be avoided. The antenatal and early postnatal periods are not times to pursue new sports. Activities can be divided into three categories (see Table 12.2). Those activities which can be continued throughout pregnancy are those where the risk of injury is limited, whereas some activities may become unsafe as pregnancy progresses, especially those which involve an extreme range of movement and balance, as well as contact sports. Activities which involve bending, twisting and stooping may increase disc compression in the spine (Adams, 1997).

Sports which involve the risk of possible injury to the mother or fetus, such as blunt or penetrating abdominal trauma, should be avoided during pregnancy. The hyperbaric conditions linked with scuba diving put the fetus at risk of air embolism during decompression and it has been suggested that there are teratogenic effects (Newhall, 1981). Diving should be discouraged, particularly during the early weeks of embryonic development. High altitude sports may interfere with uteroplacental circulation, causing fetal hypoxia; maternal hypoxia is also a risk because of the length of the acclimatisation process (Huch, 1990). Lifting weights results in a prolonged Valsalva manoeuvre, with a possible reduction in splanchnic blood flow and a rise in blood pressure, and should be avoided.

Highly trained athletes and those women who are competent in their sport are likely to be aware of the risks of pregnancy and the need to seek expert advice. Studies on well-conditioned runners and aerobic dancers found no adverse effects of fertility, spontaneous abortion, abnormal placentation, nor an increase in congenital abnormalities (Clapp, 1989).

Physiological effects of exercise in pregnancy

Cardiovascular response to exercise in pregnancy causes an increase in heart rate and cardiac output similar to those occurring physiologically at this time (20% and 40% respectively) (Hytten, 1996). During the third trimester exercise causes an additional rise, although this is not considered harmful to the mother or fetus providing the exercise is of limited duration. The safety of the mother and fetus during prolonged strenuous exercise remains to be studied (Doorn, 1992).

Exercise and pregnancy have opposing effects on regional blood flow distribution, compared to the non-pregnant state. During exercise blood is diverted to the muscles and skin, but away from the viscera, whilst during pregnancy blood is diverted towards the renal, uterine and cutaneous circulation (Hytten, 1996). The fall in splanchnic blood flow during moderate exercise is approximately 50% and there is concern that this may directly affect the delivery of oxygen to the fetus. However, the normal pregnancy changes such as the increase in plasma volume, erythrocytes and cardiac output compensate for the change in blood flow during physical activity. Indeed, an increase in uterine blood flow immediately after cessation of physical exercise has been found (Morris, 1956), but alterations in fetal heart rate have been observed, including bradycardia (Artal, 1984) and tachycardia (Collings, 1985).

From a cardiovascular perspective it would therefore appear that mild to moderate exercise during pregnancy is not harmful to the normal healthy mother or her fetus, but there is a definite need for women to include a warm-up phase before commencing exercise to facilitate blood flow to the muscles, and a cooling-down phase to enable the heart rate and cardiac output to return to the pre-exercise state. It is also important that the mother does not simply stop exercising suddenly without engaging in the cooling-down phase, otherwise a 'pooling' effect of blood in the muscles occurs, hindering the redistribution of blood to other major organs.

Pulmonary effects During exercise there is an increase in oxygen consumption, but this increases as pregnancy progresses in women indulging in mild to moderate exercise. Interestingly, oxygen consumption has been found to be considerably less in pregnant women engaging in strenuous activity, which may be attributed to a physiological rejection of hypoxia (Artal, 1986).

Aerobic capacity may be reduced as pregnancy progresses, resulting in a reduction in physical activity, although it is unclear whether this is due to the inability to transfer oxygen and carbon dioxide from the atmosphere to the cells or to a reduction in exercise intensity (Artal, 1986a). Generally pregnant women respond well to the pulmonary demands of exercise because increased ventilation occurs at this time.

Thermoregulatory effects The metabolic rate and production of heat are increased during exercise, which results in a need for greater heat dissipation; most is lost through evaporation, and by conduction if the exercise is in water. In women accustomed to exercising, core temperatures have been noted to rise between 0.1 and 1.3 degrees Celsius above the basal rate (Clapp, 1985) and should not exceed 39 degrees Celsius. Exercise programmes for pregnant women should be modified in response to increasing maternal weight, to avoid the risk of hyperthermia, and they should be advised against exercising in hot, humid conditions or during a febrile illness. (Pregnant women should also avoid saunas, for the same reasons.) Women without a previous exercise history may experience difficulty with heat dissipation if sudden exercise is undertaken, potentially leading to a reduced uterine blood flow (Oakes, 1976) and teratogenic effects (Miller, 1978). Increasing maternal temperature will also increase the demands of the fetus for oxygen and can eventually result in hypoxia and possible fetal death (Charles, 1998). Women should exercise wearing loose fitting clothing and take frequent additional fluids.

Metabolic and endocrine effects   During exercise in non-pregnant individuals glucose uptake in the muscles is increased but hypoglycaemia is prevented by an increase in the production of hepatic glucose. Fuel metabolism is also affected by an increase in glucagon, cortisol, adrenocorticotophic hormone, epinephrine and norepinephrine and a decrease in insulin levels. During aerobic activity increased insulin sensitivity in the muscles allows mobilisation and oxidation of fat, which decreases the rate of depletion of muscle glycogen.

In pregnant women glucose concentrations remain constant or decrease following exercise (Artal, 1981; Platt, 1983) and may be insufficient for fetal glucose utilisation. Artal (1981) found a rise in glucagon and a stable insulin level in women taking mild exercise, but no studies have been undertaken on the effects of high intensity exercise. Excessive catecholamine production is associated with maternal stress and is noted in exercising pregnant women. Redistribution of blood flow may occur due to the sensitivity of uterine circulation to catecholamines, which may result in hypoxia, although regular pregnancy exercise can reduce the catecholamine response (Russell, 1984) and no correlation between regular exercise and preterm labour has been found (Jarrett, 1983).

Musculoskeletal effects   Oestrogen, progesterone and relaxin hormones alter the composition of collagen, found in joint capsules, ligaments and fibrous and connective tissues, particularly the pelvic fascia and rectus abdominis muscles, and affect the elasticity and flexibility of joints, muscles and ligaments. Relaxin is thought to have a direct influence on the sacroiliac joints and symphysis pubis, increasing motility; the ribcage is also affected by increasing hormone levels, resulting in rib flaring in the third trimester.

The changing centre of gravity as pregnancy progresses affects posture by exaggerating the lumbar lordosis, causing kyphosis and hunched or rounded shoulders, and a tendency of some women to push the head and chin forwards beyond the line of the shoulder girdle (Figs 12.1, 12.2). These postural alterations can lead to lumbar and thoracic backache, head and neck ache and increased pressure on the symphysis pubis. Irrespective of whether or not the mother engages in sports and exercise she should be advised by the midwife about her posture, including correct alignment of the shoulders to the hips, pulling in of the abdominal muscles, tucking in of the buttocks to tilt the pelvis forwards and adoption of a military position of the head (Figs 12.3 to 12.5). Injury and trauma can occur from incorrect posture, coupled with overexertion, cumulative or one-off exposure to activity, or a combination.

There is a tendency for women whose abdomen is large in late pregnancy to swing excessively or 'waddle' when walking, increasing instability and the risk of additional strain on the sacroiliac joints and lumbar spine, and some sporting activities which depend on balance are contraindicated. Women may opt for non-weight bearing exercise such as swimming, although care should be taken in late pregnancy to avoid an exacerbated lumbar lordosis during breast stroke or front crawl (Fig. 12.6), particularly if the head is held out of the water and the neck hyperextended. This causes the cervical vertebrae to compress the apophyseal joints and increase intervertebral disc pressure; there is also an increase in the curvature of the thoracic spine. Further tension may be placed on the vertebrae during

Fig. 12.1. Poor standing posture.

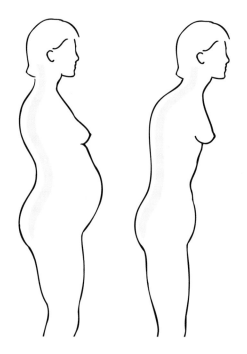

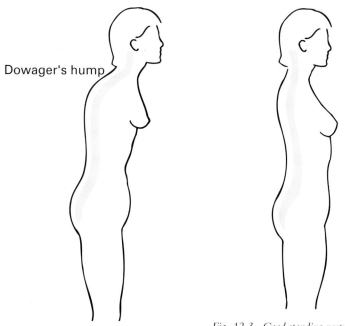

Dowager's hump

Fig. 12.2. Poor posture, illustrating chin poking and dowager's hump.

Fig. 12.3. Good standing posture.

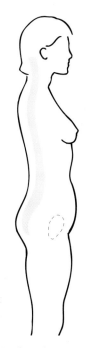

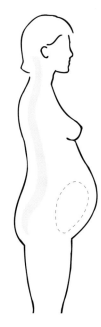

Fig. 12.4. Good standing posture, first trimester.

Fig. 12.5. Good standing posture, second and third trimester.

Fig. 12.6. Incorrect swimming posture with increased lordosis.

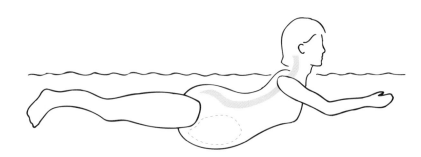

swimming in women whose abdominal muscles are weak, especially the internal and external rectus abdominis, resulting in diastasis recti (Blakey, 1992). Incorrect leg movements when using breast stroke may cause rotation of the hip joint and an increased incidence of symphysis pubis separation. The leg action should be adapted to use a flexed and extended hip action and avoiding bilateral abduction. The mother could be advised to wear goggles to ensure her head dips lower into the water when performing breast and crawl strokes, thereby reducing the risks of spinal injury and strain.

General advice regarding exercise during pregnancy

- The woman should wear good quality supportive footwear, appropriate for the activity in which she is engaged. Sports shoes provide a cushioning effect and help to avoid jarring of the joints and spinal column.
- She should wear a supportive bra, especially if she is involved in impact activities. Swimming costumes offer minimal support so a supportive bra should be worn underneath.
- Adequate amounts of clear fluids should be sipped throughout the period of exercise and following exertion.
- A warm-up phase is vital to prepare joints and muscles for exercise and to avoid muscle strain. An increase in synovial fluid in the joints will help to prevent injury during the active phase. Static stretching of the major muscle groups helps muscles to stretch more easily and become less resistant.
- During exercise the woman should work at a level where she is slightly out of breath but able to hold a conversation. She should not feel stressed, nor should her heartbeat exceed 140 beats per minute. Teaching her to take her pulse rates before and after exercise involves her in this monitoring process.
- A cool-down phase should complete the exercise session to enable heart and respiratory rates to return to pre-exercise levels. Sudden pooling of blood in the lower limbs and major muscles, which could initiate hypotension, will be prevented and the gentle reduction in intensity assists venous return to the heart. Sudden cessation of intensive activity may lead to hypotension and fainting. Static stretching of major muscle groups maintains muscle length, flexibility and mobility, preventing injury.

- If the woman feels unwell during exercise she should slowly reduce the activity to prevent further the problems already highlighted. She should seek medical advice and review her exercise programme.

Postpartum exercise Hormonal adaptations continue in the early puerperium, affecting in particular the musculoskeletal system for up to 6–8 weeks (Brayshaw and Wright, 1994), although some effects continue for 6 months (Polden and Mantle, 1990).

Before a woman resumes exercise or sport it should be ascertained that the events of pregnancy and labour do not contraindicate further physical activity. Postnatal exercises should focus on toning the pelvic, back and abdominal muscles, and many women can resume aerobic exercise safely within 10–14 days of a normal delivery, although water-based activities should be delayed until the lochial discharges have ceased. Women who have had an operative delivery should not resume exercise for at least 3–4 weeks, depending on their general condition at that time.

Methods available to the midwife Since stress is both a physical and an emotional reaction to what has happened or is happening to us, and our interpretation of those events, we can explore various therapies that deal with all aspects of coping with the symptom of stress. Some can be simply taught and learned and can be practised safely at home alone or with a partner; these include meditation, breathing techniques, relaxation exercises and visualisation. Other therapies need to be taught and supervised by a qualified therapist but are generally available, such as yoga, Alexander Technique, Tai Chi and hypnotherapy.

Clear advice, information and giving the time and space to answer questions honestly and in a way the woman feels acceptable, may be enough to reduce the anxiety of pregnancy significantly for some women. As can be seen in other chapters of this book, simple remedies may improve much of the physical stress. It may be possible for the midwife herself to offer massage or aromatherapy or reflexology, with appropriate training.

Other women will benefit from more formalised counselling to deal with problems that they feel are affecting their feelings about the pregnancy or about motherhood, or the feelings about past events that may arise in this new situation.

Counselling Counselling may be seen as a therapy complementary to conventional medicine in that so much of how we feel about ourselves affects how we feel in our bodies. Counselling as practised by a trained and qualified counsellor is a therapy that aims to help the client to clarify the problems, examine her resources for coping with them and her reasons for not feeling able to cope and to make choices for further action, in a non-judgemental and supportive atmosphere. As well as the skills required by the counsellor to maintain a relationship that is non-judgemental, warm and genuine (the three tenets of counselling relationships) the client requires time and a safe space in which to explore feelings. This may be difficult for health professionals to offer in the course of their normal work. They can, however, learn to offer a 'counselling approach'. The best outcomes of counselling are when it is client-led. That is that the aims of the client and counsellor towards change are congruent. The counsellor needs to be facilitating change, not setting the agenda for changes. The goals must be those of the client.

There is a power imbalance in the roles of the counsellor and client; the counsellor is seen as the expert help-giver and the client as the help-seeker. Street and Downey (1996) describe this as the 'medico-collaborative' model of helping, suggesting that 'it seeks to work with the client rather than on the client ... and rests upon a belief that the counsellor will try to persuade the client to accept a more hopeful or helpful view of their personal dilemma and the best course of action to take in the process of counselling. It is not being done to them but being explored with them.' The counselling model that fits this concept most closely is that of Egan (1982), described below.

The counselling approach for health professionals There are certain principles of counselling that should be observed. It needs to be more focused and purposeful than just a chat with a friend, and the needs of the client must be uppermost. The counsellor needs to maintain a therapeutic distance, that is, a lack of emotional involvement. The therapist has not to be so distant as to fail to engage with the client but to seek to avoid becoming personally affected. It the client presents problems very similar to those of the counsellor this too may prevent the therapeutic distance being maintained. If the therapist shares her own feelings or solutions this may either be seen as the counsellor requiring the client to support her or her solution being the one that the client should also adopt or risk displeasing the therapist. Avoid advice giving in the counselling alliance. This affects the power balance and can make the client dependent and reluctant to seek out her own answers, which is a central aim of the therapy. When the advice proves to be wrong, this also destroys trust in the therapy. The inexperienced counsellor should also avoid interpretation, that is explaining to the client the meaning of what she is thinking or feeling. This technique is used in some models of therapy but it has the risk of appearing judgemental and leaving the client feeling guilty or rejected.

The basis of counselling is listening and attending, valuing what the client is expressing not just in words but in the unspoken communication. The relationship between client and counsellor is a microcosm of all the relationships the client experiences, and if the counsellor appears neglectful or lacking in concern this may confirm for some clients their lack of value.

The counsellor does not have to put everything right for the client. The client may often become distressed in sessions from remembering or talking about painful issues but this is what the counsellor is working with, not trying to stop. It may be important just to acknowledge the importance of it for the client and help her to move towards a way of making it better for herself.

A model that may be helpful for the health professional counsellor is that developed by Egan (Egan, 1982). His three-stage model of the counselling relationship is as follows.

1. Identifying and clarifying the problems The client sometimes just feels sad or disturbed or confused. She has not always identified the immediate cause of the feelings, as they may have become overwhelming in themselves. To be able to work out the precipitating factors may help to clear some of the confusion. It may also give the client 'permission' to feel upset, to recognise the normalcy of the response. It also helps to lead on to the second stage.

2. Goal-setting—developing and choosing goals In this the client chooses the end point of the counselling but also sets her own final goal. It may be just to get through the day without thinking about a loss or problem or it may be that she would choose to think about something without feeling overwhelmed. It is important for the goal to be set by the client, and it may be important for the counsellor to help make the goals realistic.

3. Action—moving towards the chosen goals The client may need some guidance in working out ways of achieving her goals. These should start with the most easily attained, so that the client may grow in confidence. Again the client should feel comfortable with the methods chosen, which may be based on a behavioural programme of setting tasks to achieve or a cognitive approach of trying to think differently about a problem or situation.

These stages can be dealt with separately, although they overlap. It helps to assess the development of the relationship and the work being achieved. It also helps to keep it progressing. The fact that the client is setting the agenda is also important in helping her to recognise that she has the resources to cope and only requires the support and guidance of the counsellor.

Counselling skills can be learned and used by most health professionals, but it is important to recognise that it is a skill and not just something that anyone with the time can do. Clients can be greatly helped, but also hurt by counselling.

These principles of counselling are also part of the whole field of psychotherapy. There are different 'schools' of therapy based on differing theoretical constructs. All aim to give the client an opportunity to explore their feelings, experiences and life situation, to effect some change in how they feel. Classic analysis, based on the work of Sigmund Freud, works by 'free association', allowing the client to express her thoughts and feelings and dreams to the analyst for interpretation. It is intended as a long-term therapy only undertaken by therapists after a long and rigorous training. Clients entering a psychotherapy contract should be aware of the commitment to therapy, and the cost that may ensue as well as the painful nature of some of the work. Melanie Klein, Carl Jung and others continued the work of Freud and developed their own theories of psychological/emotional development. The work has continued through the twentieth century and includes the post-modern movement with the work of Lacan and others.

At the other end, at least in time-scale if not proven efficacy, are the short-term therapies. These may be behavioural in their approach, such as cognitive behaviour therapy (CBT) or more exploratory cognitive analytical therapy (CAT). Most theories are now being used for short-term therapy. Although this is often preferred by those wanting low-cost alternatives, outcome measures show that it is no less effective if clients are properly assessed for suitability. Recent studies have shown that clients in counselling want three main things: they want the counsellor to understand, to give practical advice about resolving their difficulties and to achieve positive change in a few sessions (Stiles et al., 1990).

The woman at risk It is important to recognise that for some women, information, advice and basic supportive counselling may not be enough. It is important also to identify areas of increased risk of abnormal psychological reaction to pregnancy and childbirth. Women for whom the pregnancy is unwanted either because of timing, her partner or their own issues; those who have experienced problem pregnancies or losses; women who are experiencing difficult concurrent life events are all more likely to be experiencing increased stress and distress. Those also at risk are the women already showing some symptoms of stress such as alcohol or drug abuse, eating disorders, agitation or depression. We cannot assume, however, that all these women will experience difficulties during pregnancy, or indeed that they will confide their anxieties to their professional carers. We must therefore be aware of the symptoms of extreme stress or psychological disorder, as well as giving women the opportunity both in time and space and in attitudes to express their feelings.

Some symptoms of disorder may be fairly obvious: paranoia, delusions, depersonalisation and de-realisation will usually be observed and referred to the psychiatric services. However, there are more subtle changes that carers who are listening to the woman may notice and act on. She may become overly anxious about the pregnancy or concerned about potential or actual harm being done to the baby. Some women are also unusually concerned about the baby being abnormal. All these feelings are normal, but become exaggerated in the woman who may be more at risk. Some women's state of mind may lead them to become obsessive, with compulsive cleaning or checking behaviour. Others may deny their pregnancy or their needs in pregnancy. All these women require time and skilled help to deal with their feelings, help which may not be available in the antenatal clinic, and they should be referred for counselling, psychotherapy or psychiatry if they are willing to accept help.

The stress of the carer

A GP described the expectations of the professionals caring for a pregnant woman to be 'to produce a perfect, healthy baby and a mother who is delighted with the outcome'. This is clearly not possible in every case and sometimes outside the ability of the carer to influence. Realistic expectations not just for the woman but also for her carers are important in reducing the feeling of failure that can result from expectations that are not achieved. The carers have their own expectations of themselves and their role, which may not necessarily coincide with those of the woman or her partner and this can lead to tension and lack of communication. Throughout her pregnancy the woman who has become 'medicalised' may expect her carers to interpret for her the condition of her baby and its needs. The lack of ability to make choices or to obtain information for herself may lead her to feel vulnerable. This vulnerability gives increased power to the carers in an area where 'knowing' gives power of itself. They may not always welcome this, but it needs to be recognised if the power balance is to be addressed. We receive information and act on it best when we feel in an adult/adult relationship with our advisers; if we are caught in a parent/child relationship, whilst it may feel supportive at some level, we are handing over responsibility to the carer.

One great value of the carer, the midwife or the wise-woman may be to provide a calm, rational space for the client when she feels agitated or uncontrolled. This may feel burdensome to the carer who is not feeling calm or controlled herself, and may produce stress of itself.

The helplessness we have discussed, being experienced by the pregnant or labouring woman, may also be experienced by health professionals if they too feel they are unable to control or affect a situation. As carers we too need to be aware of our own areas of stress and our coping mechanisms and to feel able to take action or seek help and support when appropri~

Reducing stress —self-help therapies

Earlier in this chapter it has been shown that relaxation eliminate the harmful effects of stress and tension.

Pregnancy is a stressful time for most women b tionally, and most can benefit from techniques th Here we will examine some techniques that are e safely practised by the woman alone or with a partner, from a therapist. However, midwives may appreciate a review of some of the techniques that could also be taught in parent education classes.

Breathing Breathing is automatic and usually involuntary, but it can be consciously controlled to help with mental and physical reduction of stress. Our breathing reflects our state of mind and can be controlled to improve our feelings. We sigh when we are sad, we yawn when tired and hyperventilate when anxious or excited. Our tone of voice is also changed; high on an inhaled breath in anxiety, low and exhaled when low or depressed.

When we are calm and relaxed we generally breathe abdominally, that is using the diaphragm to contract and push down, making the abdominal muscles relax and lift. The lungs can then fill easily. This creates the optimum oxygen exchange. Diaphragmatic breathing has been shown to reduce high blood pressure and increase feelings of relaxation. Costal breathing, from the chest alone, is harder work and less efficient in taking in oxygen and expelling carbon dioxide. Costal breathing is part of our fight/flight mechanism. It may be effective in helping us to run a race but will not reduce tension.

Health professionals can help women and their partners to learn effective techniques to control breathing and thus increase a feeling of relaxation. Abdominal breathing can be taught with the subject lying or sitting comfortably with one hand placed on the chest and the other on the abdomen. The midwife or helper should encourage the woman to inhale and exhale slowly, noticing where the movement comes from under the hands, and then push the abdominal muscles gently on inhalation and be aware of them pushing out again on exhalation, with little movement in the chest. The woman can be helped to be aware of breathing slowly and smoothly, and try to reduce the number of breaths to around 12 to 15 per minute. It helps if someone else can count the number of breaths until it becomes almost automatic. If the mother is breathing too fast and finds it difficult to slow down, it may help to have the midwife or helper close by breathing slowly and evenly with her, until a better rhythm is achieved.

A simple and effective exercise is known as Sigh Out Slowly: here the breath is controlled after the inhalation and released slowly and gently on a sigh until the breath is all expelled; the inhaled breath is then left to take care of itself.

Relaxation During antenatal classes the midwife can advise women to try relaxing mental tension by involving themselves in an activity which they enjoy; listening to music, going for a walk, reading a book, may all encourage a sense of calm. Women sometimes need 'permission' to actually relax and devote time to themselves. Anything that is found to be relaxing may also be helpful as a distraction during early labour. However, if women have become physically tense they may need to deal with this specifically with relaxation exercises.

These can all be safely taught and practised. It may be helpful to use background music to aid relaxation and to cut out extraneous noise. There are some cassette tapes of relaxing music available. The advantage of these is that the music itself has no particular emotion attached to it as a famous or popular tune may have. In pregnancy it is best to lie or sit comfortably in a well-supported position. There should be support under the neck and lumbar spine if semi-recumbent, and if lying on the side, a pillow under the upper knee will avoid strain on the lumbar-sacral spine. Good support prevents the woman becoming aware of discomfort and needing to keep changing position. She should choose a place that is warm and where interruption is least likely.

The midwife can help the woman to start diaphragmatic breathing with the eyes closed, and once this is settled the woman can start to think of relaxing each area of the body in turn. It is helpful to have the midwife or a helper guide the subject around the body. She may begin with the right foot and concentrate on making it feel relaxed whilst still breathing steadily, then move on to the rest of the leg, and then the left foot and leg. She may then progress to the arms, and then the spine. When the back muscles are relaxed she could try the head and neck, making sure that the teeth are not clenched and the eyes not screwed up. The client should stay as relaxed as possible and concentrate on breathing. To end the relaxation she may begin by moving the arms and legs slowly and then stretch and yawn, sit up gently and stand for a few moments before moving around.

Edmund Jacobson (Jacobson, 1938) developed the system of progressive tension and relaxation. With this method muscles are first tightened, held for a count of five, and then relaxed. Again this is used progressively through the body. This helps the awareness of relaxation but some people find it difficult to maintain regular breathing and start to hold their breath; they should be reminded of the SOS, sigh out slowly, technique.

Meditation The technique of meditation is easily learned but does require considerable practice and repetition to become effective. It can however be both suggested and taught by the midwife, offering several possible techniques for the woman to find the one that suits her best.

Meditation in one form or another has existed in almost every culture and religion and is still valued as a method of developing self-awareness and potential, as well as offering a way of finding a calm centre in life. At a physical level it has the effect of reducing the respiratory rate, cardiac output and activity of the sweat glands, thus reducing the level of tension and anxiety (Hewitt, 1978). Those who are able to meditate regularly report a great feeling of relaxation and peace.

There are several ways of meditating and it may be necessary for the individual to try them all to discover the most effective for themselves. It is important, particularly at first, to be in a quiet, comfortable place, undisturbed. The three methods of meditation examined here are breathing, mantra, and object-focus, and may be used as a guide by the midwife.

Breathing: begin by becoming as relaxed as possible, and take slow, deep breaths. Start to become aware of the breathing itself, how the air feels in the nostrils and the sensation of the air filling the lungs. The feelings may change as the focus becomes more intense. If other thoughts begin to intrude, try to return to the sensation of the breathing.

Mantra: this is the repetition of a word or phrase. It may be the name of a god or any sound that has no negative attachment, chosen by the meditator or teacher. Buddhists use the word 'om', which means, all that is, past, present and future. The sound is repeated over and over, closing out thoughts of anything else. It may be accompanied by holding an object, as with rosary beads, to aid concentration. At a simpler level the technique sometimes employed in labour of singing or tapping out a simple song repetitively is based on this concept.

Object-focus: here the image of a place or an object becomes the focus of concentration. The meditator chooses an image that feels positive and allows the mind to focus once the subject has become relaxed. A beach may be chosen, for example, and the meditator will start to explore mentally the feelings, smells and sounds associated with it. It is safest to ask the client to select their own scenario, to avoid associated fears or phobias, such as water or heights.

About one-tenth of adults are unable to hold a mental picture and this method will be unsuitable. They may be able to use an actual object on which to focus, and maintain the relaxed concentration in this way.

To become practised and effective any meditation method needs to be repeated about twice a day for 10–15 minutes, until the subject can easily become relaxed and focus with concentration. The benefits for stress reduction and peace of mind can be profound.

Visualisation This is exemplified by the phrase 'Every day in every way, I'm getting better and better'. It aims to encourage positive images about physical and mental activities and attitudes. The mind and body are so closely connected that our thoughts can affect our physical responses. Close your eyes and think of a lemon. Imagine you are holding it in your hand, smell it, squeeze it—now bite into it and suck—your mouth fills with saliva, and no lemon is required. Visualisation harnesses this response to help deal with making actual events more positive.

The subject should always begin by finding a comfortable, undisturbed position and begin to breathe slowly and steadily, and with the eyes closed try to picture a situation that the subject wants to explore. Some women are able to visualise their baby growing in the uterus, how it is looking and moving. For pregnant women, anxious about labour, visualising the birth of the baby with guidance from someone experienced may help to encourage positive images. They can concentrate on feeling relaxed and imaging the baby sliding through the birth canal gently and smoothly. Sheila Kitzinger advocated imaging the vulva in labour as a flower bud opening up.

It is sometimes helpful to begin with a simple sentence such as 'My body is good', and develop an image of the good body. This can then progress to 'my body is good and healthy'. It is important to keep the thinking in the present and keep it positive. In labour the thoughts 'I can do it, I will do it' may be positive.

Breathing as a means of relaxation, meditation and visualisation can be learned and practised alone, but other techniques need specific training and supervision, such as yoga, autogenic training, Alexander Technique and hypnotherapy.

Contraindications Although relaxation exercises are usually helpful and harmless, in certain circumstances they can be contraindicated or the midwife should be particularly aware of possible difficulties.

Those exercises requiring progressive tensing and relaxing of muscle groups may be unsuitable for anyone who should avoid raising their blood pressure, as the tensing phase can have this effect. It may be possible to do the exercises, but with a short tensing phase. Depressed women may be better advised to choose action rather than technique, to distract from negative thoughts. Midwives should also be aware that techniques involving deep breathing and breath holding can induce anxiety or panic attacks in women suffering from anxiety disorders.

Those women with extreme stress and anxiety or serious problems in their everyday life may find it very difficult to achieve any meditative state alone, and may need guidance or a partner supporting and going through the exercise with them or seek out one of the methods that involve a therapist being present. It is also important for women to recognise that although they may have done all they can to visualise a perfect birth, things can go wrong and they must not feel that they have failed to visualise it properly and therefore bear some responsibility for not helping their baby sufficiently.

Reducing the stress— supervised therapies

There are many supervised therapies that may be helpful for the reduction of stress. The choice of therapy may be one of availability or the woman's preference for an 'active' or 'passive' therapy, her previous knowledge about a particular intervention or advice from a health professional on its suitability. Elsewhere in the book there is information about hypnotherapy, which has very positive effects on the reduction of stress.

Autogenic training Developed by Schultz and popularised by Luthe (1963), and well described by Kermani (1992), this technique helps to bring about relaxation, encouraging the subject to think in a certain way. Particular phrases are learned that, with repetition, result in physical changes. For example, in a relaxed and comfortable position the subject begins to repeat 'My right arm is heavy', 'My left arm is feeling heavy', 'Both arms are feeling heavy'. This may need to be repeated for some time until there is a sensation of heaviness experienced. This in itself may be quite relaxing. The subject then moves on to use the same method for other parts of the body, for example the legs and head. Sensations are added later, such as feeling warm. Learning is progressive and should be supervised by a trained practitioner to bring about effective change, although it is practised alone.

There are other therapies that may be helpful in reducing stress; biofeedback, a way of monitoring our physical processes, enables us to become aware of them and thus make changes by applying our mind; spiritual healing is when the healer affects the energy field of the client, to make it more positive; art therapy and movement therapy may also be useful ways of getting in touch with feelings and expressing them, to help in the release of tension and anxiety.

Yoga Yoga, with its emphasis on physical and mental relaxation and control, is very suitable for pregnant women. The physical posture can be adapted throughout the changes of pregnancy and will encourage strength and suppleness. The gentle stretching exercises help maintain free movement and assist with posture. They can also help with backache and constipation. The breath control and meditation exercises help to lessen tension and increase a feeling of being in control. There are some classes especially for pregnant women, and some teachers are willing to include suitable exercises within general classes.

Environmental methods of stress reduction

Midwives working within maternity units may be able to influence the environment in order to help reduce the stress of mothers, their partners and staff.

Colour therapy is a relatively new idea in which colour is used to affect the mood of those in the environment. Blue and peach are regarded as particularly calming, and could be used as the dominant wall colouring or for coloured light bulbs. Emerald green is associated with intellect and bright yellow with logic, so that operating theatres or offices could be decorated with a predominance of these colours.

Aromas could be varied throughout the department, using refreshing but calming essential oils such as mandarin in a vaporiser through the day;

sleep-enhancing camomile on postnatal wards in the evening and rosemary and basil to stimulate and aid concentration in theatres. Care should be taken to use electrical vaporisers, which although more expensive are much safer than those based on candles.

A homely atmosphere could be planned when decorating the delivery suite, with beds more like conventional ones, rocking chairs and equipment stored behind cupboards until needed. This has long been advocated as a way of helping women to feel that a hospital birth can be as satisfying as a home birth, and it may help to reduce a mother's fear.

Staff attitudes are probably the most important means of inducing or reducing stress. A positive, friendly manner, offering women as much choice about their pregnancy and labour as possible, will result in better cooperation between staff and mothers and a feeling that they are part of a team. Many innovative units have introduced team midwifery, the named midwife concept and aspects of choice for mothers. It would appear however from the investigations that resulted in the *Changing Childbirth* document (Department of Health, 1993) that there is still a long way to go in many areas.

Many of the therapies discussed here are available through health professionals, or therapists may be contacted through national organisations.

Conclusion

The causes of stress, whilst having common elements, will be unique to the individual. Responses to stress are equally dependent on the circumstances, personality and experience of the individual. Methods of stress reduction must be appropriate, if they are to be effective.

We need to acknowledge the stress, mobilise our coping mechanisms or learn ways we can employ to develop new ones. We can never eliminate fear, anger and anxiety from our life but we can hope to learn how to minimise the damage they do.

Training

Autogenic Training: Centre for Autogenic Training, 101 Harley Street, London, W1N 1DF

Counselling: British Association for Counselling, 1 Regent Place, Rugby, CV21 2PJ Tel: 01788 578328

Healing: Guild of Spiritual Healers, 36 Newmarket, Otley, W. Yorkshire, LS21 3AE

Further details of training in various branches of complementary therapies can be found in: Maher G 1992 *Start a Career in Complementary Medicine*. Tackmart Publishing, London.

References

Adams M 1977 Biomechanics of low back pain. In: National Back Pain Association/ Royal College of Nursing *The Guide to the Handling of Patients* 4th edn. NBA/RCN, London

American College of Sports Medicine (ACSM) 1990 The recommended quantity and quality of exercise for developing and maintaining cardiorespiratory and muscular fitness in healthy adults. *Medicine and Science in Sports and Exercise* 22: 265–274

Artal R 1981 Exercise in pregnancy I. Maternal cardiovascular and metabolic responses in normal pregnancy. *American Journal of Obstetrics and Gynecology* 140: 123–127

Artal R 1984 Fetal bradycardia induced by maternal exercise. *Lancet* (2): 258–260

Artal R 1986 Pulmonary responses to exercise in pregnancy. *American Journal of Obstetrics and Gynaecology* 154(2): 378–383

Artal R 1986a *Exercise in Pregnancy*. Williams & Wilkins, Baltimore

Blakey P 1992 *The Muscle Book*. Bibliotek Books, London

Bouchard C 1994 *Physical Activity, Fitness and Health: International Proceedings and Consensus Statement*. Human Kinetics Publishers

Brayshaw E, Wright P 1994 *Teaching Physical Skills for the Childbearing Year*. Hale Books for Midwives, London

Brown G W, Harris T 1978 *Social Origins of Depression*. Tavistock, London

Bung P 1990 Maternal and fetal heart rate patterns: a pregnant athlete during training and laboratory exercise tests. *European Journal of Obstetrics and Gynaecology* 9: 232–235

Caspersen C 1985 *Physical activity, exercise and physical fitness: definitions for health related research*. Public Health Reports 100. Department of Health, London

Charles C 1998 Fetal hyperthermia risk from warm water immersion. *British Journal of Midwifery* 6(3): 152–156

Clapp F 1985 Fetal heart rate responses in running in mid-pregnancy and late pregnancy. *American Journal of Obstetrics and Gynaecology* 153: 251–253

Clapp F 1989 The effects of maternal exercise on early pregnancy outcome. *American Journal of Obstetrics and Gynaecology* 161: 1453–1457

Collings C 1985 Fetal heart rate response to maternal exercise. *American Journal of Obstetrics and Gynaecology* 151(4): 498–550

Doorn M 1992 Maternal and fetal cardiovascular responses to strenuous bicycle exercise. *American Journal of Obstetrics and Gynaecology* 166(43): 854–858

Egan G 1982 *The Skilled Helper*. Brooks/ Cole, CA, USA

Friedman M, Rosenman R 1974 *Type A Behaviour and Your Heart*. Knopf, New York

Guthrie K 1984 Maternal hypnosis induced by husbands during childbirth. *Journal of Obstetrics and Gynaecology* 4(5): 93–95

Health Education Authority 1993 *Physical activity strategic research*. Report to the HEA. HEA, London

Hedegaard M, Henrikson T B, Sabroe S, Secher N J 1993 Psychological distress in pregnancy and preterm delivery. *British Medical Journal* 307: 234–239

Hewitt J 1978 *Meditation*. Hodder & Stoughton, London

Holmes T A, Rahe R H 1967 The social readjustment rating scale. *Journal of Psychosomatic Research* 11: 213–218

Huch R, Erkkola R 1990 Pregnancy and exercise—exercise and pregnancy. A short review. *British Journal of Obstetrics and Gynaecology* 97: 208–214

Hytten F 1996 *Clinical Physiology in Obstetrics*. Blackwell Scientific, London

Hytten F, Chamberlain G 1991 *Clinical Physiology in Obstetrics*. Blackwell Scientific, London

Jabaaij L 1993 *Journal of Psychosomatic Research* 37: 361–9

Jacobson E 1938 *Progressive Relaxation*. University of Chicago Press, Chicago

Jarrett J 1983 Jogging during pregnancy: an improved outcome? *Obstetrics and Gynaecology* 61: 705–709

Kermani E 1992 *Autogenic Training*. Thorsons, London

Killoran A 1995 *Moving On: International Perspectives on Promoting Physical Activity*. Health Education Authority, London

Lazarus R 1966 *Psychological Stress and the Coping Process*. McGraw-Hill, New York

Luthe W 1963 Autogenic training: method, research and application in medicine.

American Journal of Psychotherapy 17: 174–195

Miller P, Smith D, Shephard T 1978 Maternal hyperthermia as a possible cause of anencephaly. *Lancet* I: 519–520

Morris N 1956 Effective uterine blood flow during exercise in normal and pre-eclamptic pregnancies. *Lancet* 2: 481

Newhall J 1981 Scuba diving during pregnancy: a brief review. *American Journal of Obstetrics and Gynaecology* 140: 893–894

Oakes G 1976 Uteroplacental blood flow during hyperthermia with and without alkalosis. *Journal of Applied Physiology* 41: 198–201

Palmer S 1992 Guidelines and contra-indications for teaching relaxation as a stress management technique. *Journal of the Institute of Health Education* 30: 25–30

Patel C 1987 *Fighting Heart Disease*. Dorling Kindersley, London

Platt L et al. 1983 Exercise in pregnancy II. Fetal responses. *American Journal of Obstetrics and Gynaecology* 147: 487–491

Polden M, Mantle J 1990 *Physiotherapy in Obstetrics and Gynaecology*. Butterworth Heinemann, London

Raphael-Leff J 1991. *Psychological Processes of Childbearing*. Chapman & Hall, London

Russell J 1984 The relationship of exercise to anovulatory cycles in female athletes: hormonal and physical characteristics. *Obstetrics and Gynaecology* 63: 452–456

Seyle H 1956 *The Stress of Life*. McGraw-Hill, New York

Sharma J B, Smith R J, Wilkin D J W 1993 Induction of labour at term. *British Medical Journal* 306: 1413

Sharpe D 1988 Validation of the thirty-item General Health Questionnaire in early pregnancy. *Psychological Medicine* 18: 503

Stiles W B at al. 1990 Correlation of session evaluations with treatment outcome. *British Journal of Clinical Psychology* 29: 13–21

Street E, Downey J 1996 *Brief Therapeutic Consultations*. Wiley, Chichester, UK

Wallace A 1987 The effects of aerobic exercise on the pregnant woman, fetus and pregnancy outcome: a review. *Journal of Nurse-Midwifery* 32(5): 277–290

Further reading

Bailey R, Clarke M 1989 *Stress and Coping in Nursing*. Chapman & Hall, London

Consumers' Association 1992 *Which Consumer Guides: Understanding Stress*. Consumers' Association, London

Dalton K 1989 *Depression after Childbirth*. Oxford University, Press, Oxford

Heardman H 1982 *Relaxation and Exercise for Childbirth*. Churchill Livingstone, Edinburgh

Madders J 1980 *Stress and Relaxation*. Optima, London

Mosse K 1993 *Becoming a Mother*. Virago, London

Oakley A 1991 *Social Support and Motherhood*. Blackwell, Oxford

Sutcliffe J 1991 *The Complete Book of Relaxation Techniques*. Headline, London

Watts A G 1977 *Relax—Dealing with Stress*. BBC Publications, London

Fiona Mantle, Bach Flower Remedies
Sue Mack, Alexander Technique

Chapter 13 ## Other Therapies

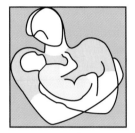

Bach Flower Remedies

Healthcare professionals who are interested in complementary therapies may well have noticed in their local health food shop, and latterly in high street chemists, a collection of small, dark brown bottles known as the Bach Flower Remedies. The story behind these remedies is a fascinating one and highlights the inspired work of one of the pioneers of complementary therapies and holistic care in this country. The healing power of plants is known worldwide, but the methodology and the discovery of this particular collection of essences was unique to Dr Edward Bach.

Bach Flower Remedies belong to the section of complementary therapies the mode of action of which is known as vibrational medicine, consisting of tinctures or essences which are charged with a particular frequency of subtle energy. This subtle, healing energy is germane to the vitalist tradition in medicine and is known as 'vital energy'. In homeopathy this is referred to as the 'spiritual vital force', which Hahnemann described as the ultimate source of health and illness and which is present in the body until death. Bach Flower Remedies are homeopathic remedies and, although they are prepared differently from other homeopathic remedies, they contain minute quantities of physical substance. The fact that water contains memory and that the vibrational characteristics of the homeopathic remedy is imprinted on the universal medium of water, which subsequently has an effect on the body cells, has been demonstrated by Davenas et al. (1988). Unlike other homeopathic remedies, Bach Flower Remedies do not undergo serial dilution, nor are they succussed; instead there are two methods of distilling the flower essences. The first is by the sun method, where the freshly picked flowers are put into a glass bowl of spring water and left in the sun for several hours. The action of the sun's rays on the plants energises the water. Following this the flower essence is then preserved in an equal amount of brandy and is known as the mother tincture. The second method is the boiling method, when the flowers are boiled in spring water for half an hour, the essence strained and as before, diluted with an equal amount of brandy.

Before describing the remedies and their influence on pregnancy and childbirth it is important to understand the life, times and philosophy of the man who discovered them.

Dr Edward Bach

Dr Bach, physician, pathologist and homeopath, was born in 1886 in the village of Moseley near Birmingham in Warwickshire. He resolved early in life to become a doctor, but hesitated to burden his parents with the fees for his training, so, on leaving school, he started work in his father's brass foundry. This early experience of working life gave him an insight into the devastating effects of physical and mental illness leading to loss of work, and resulting in the risk of very real poverty for working families. When he was 20 he entered Birmingham University, and qualified as a doctor at University College Hospital in 1912.

Throughout his training and during his early medical career, Dr Bach became more and more interested in his patients rather than in their illnesses. At the same time, he became very concerned about the harshness of some of the conventional treatments his patients had to undergo. In 1918, whilst working at the Royal London Homeopathic Hospital, he became acquainted with the works of Hahnemann and the gentle approach of homeopathy as well as its philosophy of treating the patient and not the disease. This approach to treatment was very appealing to him.

Although greatly influenced by Hahnemann's work, Dr Bach was concerned with the nature of the remedies he was prescribing, since they were themselves made out of bacteria, as well as by homeopathy's complexity and its reliance on medical supervision for an accurate diagnosis and treatment. He was aware that the cost of medical treatment was often prohibitive for working families and he longed to devise a system of emotional healing using herbs which would be understandable and available to everyone: a philosophy of patient empowerment well in advance of his time.

During the next few years, during his holidays in the countryside, he found the first three of his 38 remedies: Impatiens, Mimulus and Clematis, which he prepared using homeopathic principles. He began treating patients with the new remedies and was delighted with the results. Bach claimed to have identified 38 healing remedies corresponding to 38 negative states which influence the course of illness and well-being. The 38 remedies are commonly divided into two groups: these are referred to as 'type remedies' relative to certain personality types and 'mood remedies' focusing on a person's presenting emotional state. Bach asserted that a presenting emotion may not be permanent nor a normal part of the patient's personality, but a result of circumstances in which the patients find themselves; thus, a remedy prescribed one week may well need to be adjusted two weeks or even two days later. Prescriptions are therefore tailored to suit the patient's changing situation and their reaction at a particular point in time. The flexibility of the system allows for the fact that a prescription may not be a once-and-for-all application, but may be adapted to suit the patient's changing situation and their reaction to the remedies. For example, many of us will recognise the type of person who suffers from overwhelming guilt and constantly blames themselves for the misfortunes of others. Pine would be their 'type remedy'. However, we can all think of instances when we have had passing feelings of guilt about what we have done or said, and in this instance, Pine would be our 'mood remedy'. Scleranthus is the 'type remedy' for people who are completely unable to make up their mind even over the smallest matter: again, a temporary situation with which we can all identify.

A glance through the list of remedies often evokes the comment, 'I need all of them!' This is a perfectly sensible response since the remedies, both type and mood, relate to normal, everyday, human emotions which we all experience from time to time.

At a superficial level the remedies appear to address the trait or state approach to personality. The debate addresses the issue of whether we have enduring traits which can be measured by psychometric tests and are an ingrained part of our personality, or whether the way we present ourselves is simply a reflection of the emotional state we are in, which is the result of the circumstances in which we find ourselves. However, since the application of the remedies takes into account changes of both type and mood over time, both on a long-term and short-term basis, they can be said to subscribe to the lifespan developmental interactionalist approach. Dr Bach's concept of personality was, therefore, far in advance of the prevailing Freudian approach of the time.

In 1934, Dr Bach and his two assistants moved to the village of Brightwell-cum-Sotwell in Oxfordshire, to a house called Mount Vernon which is now the home of the Dr Edward Bach Healing Trust, and it was here that he spent the last two years of his life and discovered the final 19 remedies.

Dr Bach died in 1936, content that his system of healing was complete. He wished his work to remain as he had devised it and that no further addition to the system be made. There is no need. By careful diagnosis and the correct combination of the remedies, all presenting personality types and moods can be helped. At first glance it could be suggested, and indeed it has been, that a system of healing devised before World War II would have little application to modern living, and this criticism is occasionally voiced about the Bach Flower Remedies. However, Dr Bach's discoveries are as pertinent today as they ever were. The pressures and strains of life may be different from the 1930s but people's reaction to them is the same, whether it be the fear of tuberculosis or AIDS, loss of family, friends or jobs, or general uncertainty about the future.

Although Dr Bach's aim was for his healing method to be available for the lay public, they can be dispensed to better effect by a Registered Bach Practitioner who has a detailed knowledge of the remedies and is better able to select the best combination for the client.

The remedies, with personality types/presenting emotional states		
	Agrimony	for those who hide their feelings behind a cheerful face
	Aspen	for unidentifiable fear of the unknown
	Beech	for people who are critical and intolerant of others, perfectionists
	Centaury	for people who are unable to say 'no' and tend to be exploited
	Cerato	for people who are unable to make up their mind and seek the reassurance of others, with a marked tendency to dither
	Cherry Plum	for uncontrollable rage, and fear of losing control
	Chestnut Bud	for those unable to learn from mistakes and past experiences
	Chicory	for fussy and overprotective people who need the appreciation of others
	Clematis	for the absent-minded, inattentive, easily bored
	Crab Apple	for feelings of self-disgust, poor body image, the need to be cleansed mentally and physically
	Elm	for those who are overwhelmed with responsibility and pressure of work
	Gentian	for depression following a setback, despondency and pessimism
	Gorse	for discouragement and despair
	Heather	for obsessive self-centredness, people always talking about their own problems
	Holly	for suspicion, jealousy and hatred, feelings of being victimised
	Honeysuckle	for those who live in the past, overwhelming nostalgia
	Hornbeam	for emotional weariness at the thought of work, dread of the day ahead
	Impatiens	for the impatient personality, always in a rush, irritable with people

Larch	for those who are competent but fear failure, with great self-doubt, feelings of inferiority
Mimulus	for a shy, nervous personality, also for fear of known things such as flying, exam nerves
Mustard	for depression of unknown origin
Oak	for fighting spirits who are overwhelmed with exhaustion
Olive	for physical or mental exhaustion due to overwork or over-exertion
Pine	for self-blame, remorse and guilt even if there is no cause for blame
Red Chestnut	for those who worry excessively about family and friends, always afraid of impending disasters
Rock Rose	for terror and panic often following accidents; useful for nightmares
Rock Water	for the perfectionist, self-denying, strong willed
Scleranthus	for inability to make choices, constant vacillation between two or more options
Star of Bethlehem	for loss, bereavement, trauma
Sweet Chestnut	for complete despair, unbearable unhappiness
Vervain	for those who are perfectionists, very active with strong principles, who have pushed themselves too far
Vine	for strong, dominant personalities who are ambitious and determined, autocratic
Walnut	the remedy for change, births, puberty, divorce
Water Violet	for those who are very reserved, self-contained, liking privacy, may become isolated
White Chestnut	for constant ruminations and worries, unwanted thoughts, inability to concentrate
Wild Oak	for when a change of direction is needed, for someone at the crossroads of life
Wild Rose	for drifters who have no ambition or direction in life and take whatever life offers
Willow	for self-pity, resentment and bitterness, people who feel they have had a raw deal in life.

Perhaps the most famous of all the remedies is Rescue Remedy. This is a composite remedy consisting of Star of Bethlehem, Rock Rose, Impatiens, Cherry Plum and Clematis. As its name suggests it is used in emergencies to combat fear, panic, shock and fear of losing control. It is also available in cream form, when Crab Apple is added for its cleansing properties.

Preparing for pregnancy

Modern living for men and women involves the integration of a variety of roles and activities, which necessitates careful planning, lots of organisation and sheer physical effort. That most people manage to achieve all this is akin to a minor miracle. It is all the more devastating then when this level of organisation and achievement does not extend into childbearing and Mother Nature sees fit to throw a spanner in the works, preventing the couple's hopes of parenthood being achieved. Unlike other obstacles in everyday life which the couple have dealt with as a matter of course, the problem of infertility can result in a long saga of fertility tests and treatment which is expensive, time-consuming and emotionally draining, as well as inflicting considerable stress on their relationship. The options which are available to them might include in vitro fertilisation, artifical insemination, ovarian donation and hormone injections, and have all to be considered by the couple. Remedies which can help them through the period, which may extend into years, include: Crab Apple for the antipathy the woman may feel towards her body which has let her down, Gentian for the possible repeated disappointments which can accompany infertility treatments, Willow for feelings of self pity and resentment and Holly for the feeling of envy or jealousy towards other women who conceive without any problems. Fortunately many women are able to overcome these setbacks, become pregnant and give birth to a very precious baby.

Antenatal care

As the previous section has indicated, a successful pregnancy can have a range of antecedents and can be achieved by a variety of methods, including the most popular! Unfortunately, pregnancy is not always the happy occasion that it ought to be. Social circumstances can be such that the pregnancy is marred by health problems, family discord or work concerns over which the mother may have little control. No one can look forward to a new life and new family if either partner is working under the threat of redundancy. Similarly, the anticipated arrival of a new grandchild does not always have the hoped-for mollifying effect on in-laws who do not approve of the relationship either for social or religious reasons, whilst the possibility of losing one income can cause tensions which can strain the happiest of relationships. Occasionally, in less settled relationships, the client may find herself abandoned by her partner when she announces the pregnancy, and single parents may feel lonely and afraid, particularly if they are young or living away from home for long periods, for example airline pilots, members of the armed forces or those who have to travel overseas on business. Bach Flower Remedies can offer a great deal of help in these circumstances. For a known anxiety, for example the threat of redundancy, Mimulus is the remedy of choice, but for the vague, ill-defined anxiety about the future Aspen would be appropriate. For family relationships which involve feelings of resentment or disappointment in the choice of partner, and for the abandoned mother or for the shock to the single mother for whom the pregnancy was unplanned, Star of Bethlehem would be prescribed. For many working women the possibility of remaining at home with the baby after birth is not an option. In some professions 'time out' to have a baby can seriously impede a woman's chances of promotion or cause her to lose touch with developments in her field of work. For some mothers, the whole idea of leaving the baby in the care of a nanny or childminder can engender strong feelings of guilt for which Pine is the remedy of choice. For others the option is open and for those with feelings of indecision Scleranthus or Cerato can help them to come to a decision. Olive may be used for the accompanying tiredness.

Midwives will recognise the woman who has been used to organising her life and having it under control and is distressed and amazed at the way in which her body starts to change and produce signs and symptoms which she may not have experienced before. Having previously enjoyed an iron constitution which allowed her to breeze through the most arduous day she now finds herself rocked by nausea, tortured by backache and bewildered by her changing emotions. Some clients may even grow to hate their body, and the baby for what it is doing to them. They may experience a feeling of being out of control and express the feelings that the baby is taking over their body. For these feelings Walnut, for the change in lifestyle, Crab Apple for the feeling of anger about the body and Scleranthus for labile emotions could be suggested.

These emotions, as well as physical changes during pregnancy, can make functioning on a day-to-day basis very difficult and many clients may find that they are not able to operate at their previously high standard. This is not in any way a suggestion that women are poor workers when pregnant, but that doing a demanding job whilst feeling tired and nauseated does tend to stack the cards against them. For those who set very high standards at home and at work and find it difficult to be more relaxed and adaptable, Rock Water is suggested. Of course this applies not only to working women but also to those running a tight schedule at home with other children to care for. By contrast, other women sail through their pregnancy, positively blooming all the way and being a constant irritation to those less fortunate.

Fears during pregnancy

Along with the usual worries of modern living, pregnancy brings its own set of anxieties. Foremost in any parent's mind is the concern that the baby is going to be 'all right'. The first words said by a new mother are not usually 'What sex is it?' but 'Is it all right?' Fortunately most pregnancies proceed normally, and there is a range of screening tests which can be conducted to ensure all is well with mother and baby. However, these tests are optional and some clients may decide that because the outcome of the tests will have no influence on their desire to continue with the pregnancy they would rather do without them. However, the fact that the tests exist at all raises the issue of choice and the debate as to whether or not a mother should undergo screening tests may cause anxiety. Again Cerato or Scleranthus is prescribed for the indecision, White Chestnut for the recurrent thoughts, debates, and arguments which go round in her mind and Mimulus for known fear of a potentially handicapped baby. Other clients experience a vaguer, diffused anxiety, for which Aspen is more appropriate. Some mothers tell midwives or health visitors that they fear they will not be able to cope once the baby is born, either because their partner will be away or because they are living a long way from their own family. This is very relevant for service families overseas when husbands can be away on active service and families remain at home, where the mother will have the total responsibility for the baby. Elm is the remedy of choice for the overpowering feelings of responsibility which threaten to overwhelm them, and Larch is recommended for those clients who suffer from a general lack of self-confidence. Occasionally these feelings may give way to panic, in which case Rock Rose would be appropriate. Many clients report that the last month of pregnancy can seem longer than the previous eight months. Most women will have given up work and be anxious for the final stage of becoming a mother, and remark to the midwife or health visitor that 'I just want to get on with it.' For the irritation and frustration experienced at this difficult time, Impatiens will help to see them through. One problem which is frequently reported is the lack of sleep due to the baby's activity and the sheer bulk of the pregnancy. There is nothing to compare with lying awake at night for all manner of disturbing thoughts to start chasing round the mind, and to this end White Chestnut will help the client to stay calm and relaxed. Olive is recommended for the tiredness during this period, together with Aspen for the feeling of free floating anxiety when faced with the unknown.

Normal labour

Health professionals might suggest that in addition to the usual preparation for labour, the client might use certain Bach Flower Remedies. Judy Howard of the Bach Centre in Oxfordshire suggests Rescue Remedy for almost all of labour, and Olive for the tiredness if labour is prolonged, Gentian for setbacks such as necessary deviations from the birth plan and Walnut for the transition stage.

Postnatal help

Although the client has been pregnant for 9 months she may have only been away from work for 6 weeks, whereas in previous generations women gave up work when they got married and had a period of settling into their new, more house-bound, role before they became pregnant. Nowadays, because the transition period between working and motherhood is so short, i.e. only a few weeks, the mind and body have very little time to adjust to their new role and the shock to the system can be extreme. In the first few hours after the baby is born, Rescue Remedy will prove a great stand-by with Walnut to ease the transition from pregnant woman to mother. If the delivery has not gone as planned because of some necessary medical intervention or it was simply different from what the client expected or was led to believe, she may well feel angry and resentful. Rationalising that the baby is safe and that is all that matters does not always make up for an unsatisfying delivery, and Willow is indicated here. A bad delivery can make her feel resentful towards the baby, particularly if it was an intervention on behalf of the baby that caused the change of plan. Thankfully the myth of 'bonding' has been firmly refuted now, but even so, many mothers still feel guilty if they do not 'fall in love' with their baby on first sight. In such conditions, Pine is indicated.

It might be worthwhile at this point to stop and consider the subject of guilt. All mothers feel guilty and anxious about their children at some point, for many varying reasons. Much of this guilt and anxiety centres around the problems of crying, feeding and sleeping, frequently reducing parents and other carers to tears of frustration, helplessness and anger. Occasionally, these feelings can be so intense that they can include hatred towards the baby for making them feel so helpless. The midwife or health visitor might suggest Holly for the hatred, Gentian for the discouragement and despondency at the continual failure to soothe the baby in spite of repeated attempts, and Gorse for feelings of complete hopelessness and despair. Willow is used for resentment and Larch for the loss of confidence that this kind of situation can engender, particularly if the client is one of those who has always had her life under control. Health professionals will be alert for the mother who struggles on even when exhausted, is too proud to ask for help and subscribes to the ethos of coping at all costs. For these clients, Oak and Water Violet are indicated.

One adjustment which may have to be made at this point is the coming to terms with the 'real' baby and not the baby the parents have fantasised about for 9 months. Occasionally, mothers fear for their own sanity and are frightened that they will harm the baby. For this Cherry Plum will help, as well as Crab Apple for the self-hatred that these feelings evoke. It is often difficult for mothers to come to terms with these feelings, some of which may be quite alien to them and make them long for their pre-motherhood self which was rational and organised. So there is to a certain extent a mini-bereavement as well as a moving forward period which can be painful. Two remedies can help here. For the feeling of unreality of the new life, Clematis can help to centre the client and Honeysuckle to counter the wish to live in the past.

One thing that will certainly happen once the client has had her baby is that she will never be short of advice. Much of this is well meaning and some of it will be useful, if irritating, which can help to put things into perspective. However, it can all become overwhelming: Walnut will help to protect her from the influences of others when she is feeling vulnerable, whilst Cerato can help her to make up her own mind about which advice she is going to adopt, following her own intuition. In addition she may be inundated with visitors, who can be extremely tiring and make getting into a routine even more difficult. Olive is the remedy for tiredness but it is much more sensible for her to dismiss the visitors and get some sleep; Olive should be used judiciously, and only when it is really necessary. It is far preferable for a client to sleep if they are tired rather than press on when exhausted. If the mother lacks assertiveness because she is tired and lacking in confidence, Centaury will help her to convey her wishes firmly.

Unfortunately, not everyone is going to be delighted to see the new baby. The family pet for one may find that his normal routine (along with everyone else's) is disrupted and that he does not get as much attention as before; dogs in particular can suffer badly from jealousy and become aggressive or more demanding. Animals respond very well to Bach Flower Remedies—in fact, some practitioners work exclusively with animals. Holly would be appropriate for an animal's jealousy, with Willow or Chicory for feelings of rejection. Other siblings, however well prepared for the baby's arrival, may exhibit behaviour which suggests that they are not as accepting as was assumed at first. Often they are quite pleased initially but when the novelty wears off and they realise that the baby is not a temporary diversion from the normal routine they can become angry, resentful and disruptive. All small children are 'needy', they have a healthy egocentricity which is not necessarily shared by other people. Chicory is the remedy for possessiveness, and, again, Holly for any jealous feelings.

There is nothing more depressing for a new mother than the sight of other mothers who appear to be coping brilliantly, who do not have perineal stitches and whose breastfeeding is well established. A client in this situation would respond to Holly for the jealousy, Willow for resentment and Gentian for the setbacks which are getting her down. Other feelings often reported include those of isolation and loneliness, as well as a general feeling of disorganisation compounded by memory lapses which can be quite distressing. The drop in household standards can be very distressing to some mothers who try to stick rigidly to their pre-baby standards. Rock Water can help to encourage a greater flexibility, Gentian to combat feelings of discouragement and despondency, and Hornbeam to cope with feelings of being unable to face the day ahead.

The new baby   For the sheer shock of being born, however gentle the birth and skilled the midwife, Rescue Remedy, with Walnut for the adjustment to life outside the uterus, is appropriate. Parents soon become aware that their baby has a personality of his own. Some babies are impatient and irritable (sometimes due to birth trauma). Impatiens is suggested, whilst for the clingy, crying baby who demands a great deal of attention and will not be put down, Chicory might be suggested.

If things go wrong

Premature labour is often unanticipated and when it happens it can be devastating. The mother's first reaction is severe shock, disbelief and feelings of unreality. Midwives would find Rescue Remedy the solution of choice since it contains the main remedies for this type of trauma: Star of Bethlehem for the shock, Clematis for the feeling of unreality and denial, Rock Rose for the rising panic, Cherry Plum for fear of losing control. In addition Red Chestnut can be used for the mother's overwhelming fears for the safety of the baby and, if this has happened before, Sweet Chestnut for the utter despair that the history is repeating itself. Pine is helpful for the irrational feelings of guilt that some mothers experience at having somehow failed the baby, while Crab Apple will subdue the feelings of anger that her body has let her down. While the baby is in the special care baby unit, Red Chestnut will help for her overwhelming fear for the safety of the baby and White Chestnut will calm the worrying thoughts which will not go away.

Stillbirth or neonatal death In the sad and unfortunate event of loss of the baby, the best remedy is Rescue Remedy since it contains the essence Star of Bethlehem for shock and bereavement, Clematis for the dissociation and denial, Cherry Plum for the fear the mother may have of losing her mind. In addition to Rescue Remedy the midwife might suggest Sweet Chestnut for the feelings of utter despair as well as White Chestnut for the recurrent thoughts of 'Why me?' The bereavement process is complex, and how well people survive it depends very much on how they are treated after the tragic event. When a baby dies the parents' future dies with it. All the hopes and plans which have occupied their thoughts and have been the focus of their lives for the last 9 months lie in ruins, leaving a void, and if the baby is the first, there is a loss of their anticipated role as parents. They will benefit from Wild Rose, which addresses the emptiness and the lack of direction when the role of parenthood has been denied.

Handicapped baby If a baby is born with a physical or mental disability, whether it is genetic or caused as a result of birth trauma, the parents will go through a bereavement process in the same way as they would if the baby had died. Rescue Remedy again is indicated, with Honeysuckle to detach them from their previous images of the baby and to help them to move on. Mimulus can be used when there is fear of what the future might bring, and Red Chestnut for concern about the baby's safety. Some parents hide their torment behind a brave face and if the midwife or health visitor feels that this is the case, Agrimony might be suggested. They may feel overwhelmed by the responsibility for such a vulnerable baby, so Elm would be indicated. For some, the birth of an imperfect baby may be seen as failure, accompanied by guilt that somehow it might have been their fault; some may feel it is a form of retribution. For this guilt Pine should be suggested, with White Chestnut again for recurrent thoughts. Parents often remark that one of the hardest things to do is to tell other people about the baby. Mimulus might help, but for parents of a seriously ill baby Rescue Remedy might be preferable.

Postnatal depression It is normal for mothers to feel weepy and emotional just after the baby's birth, and Scleranthus would be helpful during this period. More severe depression can result from some of the issues which have been discussed and already addressed in this chapter, such as bad birth experiences or problems with the baby. Feelings of inadequacy and helplessness have also been highlighted and suitable remedies suggested. In addition there are three flower remedies which are specifically used for depression, and they might be suggested in addition to those which relate to the underlying cause: for the depression caused by setbacks and despondency, Gentian; for the depression which includes feelings of pessimism and lack of hope, Gorse might be suggested; with Mustard for depression which descends without warning and Sweet Chestnut for feelings of utter despair. The remedies are not suggested as a substitute for medical intervention or counselling and practical support, particularly for severe depression, but can be used as an adjunct to other treatment.

Research The continued use of the Flower Remedies, as with other therapies, indicates their effectiveness. However, as Nicholl (1995) points out, this is not generally accepted as evidence amongst the scientific community. The Research Council for Complementary Medicine database did not reveal any research studies on the remedies, though whether this is due to lack of interest or resource is not clear. Until such research is conducted it may be difficult for the remedies to gain complete acceptance into mainstream health care. Certainly a controlled trial would be an unsuitable method of research, given the individualised nature of the prescriptions, although it might be reasonable to do one on the composite Rescue Remedy. However, since the remedy is unlikely to be given in isolation the difficulty of controlling confounding variables would make outcome measurements difficult to evaluate. On the other hand, the remedies do lend themselves to the more qualitative methods of research such as a single case study design, where an in-depth analysis could be conducted of the circumstances under which the remedies were prescribed, and their outcome.

Although at present there is no research for health professionals to draw on to justify their use of the Bach Flower Remedies it is a completely safe therapy with no known contraindications, and it can be easily incorporated into routine maternity care. The remedies are not known to conflict with orthodox medication, although they are adjusted according to the client's ongoing mental state. They may be given to babies and children in the same dosage as for adults.

How the remedies are selected and dispensed

Remedies which have been suggested in this chapter as being of relevance to specific problems are intended as a guide to the use of the flower remedies. In practice a similar scenario might, following careful questioning, indicate another remedy to be more appropriate. For example, Scleranthus might be suggested for indecision but it might be that the client is actually frightened of the consequences of that decision, in which case Mimulus should be considered. Accurate prescription of the remedies relies on a careful analysis of the client's emotional state by sympathetic questioning in order to determine the underlying problem. John Ramsell (1991) uses anxiety as an example of this, suggesting that it might have a number of causes for which different remedies would be appropriate, citing Elm for someone suffering from overwhelming responsibilities and Red Chestnut for anxiety about a family member. Since the remedies are preserved in alcohol it is suggested that the remedies are dispensed by adding two drops of the prescribed remedy to 30 ml of still, spring water. Four drops of this mixture is then taken four times a day in a little liquid. For a passing mood or for day-to-day mood fluctuations two drops of the appropriate stock remedy can be added to a glass of water and sipped through the day. Up to six remedies can be prescribed at one time and if the 'wrong' remedy is used it will have no adverse effect. The remedies are completely safe and can be given to children and babies as well as animals and plants.

Training

Health professionals who are interested in using the Bach Flower Remedies can train to use them by undertaking the practitioners' course at Mount Vernon. This consists of four study days set in one of the loveliest of educational settings and followed by written assignments to be completed over a period of months. The course is aimed at health care practitioners who already have a good working knowledge of the remedies, and aims to clarify and enhance their practice. The course emphasises the philosophy behind the remedies as well as their practical application. The written assignments are aimed at consolidating knowledge and must be completed before registration can take place. Health professionals may feel more confident about incorporating the remedies into care if they have been on a recognised course.

There is no reason why Registered Practitioners should not use the remedies both in hospital and in the community in order to enhance their care of clients and patients, thereby providing a tangible help for their emotional needs.

Andrea was a health visitor who used BFR in her practice. She was visiting Susan who had just had her second baby. Susan was having difficulty in adjusting to the new baby and difficulty in establishing breastfeeding. Andrea suggested Walnut for the changes in Susan's life and Larch for her fear of failure to breastfeed, as well as Gentian to overcome setbacks. Susan also reported feeling guilty because she was impatient with Sophie, her three-year-old, and unable to give as much time to her as she would wish. Andrea suggested Impatiens and Pine for her irritability and guilt. Sophie had started to wet the bed again since her little brother was born, so Andrea suggested Walnut again, as well as Holly and Aspen for Sophie's general anxiety.

Antenatal scenario for midwives
Angela was 25 years old and eight months pregnant. This was her second pregnancy. She had lost her first baby at 5 months and because of this she was very anxious about the birth and needed constant reassurance. Her ambivalence was obvious from the fact that she had made no plans for the baby by buying clothes or equipment, and had discouraged others from doing so. Her husband Mark was very supportive but worked long hours as a builder, which left Angela alone for much of the day. She was often weepy and fearful, with anxious thoughts constantly going round in her mind. When Mark came home she unburdened all this on to him. He of course had his own worries but felt that these were not being addressed.

If you were caring for Angela antenatally, which remedies would you suggest for her?

Postnatal scenario for midwives
Susan was a 25-year-old professional woman with a high-powered job in the city. She was anxious to return to work as soon as possible. Her partner who also worked in the city was abroad, and could not get home for the birth. Susan was very resentful about this. She had attended private antenatal classes and had planned for a natural waterbirth at home. However, because of fetal distress, she was taken to hospital for an emergency Caesarean section. Now Susan had become very depressed, resentful and feeling cheated of her 'birth

*experience'. She was taking little interest in her new baby and
did not want to breastfeed him as she had originally planned.
Her family was very concerned about her and constantly
giving her advice and trying to take over.*

*If you were caring for Susan, what remedies would you
suggest?*

**Alexander
Technique**

The Alexander Technique, which has been in use for over a hundred years,
is a method for teaching people how to eliminate bad habits of body misuse
that may cause physical disorders or even emotional problems. It is not
a passive therapy but engages the client in a process of re-education,
becoming more aware of their body and how they use it in order to protect
and heal themselves.

The Alexander Technique is so named after an Australian actor, Frederick
Alexander. He suffered persistent throat problems that threatened his career,
and set out to examine his posture to see if there was a cause in the way he
held himself. He discovered that he tensed his body in such a way that
he was affecting the balance of his back, neck and head, thus affecting his
throat and voice. This tension in the neck, a tightening of the sterno-cleido-
mastoid and trapezius muscles, is very common and a frequent cause of
backaches as well as neck pain and throat problems. Alexander taught
himself to alter his posture and become aware of the muscle tension so
that he could find better control of not just his voice but his whole body.
By the beginning of this century he was so frequently asked for help that
he set up a practice in London, mainly treating other actors but gradually
training others in his methods so that his discoveries were passed on.
Alexander also began to link the mental and physical processes of the body,
recognising that it is not possible to separate them in healing. We can cause
discomfort or even damage to our bodies from unconscious tensions: these
arise from several causes. We may feel under time pressure or professional
and family demands, we may feel anxious or fearful; all this is transferred
to tension in the body. When we concentrate we may hold our breath and
tense our muscles, frown or bite a lip: anxiety can cause muscle tension so
that movements become jerky or we may feel nauseous.

Alexander talked about 'using ourselves', meaning not just the mechanical use of our bodies but the whole self, in every area including our approach
to life. We are 'using ourselves' all the time. Much of our movement and
posture is habitual, we learn an action by repetition until we no longer think
about how we do it. Learning to skate or drive are good examples of this.
They take great concentration to learn but once learnt we would often find
it difficult to isolate the particular physical or even mental skills required
to perform them. Within our early development of physical skills we learn
by copying and practice; we also learn the attitudes to life and emotional

responses such as anxiety and anger of those around us. Thus we may learn bad habits of movement or coordination from early life. We may also develop bad habits of movement as the result of trauma or illness, or affect our posture from a dislike of our bodies or a part of ourselves that we seek to hide. Sometimes a young person who has grown quickly or very tall may develop a habit of slouching that may continue long after they are no longer standing out from their friends.

Alexander believed that what he called the 'primary control' was the relationship between the head, neck and back. This is the mechanism for organizing and controlling upright posture and coordination through the whole body. This does not mean that there is a fixed position, for the body has to be free to move, but rather the alignment of the head, neck and back that is in a dynamic relationship. He believed that we should move with head leading and the spine following, which occurs with a good head–neck–back relationship. This is a key feature of the Alexander teacher's work, to establish a good head–neck–back alignment, balance and movement being achieved with a minimal amount of muscle tension, and to identify and eliminate the bad habits. What Alexander referred to as 'good use' is fluid movement with little tension and unrestricted breathing, the best functioning in all activities. Misuse interferes with the primary control and increases the amount of muscular tension required to move, which means that muscular use is uneven, some being put under excessive tension, and upright posture and movement is an effort, producing stiffness and a limited range of movement as well as breathing difficulties. Misuse may occur in minor ways such gripping an object more tightly than required, or walking in a way that puts excessive tension on a group of muscles, or it may be that anxiety may cause you to tense the muscles in your neck or shoulders or to clench your teeth.

In trying to solve his own problems, Alexander also realised that we cannot necessarily trust our own awareness of body position. Our 'kinaesthetic' sense through which we receive information about our body in space and in relation to the different parts of itself may not be reliable; chronic tension may block its ability to feed back our tension or faulty position. Thus Alexander recognised that his bad habits were unconscious and he could not trust his senses to correct them, and he needed to develop a way of becoming more conscious in controlling his body.

Alexander based his technique on two fundamental principles, inhibition and direction. He defined inhibition as 'the restraint of the direct expression of an instinct'. The instinctive response to a stimulus has to be inhibited for the bad habits to be eliminated. Alexander believed that if he stopped doing the 'wrong' thing then the 'right' one would automatically follow. The immediate response has to be inhibited and the student has to delay the action to consider the way it is performed. If you become conscious of how you rise from a chair you will find that you change the way you perform the action. The body has to be taught to change ingrained habits but we first have to become conscious of those habits.

After inhibition comes direction. The student learns to direct himself or herself consciously to affect certain muscular activity. Alexander found that his kinaesthetic sense was not enough to allow him to be aware of what he was doing wrong, so he developed 'instructions' to himself to encourage good use, such as 'Think of the whole body lengthening'.

The main directions relate to primary control: let the neck be free, the head goes forward and upward and the body lengthens and widens. There are many other directions which the teacher will use in relation to what he or she observes in the client, such as 'Think of the shoulders dropping' or 'Think about the ribcage dropping'. These will all help the client to learn good use and ease muscle tension. Alexander was not concerned with 'correct' movement but free movement.

Learning the Alexander Technique

The aim of the Alexander Technique is not to achieve a perfect posture but rather an improvement in a general way of holding and moving oneself. This makes it suitable for people with any physical condition, and particularly useful to pregnant women whose posture will change as the baby grows. Alexander lessons are gentle and unthreatening, there is no need to undress and the touch of the teacher is non-intrusive; it is a way of establishing where the tensions are, and to help the client firstly to become aware of them and then to release them. Most lessons are one-to-one for about half an hour. The number of lessons and their frequency will be discussed with the teacher. The client will be asked to lie down, to sit and stand and to walk, so that attention can be paid to the whole range of movement. Breathing is also discussed and worked on. The teacher's aim is to increase awareness of coordination and movement on the principle of head, neck and back, aiming to bring about release of tension and change habits. The client is very much part of the process.

She is taught basic procedures such as the monkey, the lunge, the squat, kneeling and all fours. These are taught to everyone, and their particular application in pregnancy will be examined later in the chapter.

Although some of the exercises can be described, it is very difficult, even with the aid of a long mirror, to check one's own posture. In pregnancy with the constantly changing body shape this is still more difficult and the Alexander teacher can see more clearly what is happening.

The monkey (Fig. 13.1) is the basic stance on which the others are built. It is the position giving the optimum use of the musculoskeletal system and should be the position we move through from sitting to standing and for activities requiring bending or lifting. It requires the least muscular effort, the head and knees going forward are counterbalanced by the bottom going back over the heels. The legs have less tension, and weight-bearing joints

Fig. 13.1. The monkey.

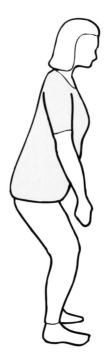

are at their mid-point. This position also expands the ribcage and allows full breathing. The lunge is the monkey with one leg in front of the other. The back is inclined forward, the knees bent and apart and one foot behind the other. The movement is used when pushing or pulling is needed, the legs and back working together, the arms hanging freely from the shoulders.

The squat (Fig. 13.2) is difficult for most adults to achieve and requires re-education of muscles and tendons. It is taught as a semi-squat monkey and then gradually deepened to a full squat. The squat may be taught

Fig. 13.2. The squat.

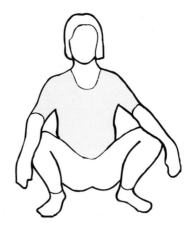

Fig. 13.3. Kneeling.

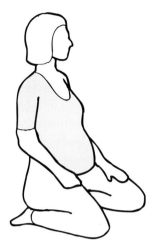

first as a semi-squat, with the client holding a rail for support until muscles are more supple.

Kneeling (Fig. 13.3) may be an alternative to squatting for activities that require you to be at floor level. With your bottom resting on your heels and a relaxed position it may be a helpful one to practise before labour. The all-fours position encourages stretching the back and is good for alleviating backache, especially when combined with a gentle rocking movement.

Alexander also recommends 'dynamic resting'. Excessive muscle tension and the force of gravity when standing up combine to compress the bones of the spine. This is the reason we are slightly taller first thing in the morning. Resting for a short period once or twice a day not only refreshes the mind but releases tension in the spine. A semi-supine position is recommended, lying on a firm surface on the back, with something firm such as a book supporting the head. The Alexander teacher will be able to help you find the best position for you as it will vary from person to person according to height and back position. This is not a good position for a woman later in pregnancy as the pressure of the uterus on major blood vessels can cause problems. The teacher will advise on more suitable resting positions. Getting up from the semi-supine position is important as you do not want to introduce unnecessary muscle tension immediately. Rolling onto the side, turning your head first in that direction and then taking the further arm across the body, will allow you to retain the correct alignment.

The use of Alexander Technique in pregnancy

Pregnancy can be a stressful time both physically and mentally. The body shape is constantly changing and poor 'use' of the body, the bad habits, will be exacerbated and the potential for aches and pains increased. Teachers recommend that the Technique is learned before conception so that good habits are already in place. However, it is possible to learn at any time as long as the teacher is aware of the pregnancy. Alexander Technique can help to develop better postural habits and reduce tension throughout pregnancy. The stress of pregnancy may also be lessened by being more aware of muscle tension and therefore better able to unwind. This has a generally beneficial affect on the nervous system and may reduce some problems such as blood pressure and heartburn. Awareness of breathing helps to reduce tension and is invaluable during labour. The consciousness that the woman develops of her body and how it responds may also help to produce a feeling of wholeness. The positive encouragement that the technique gives to dynamic resting may also help the woman take time for herself.

Misuse and good use Misuse in pregnancy is likely to be an exacerbation of general misuse and bad habits. The woman whose normal posture is over-tense may pull her head back further to compensate for the increased weight at the front, causing tension in the lower back. Someone who habitually collapses forward may do so more, making the muscles in the pelvis and legs over-tense and curving the lower back. Both postures tend to throw the weight of the baby forward and the woman compensates by hollowing her back, thus tensing the muscles, in order to maintain balance. 'Good use' in pregnancy is the same as at all times, with a slight increase in the work of the muscles that keep the body upright. This is distributed through the head, neck and back. Forsstrom and Hampson (1995) suggest that women think of the baby not sticking out in front but lying close to the spine. This way women will not throw their abdomens forward or lean over to protect the bump. The Alexander teacher can also help with pelvic floor exercises and the release of tension in the abdominal muscles that is so often present even in non-pregnant women.

Pregnancy changes the posture in everyday activities, and the Alexander Technique principles may be applied to easing the problems that arise. Standing in pregnancy can be tiring and uncomfortable, sometimes causing faintness. The woman should ensure that she stands evenly on both legs with weight distributed through the feet or slightly back on the heels. This is less likely to 'lock up' the joints in the legs. Feet should be placed hip-width apart to support the upper body, with the feet turned slightly out. Moving a little with a rocking motion of shifting the weight from foot to foot keeps the circulation going. Primary control should be maintained in walking, the head leading and the back following. Alexander Technique helps the woman to learn to walk with less tension and to avoid the 'pregnant waddle'. The vulnerability of ligaments and joints in pregnancy means that women should take extra care with lifting heavy or awkward objects. The advice is to lift from a bended knee position with the back inclined slightly forward.

Breathing correctly is an important part of learning the technique. Alexander put great emphasis on breathing, as his whole discovery arose from tension in the head and neck affecting his speech and breathing. He found that poor breathing was often the result of excessive tension interfering with the muscles, attached to the spine, which we use to breathe. This in turn affects the head–neck–back alignment. Tension in the neck and shoulders and a rigid ribcage directly affects good breathing, which then affects the tension in a circular problem. It also contributes towards the habits of breath holding or gasping, or not very fluent speech.

Alexander devised the 'whispered ah' to encourage the release of tension. The mouth is slightly open in a relaxed smile with the tongue behind the lower teeth. The throat should be relaxed but this will be affected as the technique is practised. Without taking a breath in, the client should breathe out with an open 'ah' allowing the ribcage to relax. There is then a natural breath in through the nose with the same relaxed facial position maintained. The openness of the throat will be indicated by the rounded sound of the 'ah'. It may be difficult to check how well you are doing this yourself, and the teacher's help is important.

Alexander Technique in labour

As in all stages of the pregnancy and after, Alexander Technique can help the woman to feel in control, reduce distress and help to minimise future problems. The 'conscious control' that Alexander talked about is the awareness of the body and its processes that allows the woman to relax, listen to her body and understand the mechanisms. Women who have practised the technique will be able to use 'conscious control' to maintain 'good use', relax when appropriate and keep the head–neck–back alignment. They will be able to 'listen' to their bodies and be aware of unnecessary muscle tension and to return to the relaxed state after each contraction.

During labour many women find it difficult to maintain a feeling of control and may feel fearful or just exhausted from the tension. Awareness of breathing, posture and muscle tension not only helps the physiological process by preventing the woman from tightening muscles and inhibiting breathing and free movement, it also helps her to feel more in control, able to contain some of the pain and tension and to feel less overwhelmed. Being less tense and more able to relax when possible means that she is less tired and more able to continue to feel in control even in a long labour. The relaxation described by Alexander is the release of tension in the muscles and the control of breathing, not the passive relaxation or 'letting go' of other methods.

The position the woman adopts in labour may affect not just the relative comfort or ease of the labour but also her health after the delivery. The Alexander Technique, with 'good use' as the guide, encourages the upright position, which ensures good alignment of head, neck and back and ease of breathing. The monkey, the position with least muscle tension, allows the woman freedom of movement. She can rock or sway or move her pelvis in this position and it can be maintained for some time. She can support herself by leaning her head on her folded arms against a wall or on the shoulders of a facing partner. She can also be supported from behind by someone also in the monkey position. This position requiring least muscle tension reduces fatigue in the birth partner as well as the woman in labour.

Squatting, whilst being a physiologically good position in which to give birth, is very tiring and perhaps should be kept for the second stage. The woman can be supported by a birth partner sitting in a chair while she squats on the floor. They are face to face, gripping each other's forearms, or she may be supported from behind while squatting between her partner's knees. If the woman squats on a bed she can be supported by a facing, standing partner or by a person on either side of her.

Women may find kneeling less tiring. The woman can lean against a chair or facing a birth partner who is seated.

All these positions can be learned with the Alexander teacher during pregnancy so that the woman can feel confident that she is maintaining 'good use' at each stage. If the woman has to lie down for various procedures she should try to maintain a semi-recumbent position, with her head slightly raised on a book or books and one knee raised.

Alexander Technique also helps breathing during labour. The ability to reduce the tension around the head and neck, particularly, prevents restricted breathing. Holding the breath can make the woman feel dizzy and uncomfortable, and in itself increases tension. Also controlling breathing with each contraction, listening and responding to the body, helps the woman to feel in control and reduces fear and pain.

After the birth   It is very easy for the new mother to neglect herself in the first few weeks after the baby is born. She may feel vulnerable, uncomfortable or fragile, elated, joyous or just exhausted. Taking the time to think about herself and her well-being as well as that of her child will be relaxing in itself. Alexander Technique's gentle non-invasive approach may help the woman who needs it to begin to feel comfortable with her body again. The teacher needs to be aware of the recent delivery to respect that the ligaments and muscles may still be soft and need time to recover. The woman will also benefit from the teacher's help in relating to her pre-pregnant posture and her new shape. The attention to physical and emotional needs that is encouraged by the technique may help the woman to adjust to her new self and other image. Motherhood changes so much about how a woman sees herself and is seen by other people; the self-awareness that she gains from Alexander Technique may help to re-establish her identity and boundaries.

After the birth, resting is encouraged and most teachers suggest two or three periods of rest in a semi-recumbent position for about fifteen minutes each time.

Looking after the baby

Alexander principles can help prevent backache and muscle tension from the frequent bending, lifting and carrying that looking after a baby involves. Some bad habits can arise from using the arms and shoulders and bending the back to lift and carry rather than using the stronger long muscles of the back and remembering the Alexander way of lengthening the back and opening the shoulders. The 'monkey' is again the ideal way of starting the bending and lifting movement. The 'lunge' can be employed to move forward and down. The woman must be aware of using the ankle, knee and hip joints to bend to the floor. There will be less strain and tension if the baby is carried close to the body and well supported. Carrying a baby over one shoulder may give her a better view but will tend to make the mother arch her lower back. Also carrying on one hip may twist the spine and put the body out of alignment. Advice on carrying at each stage should be sought.

Other ways to avoid back problems and bad use are to be careful about the handle height of a pram or pushchair so that you are not straining forward, and when breastfeeding to lift the baby to the breast rather than to slump forward to the baby.

Alexander Technique can be used by all ages at all stages of life. It is never too early or late to learn. It is gentle, non-invasive and does not require a prolonged learning period. Many students return to their teachers from time to time to check that they are maintaining good habits, and feel the benefits of the change in many areas of their lives.

Training

Training for Alexander Technique lasts for three years and requires about twenty hours a week in college as well as home study. Most of the courses are largely experiential with some study of anatomy and physiology. Some courses have a waiting list. You should also be aware that many courses require you to have had a year of lessons before applying to train.

References

Bach Flower Remedies

Davenas E, Beauvais F, Amara J 1988 Human basophil degranulation triggered by very dilute antiserum against IgE. *Nature* 333: 816–818

Nicholl L K 1995 Complementary therapies and nurse education—the need for specialist teachers. *Complementary Therapies in Nursing and Midwifery* 1 (3): 69–72

Ramsell J 1991 *The Bach Flower Remedies: Questions and Answers.* C.W. Daniel, Saffron Walden, UK

Alexander Technique

Forsstrom B, Hampson M 1995 *The Alexander Technique for Pregnancy and Childbirth.* Gollancz, London

Further reading

Bach Flower Remedies

Bach E 1931 *Heal Thyself.* C. W. Daniel, Saffron Walden, UK

Bach E 1933 *The Twelve Healers and Other Remedies.* C.W. Daniel, Saffron Walden, UK

Howard J 1991 *The Story of Mount Vernon: Home of the Bach Flower Remedies.* Albry Printing Co., Wallingford-on-Thames, UK

Howard J 1991 *Growing Up with Bach Flower Remedies; the Use of the Remedies During Childhood and Adolescence.* C. W. Daniel, Saffron Walden, UK

Howard J 1992 *Bach Flower Remedies Step by Step.* C. W. Daniel, Saffron Walden, UK

Weeks N 1989 *The Medical Discoveries of Edward Bach, Physician.* C. W. Daniel, Saffron Walden, UK

Alexander Technique

Brennan R 1991 *Alexander Technique.* Element, Shaftesbury, UK

Drake J 1991 *Body Know-how: A Practical Guide to the Use of the Alexander Technique in Everyday Life.* Thorsons, London

Conclusion

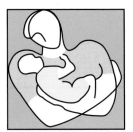

This book is intended to be an introduction to complementary medicine for the pregnant and childbearing woman and those who care for her. It is not intended as a 'how to' guide but as an overview of those therapies commonly available and their application to maternity care. There are books available that contain more detailed information, many of them noted at the end of the chapters, as well as training courses for those who seek to extend their practice. The editors hope that this book may widen the debate about the value of complementary therapies, and encourage women, and all healthcare professionals who care for them, in both conventional and complementary medicine, to seek out more information about the treatments outlined here or to explore others that may offer the pregnant and childbearing woman care, support and choice.

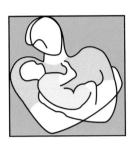

Appendix 1: Quick Reference Chart for Possible Uses of Complementary Therapies for Mother and Baby

Please refer to individual chapters for more information on safe practice.

Condition	Acupuncture	Alexander Technique	Aromatherapy	Bach Flower Remedies	Chiropractic	Herbal Medicine	Homeopathy	Hydrotherapy	Hypnotherapy
Anaemia	✓		Lemon			Herbal mineral preparation, e.g. Floradix™	e.g. Ferrum met. Arsenicum Pulsatilla Natrum mur. China		
Backache	B23, B47, B48 points	✓	Lavender Marjoram Rosemary } with caution Clary sage in labour	Rescue Remedy cream if trauma. Olive if exacerbated by exhaustion	✓	Mustard compress	Arnica if traumatic; Sepia or Nux vomica if with constipation	✓	
Breast engorgement	✓		Jasmine			Cabbage leaves (Vitamin C acts as anti-inflammatory)	e.g. Bryonia if breasts hard, early mastitis. Belladonna if breasts red, hot and tender		
Breech presentation	Moxibustion to B167 point	✓			✓		✓		
Bruising			Black Pepper	Rescue Remedy cream (not on open wound)			Arnica (not on open wound)		
Carpal tunnel syndrome	TW4, TW5, P6 & P7 points		Juniper, Cypress (Compress)		✓				
Colic (neonate)	✓		Peppermint, Fennel, Orange	Rescue Remedy to calm	✓	Dill, Camomile tea, Fennel	e.g. Chamomilla if baby angry and better if carried; Bryonia if irritable and worse when moved	✓	
Conjunctivitis (neonate)			Camomile (tea) as eyebath			Camomile tea, Eyebright			
Constipation	CV6, ST 36 points	✓	Orange, Lemon, Lime, Neroli, Grapefruit, Rosemary		✓	Mallow, Senna, Dandelion root, Garlic, Onions	e.g. Nux vomica, Bryonia, Natrum mur.		
Depression	✓	✓	Ylang Ylang, Neroli, Lavender, Bergamot	Hornbeam, Rescue Remedy, Crab Apple if a feeling of uncleanliness, Star of Bethlehem if shocked	✓	Agnus-Castus, Jasmine tea, St John's wort	e.g. Sepia if despondent, weepy. Arnica if traumatised and exhausted.	✓	
Diarrhoea	Sp16, CV6		Sandalwood, Camomile, Neroli: Tea tree if infective	Crab Apple if a feeling of uncleanliness	✓	Slippery Elm, Marshmallow root	e.g. Arsenicum, Pulsatilla, Phosphorus, China		

Massage	Nutritional Medicine	Osteopathy	Reflexology/Reflex Zone Therapy	Relaxation Techniques/Exercise	Shiatsu/ Acupressure	Tai Ch'i Gong	Yoga	Other Therapies
	Blackcurrants, Parsley, Mint, Fennel, Watercress, Horseradish							
With care around sacrum in early pregnancy		✓	Foot zones for spine, shoulders, sacro-iliac joints and general relaxation		B23, B47, B48 points; TENS in *late* pregnancy	✓	✓	
Breast massage from axilla to nipple			Breast zones on feet, good for venous engorgement		✓			
Clockwise abdominal massage (cf,ecv)		✓		Knee–chest position 20 min. daily from 32 weeks			✓	
	Buckwheat tea for rutin content							
Wrist 'wringing'		✓	Foot zones for wrists plus general relaxation zones	Splinting of hands and wrists at night	TW4, TW5, P6, P7 points		✓	
Clockwise abdominal massage (relaxes mother if she does it)	Fluids ++	Cranio-sacral therapy	Foot zones for GIT & liver + general relaxation zones	For mother	✓			
Clockwise abdominal massage	Avoid tea (tannin); artichokes for fibre. Start meals with raw food	✓	Clockwise massage of arches of both feet (5 min. each foot)	✓	CV6 point, ST36 point	✓	✓	
Full body massage for relaxation	Zinc, Vitamin B6	Cranio-sacral therapy	General relaxing reflexology	✓	✓	✓	✓	
Anti-clockwise abdominal massage	If persistent, may be due to food allergies	✓	Anti-clockwise massage of arches of feet		Sp16, CV6 points		✓	

Condition	Acupuncture	Alexander Technique	Aromatherapy	Bach Flower Remedies	Chiropractic	Herbal Medicine	Homeopathy	Hydrotherapy	Hypnotherapy
Fretful Baby			Camomile, Orange	Rescue Remedy (and for mother!)	✓	Camomile tea	Chamomilla especially if older baby, teething	✓	May help mother if fretfulness exacerbated by tense mother
Haemorrhoids	✓		Cypress, Juniper, Frankincense, Patchouli	Crab Apple in bidet. Rescue Remedy cream (if not bleeding)	✓	Witch hazel, Camomile cream	e.g. Pulsatilla; Nux vomica if constipated, Hamamelis if sore/bleeding	✓	
Headaches	GB41, LV3, GV16, GB20.5, B2 points	✓	Lavender (+peppermint if postnatal)	Impatiens, Walnut, Olive	✓	Dandelion root, Lavender tea	e.g. Arnica, Aconite		✓
Heartburn/ Indigestion	✓GV16, BG20.5 B2 points	✓	Lemon, Orange, Lavender, Neroli, Black Pepper			Slippery Elm, Ginger, Dandelion root	e.g. Nux vomica if acid reflux. Sulphur if worse late a.m. or with milk		✓
Hypertension	✓GV16, BG20.5, B2 points	✓	Ylang Ylang, Rosewood, Lavender, Lemon, Melissa	Rescue Remedy, Walnut, Olive, Crab Apple	✓		e.g. Belladonna if slow onset, sensitive to noise; Gelsenium if slow onset, weary, exhausted	✓	✓
Induction/ acceleration of labour	GB21, GB27–34, B67 points	✓	Lavender, Jasmine, Clary sage, Nutmeg	Rescue Remedy, Mimulus if fearful of labour, Walnut for protection	✓	Raspberry leaf tablets or tea to tone uterus from 32 weeks	e.g. Caulophyllum if post dates. Aconite if fearful of labour	✓	✓
Infertility	✓	✓	Ylang Ylang, Mandarin, Frankincense to reduce stress but *not periconceptional*	Pine, Walnut, Cerato, Elm, Gentian	✓	St John's wort to improve pelvic circulation or Chasteberry to regulate menstrual cycle	Constitutional remedy or e.g. Silica, Phosphorus, Natrum. mur.		✓ for relaxation
Insomnia	✓	✓	Camomile (tea), Lavender, Ylang Ylang	Olive, Rescue Remedy	✓	Camomile, Hop pillow, Lavender tea, Lime flower	e.g. Coffea if mind too active, aconite if anxious and afraid	✓	✓
Lactation/ insufficient	LU1, ST16, P1 points		Geranium, Jasmine?, Lemon Grass, Fennel (tea)	Rescue Remedy if psychological inhibition	✓	Fennel tea	e.g. Aconite, Bryonia, Phytolacca	✓	✓ for relaxation
Nausea/ vomiting	P6 (Neiguan) point	✓	Ginger, Lime, Camomile, Bergamot, Mandarin, Petitgrain; Peppermint in labour but *not* first trimester	Crab Apple, Rescue Remedy	✓	Ginger, Yoghurt, Lemon balm, Camomile or Black Horehound tea	e.g. Ipecacuanha if constant, worse for smell of food; Nux vomica if worse in morning, pulsatilla if worse in evening and better at night		✓

Massage	Nutritional Medicine	Osteopathy	Reflexology/Reflex Zone Therapy	Relaxation Techniques/Exercise	Shiatsu/Acupressure	Tai Ch'i Gong	Yoga	Other Therapies
General full body massage for relaxation; teach mother to do it	✓	Cranio-sacral therapy	General relaxation reflexology	✓ for mother	✓		May help mother if her tension exacerbates baby's condition	
	High fibre foods; see also constipation	✓	Suppression of zones for rectum	✓ at time of defecation	✓	✓	✓	
Head massage in 'hairwashing' action. Temple massage. Indian head massage	Avoid caffeine + E200s range of additives	✓	Foot zones for head, neck, shoulders plus any other symptomatic zones	✓	Sub-occipital points—GV16, GB20, also B2 + GV24.5 points	✓	✓	
Abdominal and chest massage, back massage	Avoid tea & coffee, sugar, alcohol, additives E276. Garlic—raw or capsules	✓	Foot zones for oesophagus, cardiac sphincter, stomach plus general relaxation zone	✓	✓	✓	✓	
General relaxing back or full body massage		✓	General relaxing reflexology	✓	✓	✓	✓	
General relaxing. Nipple stimulation	✓	✓	Foot zones for pituitary gland, uterus plus general relaxation techniques	Breathing and relaxation exercises	GB21, BL67, GB27–43 points	✓	✓	Sexual intercourse to stimulate local release of prostaglandins
Full body massage for relaxation	Vitamin & mineral supplement as appropriate, zinc, magnesium, selenium	✓	✓	✓	✓	✓	✓	
General full body or back massage for relaxation	Avoid all stimulants	✓	General relaxing reflexology	✓	General shiatsu massage for relaxation	✓	✓	
Breast & nipple massage to encourage oxytocin output	Fluids ++, well balanced diet	✓	Stimulation of foot and hand zones for breast and pituitary gland	✓	LU1, ST6, P1 points	✓	✓	
May aid relaxation, e.g. feet or neck + shoulders	Reduce tea, coffee, alcohol, fatty, spicy foods; Vitamins B6 & zinc supplements, also chromium especially if previously on contraceptive pill	✓	General relaxation techniques. Suppression of foot zones for GIT & Liver	✓	P6 point acupressure wrist bands —'Sea Bands'™	✓	✓	

Condition	Acupuncture	Alexander Technique	Aromatherapy	Bach Flower Remedies	Chiropractic	Herbal Medicine	Homeopathy	Hydrotherapy	Hypnotherapy
Nipples, sore			Camomile (teabags), Geranium (leaves)	Rescue Remedy Cream		Calendula, Camomile tea bags, applied to nipples, Geranium leaves	e.g. Aconite, Arnica cream, Arsenicum, Bryonia, Graphites, Pulsatilla		
Oedema	✓	✓	Cypress, Juniper, Geranium, Patchouli	Olive & Rescue Remedy in foot bath	✓	Dandelion, Olive leaf compress, Cabbage, Geranium or Rhubarb Leaves	✓	✓	
Pain relief in labour	GB21, , GB27–34 B167 point	✓	Clary sage, Lavender, Nutmeg, Orange, Black Pepper, Jasmine	Mimulus, White Chestnut, Rescue Remedy	✓	Raspberry leaf, Motherwort, St John's wort, Blue Cohosh, Black haw	e.g. Arnica, Caulophyllum, Cimicifuga, Belladonna, Aconite, Lycopodium	✓	✓
Perineal discomfort			Lavender, Camomile, Thyme, Geranium	Rescue Remedy & Crab Apple added to bidet		Witch hazel	e.g. Arnica (no cream on open wounds), Calendula, Causticum, Staphysagria	✓	
Postnatal depression	✓	✓	Ylang Ylang, Jasmine, Neroli, Rose	Walnut, Mustard, Sweet Chestnut, Gentian, Pine, Cherry Plum	✓	Lavender tea	e.g. China, Cimicifuga, Natrum mur, Pulsatilla, Sepia	✓	✓
Retained placenta	B167 ✓		Lavender, Nutmeg, Clary sage, Jasmine, Basil		✓		e.g. Belladonna if with PPH, Caulophyllum, Secale if grande Multipara		
Retention of urine	✓		Sandalwood		✓		e.g. Aconite, Arnica, Lycopodium, Staphysagria		
Sciatica	✓	✓	Rosemary, Petitgrain		✓		e.g. Phytolacca, Bellis perennis, Causticum	✓	✓
Sinus congestion	B2, ST3, LI20 point		Eucalyptus, Tea tree, Thyme, Frankincense		✓	Peppermint tea, Dandelion root			
Stress & anxiety	✓	✓	Bergamot, Camomile, Marjoram, Lavender, Jasmine, Rose, Ylang Ylang	Rescue Remedy, Mimulus, Aspen, Hornbeam, Crab Apple, Gentian, Sweet Chestnut, Cherry Plum	✓		e.g. Aconite, Calcarea carb., Gelsenium, Opium, Pulsatilla	✓	✓
Subinvolution	✓		Lavender, Clary sage, Nutmeg with care	Crab Apple	✓	Raspberry leaf	e.g. Arnica, Caulophyllum, Pulsatilla, Nux vomica		

Massage	Nutritional Medicine	Osteopathy	Reflexology/Reflex Zone Therapy	Relaxation Techniques/Exercise	Shiatsu/ Acupressure	Tai Ch'i Gong	Yoga	Other Therapies
To ease any engorgement				✓			✓	
Bimanual upwards massage of legs	Add parsley, garlic and onions to diet	✓	General reflexology procedure to tone and stimulate circulation	Leg exercises, roll feet over milk bottles to encourage circulation	Sp9, SP6, K9, K2 points	✓	✓	
General relaxing massage. Sacral and suprapubic massage. Light abdominal effleurage. Foot massage		✓	General relaxing reflexology plus zones for pituitary gland, uterus, etc. Heel pressure	Breathing, relaxation, mobility postural changes	GB21, GB27–34, B167 points; TENS to acupuncture points	✓	✓	
Antenatal perineal massage may prevent need for episiotomy	Vitamin C, B6 + zinc		Suppression of foot zone for vagina & perineum with care—precise location	For general relaxation			✓	
General relaxing massage	Well balanced diet. Avoid stimulants. Vitamin C, B6 + zinc supps. to aid healing	Cranio-sacral therapy	General relaxing reflexology procedure	✓	General shiatsu massage	✓	✓	
Gentle abdominal massage (fundal); nipple stimulation		✓	Stimulation of foot zones for pituitary gland & uterus	✓	B167			
		✓	Stimulation of kidney, ureter and bladder zones on feet	✓	✓			
Avoid massage unless cause is known		✓	Suppression of zones for spine and sciatic area, *with care*	Simple back and leg exercises under physio supervision	✓	✓	✓	
Head massage	Avoid dairy products— mucus increases	✓	Stimulation & expression of facial and chest zones	Deep breathing exercises	B2, ST3, LI 20 points			
General relaxing massage	Avoid stimulants, e.g. tea, coffee, alcohol	✓	General relaxing reflexology and solar plexus when acute	✓	General shiatsu massage & K1 points when acute	✓	✓	
Abdominal massage of uterine fundus		✓	Stimulation of zones for pituitary gland & uterus	✓	✓			

Condition	Acupuncture	Alexander Technique	Aromatherapy	Bach Flower Remedies	Chiropractic	Herbal Medicine	Homeopathy	Hydrotherapy	Hypnotherapy
Symphysis pubis pain	✓	✓	Lavender		✓		e.g. Arnica	✓	
Thrush			Tea tree Oil (diluted) or pessaries	Crab Apple in bidet		Garlic cloves Live natural yoghurt on tampon Marigold tea, Thyme tea, Cranberry juice	e.g. Candida, Acidophilus, Sepia	May ease discomfort at meatus	
Urinary tract infection			Sandalwood, Benzoin, Frankincense, Bergamot		To ease frequency of micturition	Dandelion leaf, Garlic	e.g. Arsenicum, Belladonna, Sepia	May ease discomfort at meatus	
Varicose veins	✓	✓	Cypress, Juniper berry, Lavender, Lemon	Olive to ease feeling of 'weary' legs	✓	Yarrow, Witch hazel compress	e.g. Bellis perennis (vulval), Lycopodium (legs and vulva), Pulsatilla (legs), Hamamelis virginica		

Massage	Nutritional Medicine	Osteopathy	Reflexology/Reflex Zone Therapy	Relaxation Techniques/Exercise	Shiatsu/ Acupressure	Tai Ch'i Gong	Yoga	Other Therapies
General relaxing massage		✓	Gentle work on foot zone for symphysis pubis	✓	✓	✓	✓	
	Avoid yeast products and sugar							
	Avoid acidic foods	To ease frequency of micturition	Treat zones for urinary tract to encourage diuresis					
Avoid *direct* massage of varicosed areas		✓	General relaxing reflexology procedure	✓	✓	✓	✓	

Ainsworth's Homeopathic Pharmacy, 38 New Cavendish Street, London W1M 7LH. Tel: 0171 935 5330

Anglo-European College of Chiropractic, 13–15 Parkwood Road, Bournemouth BH5 2DF. Tel: 01202 436200

Aromatherapy Database, Bob Harris, 2 Ruelle du Tertre, St Germain le Guillaume, Butet 53240, France. Tel: (33) 243027728

Aromatherapy Organisations Council, 3 Latymer Close, Braybrooke, Market Harborough LE16 8LL. Tel: 01858 434242

Association of Reflexologists, 27 Old Gloucester Street, London WC1 3XX. Tel: 0990 673320

British Acupuncture Council, Park House, 206–208 Latimer Road, London W10 6RE. Tel: 0181 964 0222

British Association for Counselling, 1 Regent Place, Rugby, Warks CV21 2PJ. Tel: 01788 578328

British Chiropractic Association, Blagreave House, 17 Blagreave Street, Reading, Berks RG1 1QB. Tel: 0118 950 5950 Fax: 0118 958 8946

British Complementary Medicine Association, 249 Fosse Road South, Leicester LE3 1AE. Tel: 0116 282 5511. Fax: 0116 282 5611

British Diastasis Symphysis Pubis Support Group, Mont Hamel House, 2 Chapel Road, Ramsgate, Kent CT11 9RY. Tel: 01843 587356

British Holistic Medicine Association, St Marylebone Parish Church, Marylebone Road, London NW1 5LT. Tel: 0171 262 5299

British Homeopathic Association, 27a Devonshire Street, London W1N 2RJ. Tel: 0171 935 2163

British Hypnotherapy Association, 1 Wythburn Place, London W1H 5WL. Tel: 0171 262 8852

British Massage Therapy Council, Greenbank House, 65a Adelphi Street, Preston PR1 7BH. Tel: 01772 881063

British School of Osteopathy, 275 Borough High Street, London SE1 1JE. Tel: 0171 407 0222. Fax: 839 1098

British School of Reflex Zone Therapy, 23 Marsh Hall, Talisman Way, Wembley Park, Middlesex HA9 8JJ. Tel: 0181 904 4825

British Shiatsu Council, 121 Sheen Road, Richmond, Surrey TW9 1YJ. Tel: 0181 852 1080

British Society for Nutritional Medicine, PO Box 3AP, London W1A 3AP. Tel: 0171 436 8532

British Wheel of Yoga, 1 Hamilton Place, Boston Road, Sleaford, Lincolnshire NG34 7ES. Tel: 01529 306851

Centre for Autogenic Training, 101 Harley Street, London WIN 1DF.

Centre for Complementary Health Studies, University of Exeter, Streatham Court, Rennes Drive, Exeter EX4 4PU
Tel: 01392 433828/263263

Complementary Therapies in Maternity Care National Forum, c/o Denise Tiran (Chair), School of Health, University of Greenwich, Honeycombe Building, Mansion Site, Avery Hill Campus, Avery Hill Road, Eltham, London SE9. Tel: 0181 331 8000

Complementary Therapies in Nursing and Midwifery Journal, Churchill Livingstone, 24–28 Oval Road, London NW1 7DX
Tel: 0171 424 4200

Council for Complementary and Alternative Therapy, Park House, 206–208 Latimer Road, London W10 6RE. Tel: 0181 968 3862

Faculty of Homeopathy Royal London Homeopathic Hospital, Great Ormond Street, London WC1N 3HR. Tel: 0171 837 8833

General Council and Register of Consultant Herbalists, Grosvenor House, 40 Sea Way, Middleton on Sea, West Sussex PA22 7AA

General Council and Register of Naturopaths, Lief House, 120–122 Finchley Road, London NW3 5HR. Tel: 0171 435 6464
Fax: 0171 431 3630

General Osteopathic Council, 10 Greycoat Place, London SW1P 1SB. Tel: 0171 799 2442. Fax: 0171 799 2442

Guild of Spiritual Healers, 36 Newmarket, Otley, West Yorkshire LS21 3AE

Helios Homeopathic Pharmacy 97 Camden Road, Tunbridge Wells TH1 2QP. Tel: 01892 536393

Holistic Association of British Reflexologists, 92 Shearing Road, Old Harlow, Essex CM17 0JW. Tel: 01279 429060

Homeopathic Trust, Hahnemann House, 2 Powis Place, Great Ormond Street, London WC1N 3HT. Tel: 0171 837 9469

International Federation of Aromatherapists, Stamford House, 2–4 Chiswick High Road, London W4 1TH. Tel: 0181 742 2605

International Journal of Aromatherapy, 65 Church Road, Hove, East Sussex BN3 2BD

International Society of Professional Aromatherapists, ISPA House, 82 Ashby Road, Hinckley, Leicestershire LE10 1SN. Tel: 01455 637987

Institute for Complementary Medicine, PO Box 194, London SE16 1QZ. Tel: 0171 237 5165

Institute for Optimum Nutrition, 5 Jerdan Place, London SW6 1BE. Tel: 0171 385 7984

International Therapy Examination Council (ITEC), James House, Oakelbrook Mill, Newent, Gloucestershire GL18 1HD. Tel: 01531 821875

McTimoney Chiropractic Association, 21 High Street, Eynsham, Oxford OX8 1HE. Tel: 01865 880974

National Consultative Council for Alternative and Complementary Medicine, 39 Prestbury Road, Cheltenham, Gloucestershire GL52 2PT

Osteopathic Information Service, Premier House Room 432, 10 Greycoat Place, London SW1P 1SB. Tel: 0171 799 2559 Fax: 0171 799 2332

Research Council for Complementary Medicine, 60 Great Ormond Street, London WC1. Tel: 0171 833 8897

Society of Homeopaths, 2 Artizan Road, Northampton NN1 4HU Tel: 01604 214000

Society of Reflexologists, 2 Chelmsford Avenue, Warden Hill, Cheltenham, Gloucestershire GL51 5DN

Society of Teachers of the Alexander Technique, 10 London House, 266 Fulham Road, London SW10 9EL. Tel: 0171 351 0828

Glossary

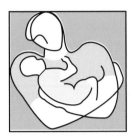

abortifacient induces abortion

carminative a property of certain essential oils or herbal remedies causing expulsion of gas from the intestines

caudal literally towards the tail

chi see Ki

concomitants accompanying sensation or pain/disorder reported at the same time as the principal complaint

circumduction to move a joint through a circular range of movement

constitutional remedy remedy most appropriate to an individual's constitution

cun a Chinese unit of measurement used to locate the acupuncture points. Sometimes described as 'Chinese inch'. One cun is the width of the inter-phalangeal joint of the patient's thumb, three cun is the width of the four fingers together at the level of the dorsal skin crease of the proximal inter-phalangeal joint of the middle finger

cupping A therapy in which a glass cup or bamboo jar is attached to the skin surface by suction to cause local congestion through negative pressure. Cupping has the function of warming and promoting the free flow of Qi and Blood in the meridians in traditional Chinese medicine theory, and to diminish swellings and pain. It is mostly used for conditions such as backache, general musculoskeletal pain, stomach-ache and asthma

demulcent a soothing substance

de-personalisation a psychiatric term for the symptom which leads a person to complain that he or she feels unreal

de-realisation a psychiatric term for the symptom which leads a person to complain that the world seems unreal

disease (homeopathy) an alteration in the state of health expressed in morbid signs, the derangement of the life energy trying to correct itself

effleurage a light, superficial massage

emmenagogue encourages menstruation

enfleurage expensive method of extracting essential oils from delicate flowers, e.g. jasmine

erector spinae muscles two large muscles which fill the grooves on either side of the vertebral column. In the lumbar spine belly is a large fleshy mass which gradually diminishes in size in the thoracic spine

galactogue encourages lactation

innervation the nerve supply to any organ or part of the body

Ki the Chinese 'Qi' or 'Chi' or Japanese 'Ki' meaning energy or motive force of life

law of cure an evaluation system to assess decline of disease from above downwards, inside to outside, important to less important organ and reverse order of appearance

law of similars the symptoms caused by too much (overdose) of a substance are the symptoms that can be cured with a small dose of that substance

modalities what makes a symptom better or worse, e.g. heat, movement, time of day. This makes a symptom complete and aids differentiation of remedies

moxa the Chinese name for the herb mugwort or 'St John's herb'

moxibustion the burning of moxa to apply heat to an area for therapeutic effect

osteochondrosis non-inflammatory condition affecting the epiphyseal plates in some young people. Necrosis followed by regeneration. Occurs in the ring epiphyses of the dorsal vertebral bodies, leads to reduced mobility and possible kyphosis

posology the study of the quantities in which drugs should be administered

potency strength of medicines produced by potentization on varying scales, e.g. decimal or centessimal

potentisation a process used to prepare remedies by dilution and shaking to make more 'potent'

proprioceptive control to be aware of the position, balance and movements of the body due to the reflex action of proprioceptors in muscles, tendons and joints

proving method of ascertaining the curative potential of substances in homeopathic practice

Qi see Ki

Qi-gong Chinese name for the slow-moving, gentle martial art-style exercise, designed to maintain and strengthen health through the building up of Qi

repertory a reference guide to the *Materia Medica*, alphabetically listing symptoms and remedies

sitz bath a means of treating vulval or anal conditions by immersion of the affected area in a container of water to which is often added essential oils or herbs

spasm in piriformis sudden involuntary contraction of the piriformis muscle. This muscle extends from the front of the sacrum, passes out of the pelvis through the sciatic foramen and is inserted into the greater trochanter

synergistic effect when the combined effect of two or more essential oils is greater than the sum of the individual oils

thenar eminence the radial side of the anterior aspect of the hand—the 'ball' of the thumb

totality of symptoms all principal signs and symptoms experienced, including aetiology and modalities and guides to the selection of a remedy

vermifuge anti-worm property

version the term applied when an alteration in the lie of the fetus in utero is brought about, or the location of its upper and lower poles reversed. It may occur spontaneously or by manipulation

vital force (homeopathy) the life energy that animates, guides and balances the organism in health and disease

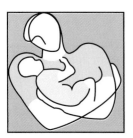

Index